Research on Immunology

Research on Immunology

Published by iConcept Press

Research on Immunology

Publisher: iConcept Press Ltd.

ISBN: 978-1-922227-91-1

Printed in the United States of America

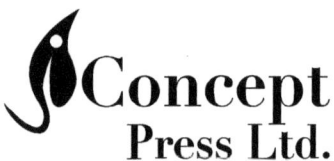

𝕀Concept
Press Ltd.

www.iconceptpress.com

Contents

Preface

Immunology is a branch of biomedical science that covers the study of immune systems in organisms. Many components of the immune system are typically cellular in nature and not associated with any specific organ; but rather are embedded or circulating in various tissues located throughout the body. *Research on Immunology* covers some of the latest aspects of the study of the immune system. It encompasses pathophysiology and physiology in health.

There are totally 11 chapters in this book. Chapter 1 presents a real-world analysis using cancer registry linked to medical claims data evaluated treatment patterns and outcomes among elderly, medically unfit, chronic lymphocytic leukemia (CLL) patients. The results suggest that chemoimmunotherapy is more effective than chemotherapy alone in elderly CLL patients with a high prevalence of comorbidity, and this supports conclusions from clinical trials in younger, medically fit patients. Chapter 2 discusses the role of the leukocyte adhesion cascade for the pathophysiology of nasal polyps in chronic rhinosinusitis patients, with a special view to the predominant immune imbalance within nasal polyps. Chapter 3 discusses the efficiency and safety of the combination of DC/CIK cytotherapy with TRT in advanced NSCLC. The authors found that this novel strategy is a potentially viable option for patients with advanced NSCLC. Chapter 4 reviews the innate and adaptive components of the human immune system that mediate allergic reactions as well as immune tolerance toward cow's milk proteins. Possible therapeutic strategies to induce immune tolerance in subjects with a risk to develop cow's milk allergy are discussed. Mechanistic interactions between cow's milk allergy and other inflammatory diseases are analysed as well.

Chapter 5 discusses the importance of immune reactions in the current understanding of the molecular pathogenesis of non-alcoholic fatty liver disease and potential immune-related treatments to be considered in future therapeutic paradigms. Given that this disease entity is still not completely understood, therefore efforts should be made to fully investigate the pathogenesis and treatment strategies. Chapter 6 discusses the discovery about the cytokine immunopathogenesis of enterovirus 71 infection and insights into agents, IVIG and milrinone, modulate the cytokine storm. Chapter 7 presents studies that: (i) characterize the L1 genetic variability of HPV 16 and HPV 18 genotypes, working with both single infection and multiple HPV infection samples, (ii) assess the prevalence of HPV variants in our region and (iii) analyze the relationship between variants and type of cervical lesion. Chapter 8 discusses various nanosystems which have shown the ability to simplify drug regimens, enhancing antiretroviral activity, while reducing their toxicity and increasing patient's compliance, preventing development of drug resistance.

Chapter 9 presents an update on the West Nile virus Infection (epidemiology, etiology, parthenogenesis, clinical aspects and treatment) and also the association with Opsoclonus Myoclonus Syndrome (a pluri-ethiological neurological disorder) through the personal experience of the authors. Chapter 10 proposes a histological image mosaicing approach to create the panoramic image automatically by mosaicing all the images acquired from a specimen. It effectively compensates for the congenital narrowness in field of views. Chapter 11 reviews the problems related to phylogenetic tree searches, sequence alignment, and phylogenetic uncertainty estimation. In addition, parallel approaches to these issues are outlined, and examples are provided of their use with microbial datasets.

Editing and publishing a book is never an easy task. Each chapter in this book has gone through a peer review, a selection and an editing process so as to guarantee its quality. Without the supports and contributions of the authors and reviewers, this book can never be able to complete. We would like to thank all of the authors in this book and all of the reviewers who participated in the reviewing process: Margarida Bastos, Angelo Calado, Juan D Canete, Chris Dardis, Luis Adrián Diaz, Magdalena Dutsch-Wicherek, Cristiano Ferlini, Keishi Fujio, Sergio Galvez, Fabiana Geraci, Noboru Hattori, Kazuya Hokamura, Tokumasa Horiike, Christo D. Izaaks, Alain Jacquet, Bae Kwon Jeong, Barbara Jezersek Novakovic, Mats W. Johansson, Kyung-Yil Lee, Bingyun Li, Hai Lin, Yasuhiro Matsumura, Ernesto Moro-Rodriguez, Hiroshi Nishina, Ryota Nomura, yan pang, Daniel R?žek, Ivan Sabol, Vittorio Sambri, Katharina Schindowski, Josef Spidlen, Eileen M Stock, Wenchao Sun, Jolien Suurmond, Cristiana Pistol Tanase, Yasuo Terauchi, Guido Vanham, Penghua Wang, Tiffani L Williams, Wei Xu, Keisuke Yusa and Massimiliano Zanin. We hope that you, the reader, will find this book interesting and useful. Any advices please feel free and are always welcome to tell us.

iConcept Press Editorial Office
August 2016

Chapter 1

Chemoimmunotherapy or Immunotherapy versus Chemotherapy among Elderly Chronic Lymphocytic Leukemia Patients

Sacha Satram-Hoang[1], Carolina Reyes[2,3], Sandra Skettino[4], Khang Q. Hoang[5]

1   Introduction

Chronic lymphocytic leukemia (CLL) is a lymphoproliferative disorder and the most common form of leukemia in adults. It predominantly affects the elderly with a median age at diagnosis of 72 years, and with almost 70% of new cases diagnosed in individuals 65 years or older (Howlader N, 2011; Siegel *et al.*, 2012). The clinical course of CLL is extremely variable in which certain patients may have indolent disease not require treatment for many years while others have rapid progressive disease requiring immediate treatment (Carney & Mulligan, 2009; Dighiero & Hamblin, 2008).

Loss of organ reserve and the comorbidities associated with aging are considered important determinants of patients' ability to tolerate the side effects of cancer therapy (Yancik, 1997; Zent, 2010). Among elderly CLL patients, 46% have major comorbidities present (Thurmes *et al.*, 2008). However, the majority of CLL clinical trials primarily enroll younger, medically fit patients who are better able to tolerate treatment-related adverse events (Byrd *et al.*, 2005; Eichhorst, Goede, & Hallek, 2009; Hallek *et al.*, 2010;

[1] Department of Epidemiology, Q.D. Research Inc., USA

[2] Department of Health Economics & Outcomes Research, Genentech Inc., USA

[3] Department of Clinical Pharmacy, University of California, San Francisco, USA

[4] U.S. Medical Affairs, Genentech Inc., USA

[5] Medical Affairs, Q.D. Research Inc., USA

Smolej, 2010). The underrepresentation of elderly patients in clinical trials makes optimal treatment strategies and disease management unclear for typical CLL patients.

For over three decades, chlorambucil (CLB), an alkylating drug was the main treatment for CLL (Han, Ezdinli, Shimaoka, & Desai, 1973; Knospe, Loeb, & Huguley, 1974). In the last decade, combinations of purine analogues with alkylating drugs such as fludarabine and cyclophosphamide were shown to improve outcomes other than overall survival (Catovsky *et al.*, 2007; Eichhorst *et al.*, 2006). Chemoimmunotherapy (the addition of monoclonal antibodies to chemotherapy) presented a major breakthrough in the treatment of CLL. Rituximab, a chimeric monoclonal antibody directed against the CD20 antigen, combined with chemotherapy (fludarabine and cyclophosphamide; FCR) demonstrated significantly improved progression-free survival (PFS) and overall survival (OS) when compared to FC alone in treatment naïve CLL patients (Hallek *et al.*, 2010). Another large randomized study in previously treated CLL patients showed an association with the FCR regimen and improved PFS, response rate, and complete remission (Robak *et al.*, 2010). Therefore, FCR is currently the standard of care for medically fit CLL patients.

Among older patients who are frail or medically unfit however, fludarabine-based chemoimmunotherapy is generally less well tolerated (Gribben, 2010). Chemoimmunotherapy is often withheld or physicians may opt to reduce dosage in order to decrease the risk of occurrence and/or severity of adverse events (Foon *et al.*, 2009). A number of other treatment approaches are employed for older patients with comorbidity or other age-related organ function decline. These treatments may include chlorambucil, rituximab monotherapy, fludarabine monotherapy or bendamustine (Leporrier, 2004; Smolej, 2012). However, because the age of patients participating in clinical trials are not representative of the disease, there is limited information available on these treatment approaches in elderly or medically unfit CLL patients. The objectives of this study was to identify patient characteristics associated with receiving treatment and to evaluate the impact of these treatments on clinical outcomes in a real-world cohort of elderly, demographically diverse CLL patients.

2   Methods

2.1   Data Sources

Details of the Surveillance Epidemiology & End Results (SEER)-Medicare database have been published previously (Warren, Klabunde, Schrag, Bach, & Riley, 2002). Briefly, the database is a collaborative effort between the National Cancer Institute (NCI), the SEER registries and the Centers for Medicare & Medicaid Services. The SEER registries are representative of about 26% of the United States (US) population and routinely collect cancer incidence and survival data from 18 population-based cancer registries from diverse geographic areas in the US. The database includes information on patient demographic, tumor characteristics, disease stage, first course of treatment and follow-up for vital status. Ninety-four percent of patients aged 65 years or older in the SEER files are successfully cross-matched to their Medicare claims files (Potosky, Riley, Lubitz,

Mentnech, & Kessler, 1993). Inpatient care, skilled nursing care, home healthcare, and hospice care are covered services under Medicare Part A, while Part B reimburses for physician and outpatient care. The SEER-Medicare linkage used in this study includes all Medicare-eligible persons reported to SEER through 2007 and their Medicare claims for Part A and Part B through 2009. Institutional review board approval was waived because there are no personal identifiers in the SEER-Medicare database.

2.2   Study Design

This was an observational retrospective cohort analysis of incident CLL cases receiving treatment in routine clinical oncology practice.

2.3   Study Population

The SEER-Medicare dataset contained 30942 patients diagnosed with CLL at any time and in any order (if patients had multiple cancers). The study inclusion criteria required that patients be diagnosed with CLL as their first primary cancer (n = 29226), between the years 1998–2007 (n = 16707), aged 66 years or older (n = 12723), to have survived the month of diagnosis (n = 12034), continuously enrolled in both Medicare Parts A and B with no HMO coverage in the 12 months preceding diagnosis (n = 8608), and received treatment with any oral or infused chemotherapy or immunotherapy between the years 2001 to 2009 (n = 2985). Given the very low incidence of rituximab in the first few years of the study (< 10% from 1998–2000) and the fact that the first CLL rituximab trials were published in 2001, we restricted the time period of treatment initiation to 2001–2009 to have sufficient sample size in each comparative treatment group. See Figure 1 for the schematic of inclusion/exclusion process.

2.4   Study Variables

2.4.1   Demographic Characteristics

The SEER program routinely collects data on patient demographics including age, race/ethnicity, residence, and socioeconomic status based on income and education. Patient age at diagnosis was stratified into four groups: 66–70; 71–75; 76–80; and > 80. Race/ethnicity was defined using the SEER recoded race variable and categorized into three mutually exclusive groups White, non-White, and Other/Unknown. Median annual household income at the census tract level and percentage of the adult population who completed specific levels of education at the zip code level were used as a proxy for socioeconomic status.

2.4.2   Clinical Characteristics

The SEER program also collects data on primary tumor site, tumor morphology, and disease stage. Identification of CLL was based on site code 75 or ICD-O-3 code 9823 in the SEER data. Stage at diagnosis is not available for CLL in the SEER database. A proxy

CLL Diagnosis (N=30942)
⇩
First primary CLL (N=29226)
⇩
Diagnosed between January 1, 1998 - December 31, 2007 (N=16707)
⇩
≥ 66 years at diagnosis (N=12723)
⇩
Survived month of diagnosis (N=12034)
⇩
Medicare Parts A and B in the 12 months prior to diagnosis (N=11331)
⇩
No HMO coverage in the 12 months prior to diagnosis (N=8608)
⇩
Initiated chemotherapy after diagnosis (N=3366)
⇩
Initiated therapy between January 1, 2001 - December 31, 2009 (N=2985)

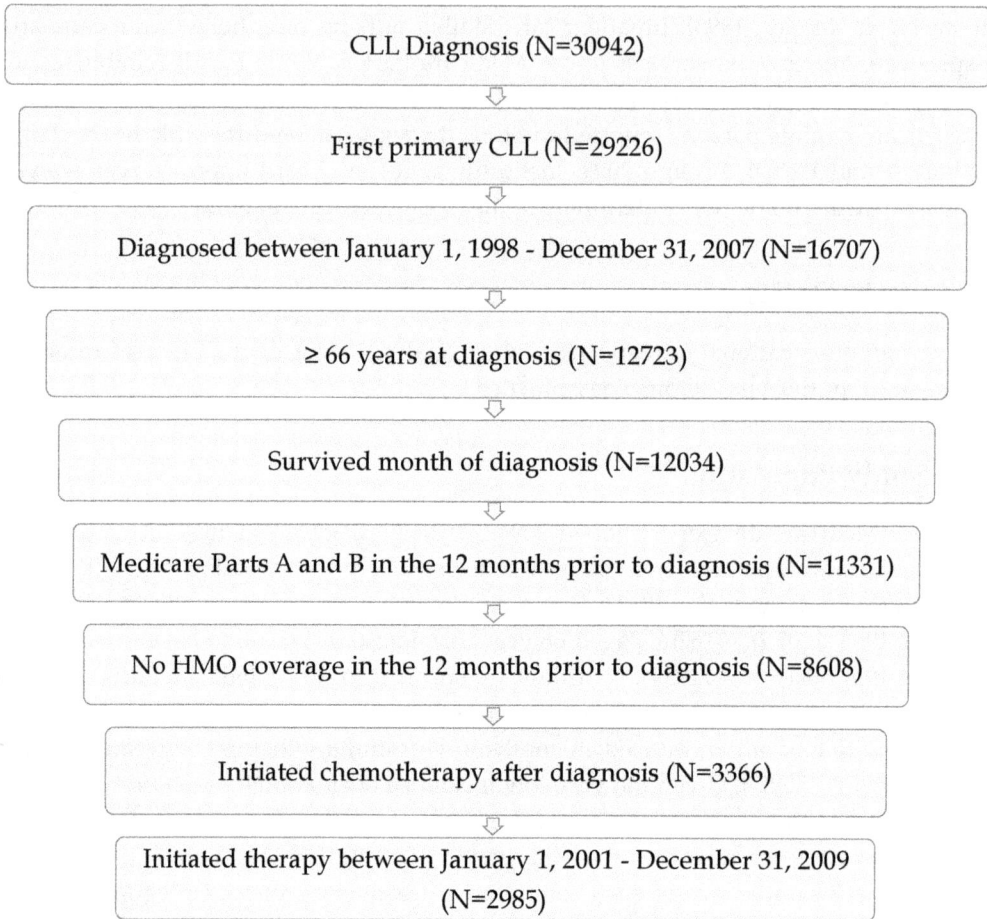

Figure 1: Schematic of Inclusion/Exclusion Process.

for stage was based on the Rai and Binet (Binet *et al.*, 1981; Rai *et al.*, 1975) staging systems with patients classified as "advanced stage" if anemia and/or thrombocytopenia were present in the claims data (Danese *et al.*, 2011).

The NCI comorbidity index (Klabunde, Legler, Warren, Baldwin, & Schrag, 2007) was calculated for each patient using diagnosis and procedure codes in Medicare Part A and B claims files to identify the 15 non-cancer comorbidities from the Charlson Comorbidity Index (Charlson, Pompei, Ales, & MacKenzie, 1987). A weight is assigned to each condition based on its potential to influence 2-year mortality and these weights are summed to obtain an index for each patient. The index accounts for the number and severity of the conditions, with higher scores indicating a greater burden of comorbid disease.

Comorbidity was also examined using the number of involved organs systems in the Cumulative Illness Rating Scale (CIRS) (Linn, Linn, & Gurel, 1968; Parmelee, Thuras, Katz, & Lawton, 1995). CIRS assesses patient comorbidity by specifying the presence or absence of pathology in each of the 14 organ systems and the severity of impairment in each involved system. Given that disease severity data were not available in this claims-based analysis to calculate a total CIRS score for each patient, we presented the number of involved CIRS organ systems. The number of involved CIRS organ systems was quantified using diagnosis and procedure codes in the Medicare Part A and B claims files to identify specific conditions that relate to each organ system category.

The NCI Comorbidity Index and the CIRS are among the most valid and reliable measures of multi-morbidity (de Groot, Beckerman, Lankhorst, & Bouter, 2003; Hines *et al.*, 2009). For both comorbidity definitions, Medicare claims during the year preceding the diagnosis were evaluated to determine the baseline comorbidity burden for each patient. Specific conditions were required to appear on at least 2 different claims that were more than 30 days apart to ensure that "rule out" diagnoses were not counted as comorbid conditions.

2.4.3   Treatment

Data were abstracted from 5 merged SEER-Medicare files to identify claims for chemotherapy or immunotherapy administration. (Warren, Harlan, *et al.*, 2002) These included the Medicare provider analysis and review (MEDPAR), carrier claims (NCH), outpatient claims (OUTSAF), durable medical equipment (DME), and the prescription drug event (PDE) files. Each of these files provides calendar year summaries of reimbursed services.

In July 2006, Medicare coverage was expanded to include prescription drugs under Medicare Part D. Chlorambucil is covered under Medicare Part D and data for its use were only available from 2007 to 2009 in the PDE claims file. Chemotherapy and immunotherapy was characterized and quantified using the International Classification of Disease (ICD) diagnosis codes, ICD procedural codes, Current Procedural Terminology (CPT) codes, Healthcare Common Procedure Coding System (HCPCS) codes, and revenue center codes. Chemotherapy claims were searched for specific drug codes to identify the type of chemotherapy administered to patients. The absence of these claims was interpreted as evidence of no treatment. The first chemotherapy claim after diagnosis indicated the start of therapy. Patients were classified into 1 of 4 treatment groups based on all chemotherapy administered during the first 60 days following initiation of treatment. The four treatment groups defined for this analysis include chlorambucil (CLB), rituximab monotherapy (R-mono), rituximab and intravenous chemotherapy (R+IV Chemo), and intravenous chemotherapy alone (IV Chemo-only).

Given that patients receiving R-mono and CLB appeared to be preferentially selected for treatment based on patient characteristics (age and comorbidity) and National Comprehensive Cancer Network (NCCN) treatment guidelines recommend CLB and R-mono for older CLL patients with comorbidities; we separated the survival analyses into two comparisons using appropriate comparator treatment groups: R-mono versus CLB during the time period 2007–2009 since this is the time period during which CLB was available in the dataset; and R+IV Chemo versus IV Chemo-only during the time period 2001–2009.

2.4.4   Mortality and Censoring

The date of death was determined by using the Medicare date or the SEER date of death if the Medicare date was missing. All other patients were assumed to be alive at the end of the follow-up period on December 31, 2009, although they may have been censored earlier for other reasons such as development of a second primary cancer or Medicare claims no longer available.

2.5   Statistical Analysis

All statistical analyses were performed using SAS software, version 9.1.3 (SAS Institute Inc., Cary, North Carolina). Demographic and clinical baseline characteristics among the patients initiating treatment between 2001–2009 (excluding CLB) and 2007–2009 (the period for which CLB data were available) were summarized descriptively. The Chi-square test for categorical variables and analysis of variance or t-tests for continuous variables were performed to determine differences between treatment groups. We considered a p-value < 0.05 to be statistically significant.

We used two methods to determine the predictors of receiving treatment within the first year after diagnosis. The Cox Proportional Hazards regression modeled time to treatment and the logistic regression modeled the odds of receiving treatment. Predictor variables in the models were selected from demographic and clinical characteristics.

The survival analyses compared CLB to R-mono from 2007 to 2009 because this was the time during which Part D Medicare claims data on CLB were available. Patients initiating treatment with R+IV Chemo and IV Chemo-only from 2001–2009 were compared. The survival analyses to assess overall risk of death were based on a comparison of two approaches as a sensitivity exercise which included the Cox proportional hazards regression and the propensity score-weighted Cox proportional hazards regression model. The traditionally adjusted Cox proportional hazards regression model allowed us to explore independent predictors of mortality, while the propensity score-weighted model is limited to assessing the effect of treatment. A comparison of these two models yielded almost identical results of treatment effect.

In the Cox proportional hazards regression, we adjusted the model for confounders that were selected from demographic and clinical characteristics using the backward elimination strategy (Greenland S, 1998). In the propensity score weighted model, we used multinomial logistic regression to calculate a propensity score, which represents the conditional probability that a patient would receive a specific treatment given each patient's pretreatment variables such as age, gender, and comorbidities (Kurth *et al.*, 2006). Follow-up was calculated from the date of treatment initiation until the first occurrence of a censoring event including date of death, development of a second primary tumor, the last date for which Medicare claims were available, or the end of the follow-up period on December 31, 2009. Kaplan-Meier survival curves and corresponding log-rank tests examined unadjusted OS by treatment group.

3   Results

3.1   Treatment Patterns

Of the patients who met the study eligibility criteria, 594 (20%) were administered R-mono, 696 (23%) were treated with R+IV Chemo, 1544 (52%) received IV Chemo-only and 151 (5%) received CLB in the first-line setting. Table 1 shows the distribution of the specific types of therapies received in the cohort.

Treatment Type		N	%
CLB		151	100
R-Mono		594	100
R + IV CHEMO	R + CHOP	46	6.6
	R + CVP	76	10.9
	R + FC	192	27.6
	R + F	303	43.5
	R + C	62	8.9
	R + Other	17	2.4
	Total	696	100
IV CHEMO-ONLY	CHOP	82[6]	5.3
	CVP		
	FC	63	4.1
	F	423	27.4
	C	22	1.4
	Other Chemo	345	22.3
	Unknown Chemo	609	39.4
	Total	1544	100

Table 1: First-line therapy initiated from 2001–2009.

Of the patients receiving R+IV Chemo, 495 (71%) received a regimen including fludarabine (F) and 376 (54%) received a regimen containing cyclophosphamide (C). There were 192 (28%) patients identified as receiving both F and C with rituximab and are included in the estimates of the two groups. Of the 1544 patients receiving IV Chemo-only, 486 (31%) received a regimen including F and 167 (11%) received a regimen containing C. There were 63 (4%) patients identified as receiving both F and C and

---

[6] Cells with counts of less than 11 are combined in compliance with the National Cancer Institute data use agreement for small cell sizes.

are included in the estimates of both groups.

Treatment with rituximab increased during the study time period until 2007 before CLB was introduced in the dataset (Figure 2). During the period of availability of all four treatment groups (2007–2009); the rate of IV Chemo-only use in first-line treatment was 41%, R+IV Chemo was 24%, R-mono was 20%, and oral CLB was 16%.

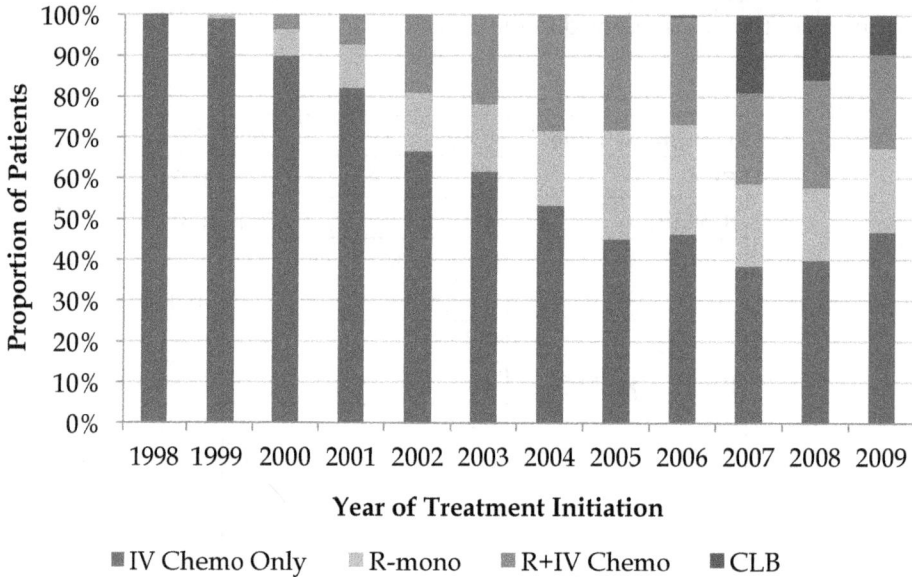

Figure 2: Distribution of therapy by year of initiation.

3.2   Predictors of Treatment

In the Cox multivariate regression analysis of time to treatment within the first year after diagnosis (Table 2), the treatment rate was significantly lower among patients > 80 years old, females, and with increasing comorbidity score. Compared to patients diagnosed at an earlier stage disease, advanced stage patients had a significantly higher treatment rate (HR = 1.48; 95% CI = 1.37–1.60). Findings from the logistic regression analysis of treatment within the first year after diagnosis were generally consistent with those from the Cox regression analysis.

3.3   Demographic and Clinical Characteristics

Table 3 shows patient baseline characteristics among the patients initiating treatment between 2001–2009 (excluding CLB) and 2007–2009 (including CLB). Patients treated with CLB (mean age 77), R-mono (mean age 77) and IV-Chemo only (mean age 76) were older at diagnosis compared to those administered R+IV Chemo (73 years; $p < 0.0001$). However, looking at the oldest age category (> 80), almost one-third (32%) of patients

	Covariates	N	Cox Model of Time to Treatment		Logistic Regression of Treatment	
			HR	95% CI	OR	95% CI
Age at Diagnosis	66–70	1661	ref		ref	
	71–75	1917	0.96	0.87–1.07	0.94	0.83–1.08
	76–80	1996	0.90	0.81–1.00	0.87	0.76–1.00
	> 80	2769	0.49	0.44–0.54	0.41	0.36–0.48
Sex	Male	4521	ref		ref	
	Female	3822	0.85	0.79–0.92	0.83	0.76–0.92
Race/Ethnicity	Non-White	645	ref		ref	
	White	7698	0.94	0.82–1.08	0.89	0.75–1.07
Stage[a]	Non-advanced	4130	ref		ref	
	Advanced	4213	1.48	1.37–1.60	1.47	1.34–1.63
NCI Comorbidity Score	0	4815	ref		ref	
	1	2010	0.93	0.85–1.02	0.90	0.81–1.02
	2	872	0.80	0.70–0.91	0.74	0.64–0.88
	≥3	646	0.67	0.57–0.78	0.60	0.50–0.73
Geographic Region	Midwest	1077	ref		ref	
	Northeast	533	1.23	1.03–1.46	1.32	1.06–1.66
	South	3760	1.20	1.06–1.35	1.27	1.10–1.48
	West	2973	1.12	0.99–1.27	1.15	0.99–1.34
Median Income Quartiles	1-Low	2166	ref		ref	
	2	2059	1.04	0.93–1.15	1.02	0.90–1.17
	3	2061	1.12	1.00–1.24	1.13	0.99–1.30
	4-High	2057	1.11	1.00–1.24	1.14	1.00–1.31

Table 2: Multivariate analysis of treatment within the first year after diagnosis.

treated with R-mono were older than 80, followed by 28% for CLB, 24% for IV-Chemo only and 7% for R+IV Chemo ($p < 0.0001$). Significantly more patients treated with CLB and R-mono were female compared with the other two treatment groups ($P < 0.05$). Patients receiving R-mono were more likely to have advanced stage disease (59%) compared to the other treatment groups (45–48%; $p < 0.05$). R-mono patients also had the highest comorbidity burden while R+IV Chemo patients had the lowest comorbidity burden ($p < 0.001$). Forty-eight percent of R-mono patients had ≥4 organ systems affected by comorbidity and 44% had an NCI score ≥ 1; while 31% of R+IV Chemo patients had ≥4 organ systems affected by comorbidity and 28% had an NCI score ≥ 1. CLB patients were also more likely to be non-white and resided in areas of lower income and

		Initiating Therapy 2001 – 2009				Initiating Therapy 2007 – 2009				
		R-mono (N = 594) %	R + IV Chemo (N = 696) %	IV Chemo-only (N = 1,544) %	P	CLB[2] (N = 151) %	R-mono (N = 186) %	R + IV Chemo (N = 224) %	IV Chemo-only (N = 386) %	P
Age at Diagnosis	66 – 70	19.9	35.9	20.8	< 0.0001	17.9	24.2	35.3	19.9	< 0.0001
	71 – 75	23.9	28.7	27.3		22.5	23.1	32.6	26.7	
	76 – 80	24.9	25.0	27.7		31.8	21.0	25.0	29.8	
	> 80	31.3	10.3	24.2		27.8	31.7	7.1	23.6	
Sex	Male	54.0	61.9	59.1	0.0150	45.7	48.9	58.5	56.5	0.0313
	Female	46.0	38.1	40.9		54.3	51.1	41.5	43.5	
Race/ Ethnicity	White	92.4	92.2	92.1	0.9726	83.4	93.5	92.4	93.8	0.0008
	Non-white	7.4	7.6	7.7		16.6	6.5	7.6	6.2	
Stage[8]	Non-advanced	36.9	52.0	4.0	< 0.0001	51.7	40.9	54.9	52.3	0.0261
	Advanced	63.1	48.0	53.0		48.3	59.1	45.1	47.7	
Number of Involved CIRS Organ Systems	0	9.4	15.7	12.1	< 0.0001	9.3	8.6	10.7	8.3	0.0292
	1 – 3	45.3	53.9	51.2		53.0	43.5	58.5	49.5	
	≥ 4	45.3	30.5	36.7		37.7	47.8	30.8	42.2	

Continued on next page…

[7] Part D chlorambucil data were only available for the 2007 to 2009 time period.

[8] Advanced stage disease was approximated by the presence of anemia and/or thrombocytopenia in the claims data

...Continued from previous page

NCI Comorbidity Score	0	55.4	69.4	59.5		62.3	54.8	71.9	60.4	
	1	25.9	20.8	24.7	< 0.0001	19.2	23.1	21.0	23.8	0.0008
	2	10.9	6.5	9.5		9.3	11.3	7.1[9]	8.8	
	≥ 3	7.7	3.3	6.3		9.3	10.8	7.0	7.0	
Geographic region	Midwest	12.3	12.4	11.9		7.9	16.1[9]	11.6	8.3	
	Northeast	5.4	7.0	6.5	0.0059	9.9		7.1	6.5	0.0900
	South	40.4	44.0	48.6		52.3	43.0	47.8	47.2	
	West	41.9	36.6	33.0		29.8	40.9	33.5	38.1	
Median Income Quartiles	1-Low	19.4	23.6	24.9		31.1	17.7	22.8	24.9	
	2	23.6	22.4	24.0	0.0560	26.5	23.1	22.3	21.0	0.0959
	3	27.8	24.1	25.5		23.2	28.5	25.9	23.6	
	4-High	28.3	28.7	24.4		18.5	30.6	28.1	29.0	
Education	% Less than high school	16.67	17.33	17.92	0.0695	20.01	16.83	16.73	17.03	0.0272
	% High school only	26.55	26.58	27.87	0.0024	29.74	26.36	26.08	26.59	0.9135
	% Some college	28.38	28.07	27.62	0.0648	26.34	27.68	27.64	27.95	0.0009
	% At least a college degree	28.22	28.03	26.60	0.0597	23.91	29.13	29.55	28.42	0.9387

Table 3: Baseline characteristics for the population initiating therapy during the period 2001–2009 and 2007–2009.

[9]Cells with counts of less than 11 are combined in compliance with the National Cancer Institute data use agreement for small cell sizes.

educational levels compared to the other three groups. There were similar proportions of patient characteristics for R-mono, R+IV Chemo and IV Chemo-only when looking at the 2001–2009 cohorts.

3.3   Comorbidity Burden

The most common specific comorbidities were hypertension (53%), hyperlipidemia (38%), coronary artery disease (24%), diabetes (21%), and osteoarthritis (21%). More than half of the patients had comorbidities involving the Blood Pressure System, followed by the Vascular System and/or the Heart System (Table 4). In general, patients receiving R+IV Chemo had fewer proportion of affected organ systems compared to other treatment groups while patients receiving R-mono had higher rates of affected organ systems.

3.4   Overall Survival

The survival analyses compared CLB with R-mono for the time period 2007 to 2009 and R+IV Chemo with IV Chemo-only from 2001 to 2009. The unadjusted overall survival was higher for patients administered R-mono compared with CLB (log rank p = 0.0478; Figure 3). Although the median survival was not reached after 1 year of follow-up, the proportion of patients surviving were 95% (standard error [SE] = 0.79) in the R-mono group and 89% (SE = 0.88) in the CLB group.

The multivariate Cox regression survival analysis (Table 5) revealed a non-significant decrease in mortality risk among patients treated with R-mono compared with CLB patients (HR, 0.466; 95% CI, 0.21–1.05). This finding was confirmed in the propensity weighted Cox regression. The full Cox regression model included age, sex, race, stage, NCI comorbidity score, geographic region, income, and year of diagnosis. The risk estimates were unchanged when replacing NCI comorbidity score with number of involved CIRS organ systems in the model.

The unadjusted overall survival was significantly higher for R+IV Chemo compared with the IV Chemo-only group (log rank p < 0.0001; Figure 4) with 5-year overall survival rates of 73% (SE = 1.08) for R+IV Chemo compared with 56% (SE = 0.94) for IV Chemo-only.

The multivariate Cox regression survival analysis adjusted for age, gender, race, stage, comorbidity, income, diagnosis year and geographic region revealed a 27% lower risk of death for R+IV Chemo patients compared with IV Chemo-only patients (Table 6). This finding was confirmed in the propensity weighted Cox regression with almost identical rates. Increasing age, increasing NCI comorbidity score were associated with significantly higher risks of death, while female gender and white race had significant protective effects on mortality. The risk estimates were unchanged when replacing NCI comorbidity score with number of involved CIRS organ systems in the model.

Several sensitivity analyses were conducted to explore factors affecting the main results. To confirm that the reduction in mortality was significant for specific treatment groups within the broader R+IV Chemo versus Chemo-only groups, we restricted the

	Initiating Therapy 2001 – 2009				Initiating Therapy 2007 – 2009				
	R-mono (N = 594) %	R+IV Chemo (N = 696) %	IV Chemo-only (N = 1,544) %	P	CLB[10] (N = 151) %	R-mono (N = 186) %	R+IV Chemo (N = 224) %	IV Chemo-only (N = 386) %	P
Blood Pressure	59.1	47.6	53.7	0.0002	62.3	58.6	50.9	60.1	0.0900
Vascular	49.2	42.8	44.0	0.0491	47.7	58.1	46.0	51.8	0.0807
Heart	42.8	31.8	41.1	< 0.0001	35.1	42.5	30.4	42.7	0.0108
Endocrine/Metabolic	32.5	27.0	29.3	0.0979	26.5	32.3	26.3	31.1	0.4099
Genitourinary	28.3	25.7	31.1	0.0304	31.8	29.0	25.0	32.9	0.2110
Musculoskeletal	31.5	24.3	27.1	0.0145	31.1	33.3	25.4	31.6	0.3010
Respiratory	21.0	16.5	21.0	0.0345	20.5	18.3	16.1	21.2	0.4397
Neurological	15.5	9.5	13.5	0.0037	15.2	18.8	7.6	16.1	0.0065
Upper GI	15.8	11.5	11.8	0.0257	12.6	14.0	9.8	15.0	0.3203
Lower GI	15.3	9.1	9.1	0.0001		18.3	10.3	13.0	0.0144
Psychiatric	7.6	3.6	4.6	0.0028	12.6[11]	8.1	18.7[11]	6.0	0.5717
Ear/Nose/Throat	8.8	8.9	6.1	0.0200	7.9	8.6		6.2	0.5123
Renal	5.9	3.7	3.5	0.0375					0.0287
Liver	2.0	1.7	2.2	0.7599	9.3[11]	10.8[11]		6.5[11]	0.7801
No CIRS Comorbidity	9.4	15.7	12.1	0.0028	9.3	8.6	10.7	8.3	0.7833

Table 4: Cumulative Illness Rating Scale organ system type by treatment status. [4] Part D chlorambucil data were only available for the 2007 to 2009 time period.

[10] Part D chlorambucil data were only available for the 2007 to 2009 time period.
[11] Cells with counts of less than 11 are combined in compliance with the National Cancer Institute data use agreement for small cell sizes.

Product-Limit Survival Estimates

With 95% Confidence Limits

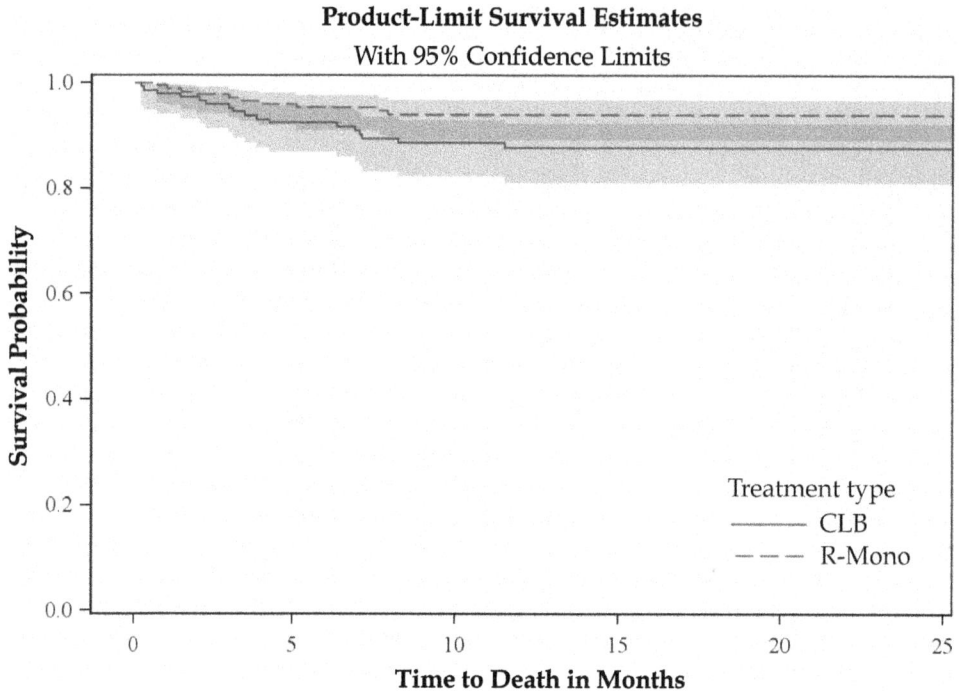

Figure 3: Unadjusted Overall Survival of CLB vs. R-mono (2007–2009).

	Covariates		Multivariate Cox Regression Reduced Model[12]		Propensity-weighted Cox Regression[13]	
		N	HR	95% CI	HR	95% CI
Treatment	CLB (ref)	151				
	R-Mono	186	0.47	0.21–1.05	0.55	0.27–1.12
Age at Diagnosis	71–75 (ref)	77				
	76–80	87	2.93	0.89–9.65		
	> 80	101	3.41	1.06–10.95		
NCI Comorbidity Score	0 (ref)	196				
	1	72	2.37	0.83–6.78		
	2	35	2.57	0.90–7.32		
	≥ 3	34	3.06	0.94–9.90		

Table 5: Adjusted Overall Survival, CLB vs. R-mono (2007–2009)

---

[12] Reduced model by backward elimination. Full model included age, sex, race, stage, comorbidity score, geographic region, income, and year of diagnosis

[13] Propensity score weighted for age, sex, race, stage, comorbidity score, geographic region, income, and year of diagnosis

Product-Limit Survival Estimates
With 95% Confidence Limits

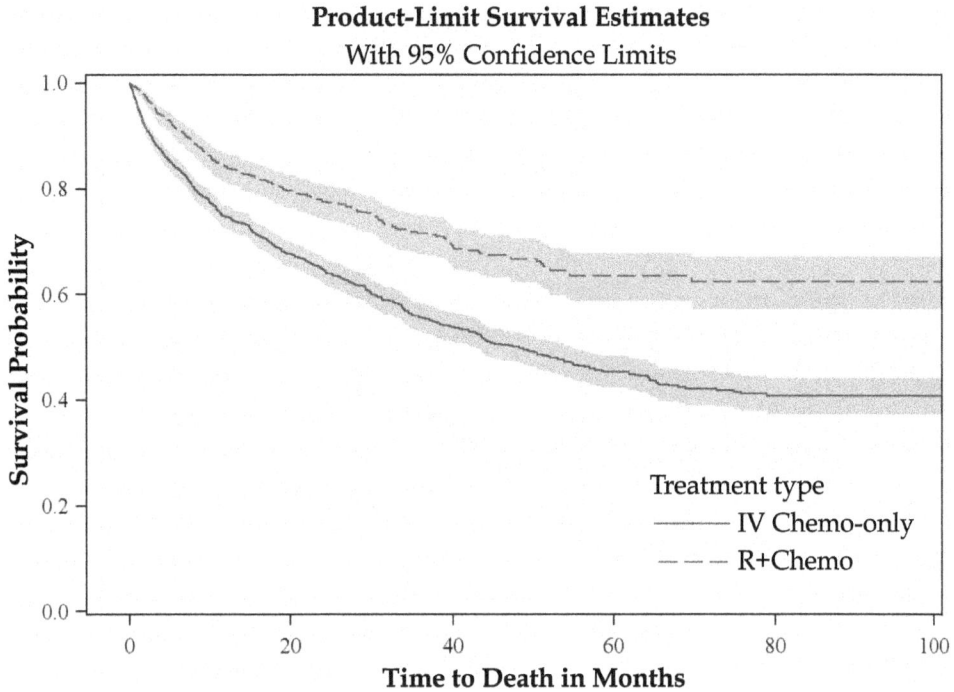

Figure 4: Unadjusted Overall Survival of IV Chemo-only vs. R + IV Chemo (2001–2009).

primary analysis to patients receiving R+F versus F-only and R+FC versus FC. R+F was associated with a 44% reduction in mortali ty compared to F-only (HR = 0.56; 95% CI, 0.43–0.73), adjusting for all other covariates in the model (Table 7). Although results were directionally similar to the primary model with a 29% reduction in mortality for R-FC compared to FC, the findings were not statistically significant due to the small sample of patients receiving FC ($n = 63$).

In a subgroup analysis by age ($\leq$ 75years old), almost identical mortality risk reductions were observed with R+IV Chemo relative to IV Chemo-only as in the overall population (Table 8). Patients > 75 years receiving R+IV Chemo exhibited an even higher 34% reduction in mortality compared to patients receiving IV Chemo-only.

We also stratified the analyses by different categories of comorbidity burden. In the subpopulation of patients with NCI comorbidity score of 0, there was a 27% reduction in mortality with R+IV Chemo compared to Chemo-only (Table 9). R+ IV Chemo was particularly effective among patients with an NCI comorbidity score of 1 showing a 41% reduction in mortality. Although the mortality risks were also lower in patients with an NCI comorbidity score of $\geq$ 2 (HR = 0.91; 95% CI = 0.58–1.46), the sample is small and the confidence interval is wider showing no statistical significant difference.

	Covariates	N	Multivariate Cox Regression Reduced Model[14]		Propensity-weighted Cox Regression[15]	
			HR	95% CI	HR	95% CI
Treatment	IV Chemo-only (ref)	1544				
	R+ IV Chemo	696	0.73	0.62–0.87	0.75	0.64–0.87
Age at Diagnosis	66–70 (ref)	571				
	71–75	621	1.25	1.03–1.53		
	76–80	602	1.44	1.19–1.76		
	> 80	446	2.22	1.81–2.71		
Sex	Male (ref)	1343				
	Female	897	0.81	0.70–0.93		
Race/ethnicity	Non-white (ref)	172				
	White	2068	0.72	0.57–0.90		
NCI Comorbidity Score	0 (ref)	1401				
	1	526	1.10	0.94–1.30		
	2	192	1.37	1.09–1.72		
	≥ 3	121	1.76	1.37–2.28		

Table 6: Adjusted Overall Survival, IV Chemo-only vs. R+IV Chemo (2001–2009).

		Multivariate Cox Regression Reduced Model		
		N	HR	95% CI
Treatment[16]	F-Only (ref)	423		
	R + F	303	0.56	0.43–0.73
Treatment[17]	FC (ref)	63		
	R + FC	192	0.71	0.44–1.12

Table 7: Adjusted Overall Survival, F Only vs. R+F (2001–2009) and FC Only vs. R+FC (2001–2009).

---

[14] Reduced model by backward elimination. Full model included age, sex, race, stage, comorbidity score, geographic region, income, and year of diagnosis.

[15] Propensity score weighted for age, sex, race, stage, comorbidity score, geographic region, income, and year of diagnosis.

[16] Model also includes age, sex, race, comorbidity score, geographic region, and year of diagnosis

[17] Model also includes age, sex, race, comorbidity score, geographic region, and year of diagnosis

		Multivariate Cox Regression Reduced Model		
Age	Treatment	N	HR	95% CI
≤ 75[18]	IV Chemo-only (ref)	742		
	R+ IV Chemo	450	0.73	0.59–0.91
> 75[19]	IV Chemo-only (ref)	802		
	R+ IV Chemo	246	0.66	0.52–0.85

Table 8: Adjusted Overall Survival, IV Chemo-only vs. R+IV Chemo (2001–2009) by Age at Diagnosis.

		Multivariate Cox Regression Reduced Model[20]		
NCI Comorbidity Score	Treatment	N	HR	95% CI
0	IV Chemo-only (ref)	918		
	R+ IV Chemo	483	0.73	0.59–0.89
1	IV Chemo-only (ref)	381		
	R+ IV Chemo	145	0.59	0.41–0.85
≥2	IV Chemo-only (ref)	245		
	R+ IV Chemo	68	0.91	0.58–1.46

Table 9: Adjusted Overall Survival, IV Chemo-only vs. R+IV Chemo (2001–2009) by NCI Comorbidity Score.

4   Discussion

This large real-world study of Medicare beneficiaries with CLL support findings from clinical trials in younger medically fit patients, in which receipt of chemoimmunotherapy was associated with favorable survival outcomes (Byrd *et al.*, 2005; Hallek *et al.*, 2010) while those who are less medically fit may not be able tolerate the toxicities associated with it (Eichhorst *et al.*, 2009). The pivotal trial by the German CLL Study Group of 781 previously untreated CLL patients (median age of 73) with coexisting conditions demonstrated that rituximab–chlorambucil compared to chlorambucil monotherapy increased response rates and prolonged progression-free survival (Goede *et al.*, 2014). Even greater improvements with the novel anti-CD20 agent obinutuzumab (GA101) plus chlorambucil compared to chlorambucil monotherapy were also reported. The ad-

---

[18] Model also includes sex, race, comorbidity score, and year of diagnosis
[19] Model also includes sex, race, comorbidity score, and year of diagnosis
[20] Model also includes age, sex, race, geographic region and year of diagnosis

justed multivariate analysis for R+IV Chemo and IV Chemo-only revealed a significantly lower risk of death for R+IV Chemo patients, even among the subset of patients > 75 years old and those with an NCI comorbidity score of 1. This suggests that chemoimmunotherapy is a more effective treatment regimen even in this cohort of older patients, many of whom had significant comorbidities (Byrd *et al.*, 2005; Hallek *et al.*, 2010). Although our follow-up time was short, there was a non-significant trend for higher unadjusted overall survival rates for patients receiving R-mono (95%) compared with CLB (89%) and a non-significant trend toward decreased mortality risk in R-mono patients. A longer follow-up period would shed more light on this finding.

We show that first-line therapy selection varied by clinical and demographic characteristics of patients. Notably, patients receiving single agent rituximab or CLB were the oldest and had the highest comorbidity burden while those receiving R+IV Chemo were the youngest and had the lowest comorbidity burden at diagnosis. The high level of R-mono usage among the very elderly in actual clinical practice is an important finding and also supports the NCCN guidelines that recommend treatment with oral therapy (chlorambucil) ± rituximab or with single-agent rituximab for patients in this age group or for those with significant comorbidity although there is a scarcity of data on this therapeutic approach (Byrd *et al.*, 2001; Huhn *et al.*, 2001; Wierda, 2006). Prior to 2007, rituximab may have been used in combination with CLB. However, this could not be confirmed because CLB use was not available in the SEER-Medicare dataset during that time period.

Another interesting finding was that patients receiving R-mono were also more likely to present with advanced disease and this may have been a consequence of the medical fitness of the patient as indicated by the older age at diagnosis and higher comorbidity burden rather than tumor burden *per se*. Co-existent renal disease may also contribute to the underutilization of IV Chemo-only or R+IV Chemo in patients with advanced disease given that fludarabine use is contraindicated in patients with severe renal impairment. In the current study, we report that < 4% of IV Chemo-only or R+IV Chemo patients had renal impairment whereas the rate was 9% and 7% in patients receiving R-mono and CLB, respectively. Further, some clinicians may inappropriately consider marrow failure (manifested by the development or worsening of anemia and/or thrombocytopenia) as an indication for caution and may opt to dose reduce or avoid chemotherapy, rather than treat (Foon *et al.*, 2009; Forconi *et al.*, 2008; Hallek *et al.*, 2008). However, even though both older age and comorbidities are significant negative prognostic factors on survival in CLL patients (Smolej, 2010; Thurmes *et al.*, 2008), the survival benefit with receipt of R+IV Chemo compared to IV Chemo-only persisted among patients older than 75 years old and in those with NCI comorbidity score of 1.

In addition to age and comorbidities, treatment selection also varied by sex, race, income, and education, similar to patterns observed in prior oncology research (Shavers & Brown, 2002; Wang, Burau, Fang, Wang, & Du, 2008). In our study, patients receiving CLB and R-mono were more likely female and this was perhaps even more notable given that females were less likely to receive any therapy versus males. Patients receiving CLB were also more likely to be non-white and lived in areas of lower socioeconomic status compared to the other treatment groups. Reducing the disparity of nonclinical factors on the receipt of cancer therapy may reduce the adverse impact on outcomes among these patients. Further research is warranted to better quantify the full spectrum of nonclinical factors that contribute to receipt of cancer therapy in order to develop strategies that facilitate appropriate cancer care for all patients.

In regards to treatment trends over our study time period, the most frequently administered regimen was IV Chemo-only followed by rituximab with or without chemotherapy. Notably, the use of rituximab increased during the study interval from 11% in 2000 to 44% in 2009. Such an increase was also reported in another SEER-Medicare analysis with a shorter follow-up period (Danese *et al.*, 2011). The higher rituximab treatment rates in the current study may be due to the extension of the follow-up period to 2009 as the evidence for the efficacy of rituximab grew (Byrd *et al.*, 2005; Hallek *et al.*, 2010; Keating *et al.*, 2005; Lamanna *et al.*, 2006; Robak *et al.*, 2006) and increasing numbers of clinicians opted to treat patients with rituximab-based regimens.

5   Strengths and Limitations

This study has several strengths, including the large sample size from a population-based registry that includes a wide geographic representation of patients with a diagnosis of CLL in the United States. The database includes information about inpatient and outpatient claims, covered services, all claims regardless of residence or service area, and longitudinal data with claims for services from the time a person is eligible for Medicare until the date of death. To our knowledge, this is the first study to include real-world treatment patterns and outcomes for CLB in an elderly population of CLL patients. However, several factors need to be considered in interpreting the findings.

First, Medicare only began to offer the Part D benefit for pharmacy claims on January 1, 2006. Therefore, it is possible that patients may have received CLB prior to their first claim recorded in the Medicare Part D claims files and our results may underestimate the number of patients who were treated with CLB. Medicare claims data may also more accurately identify agents that are intravenously administered since oral agents are covered under Medicare Part D (Lund *et al.*, 2013) and it is estimated that only 53% of Medicare beneficiaries with a first primary of any cancer were enrolled in Medicare Part D in 2009 (National Cancer Institute., 2012).

The SEER registry does not collect staging information for leukemia and our surrogate for stage (including claims for anemia and thrombocytopenia as a marker of disease severity) may not adequately assess stage in all patients in our study. Further, the use of anemia as a surrogate for advanced disease may be subject to bias as there are multiple causes of anemia in the elderly patient. Foremost among these is renal impairment which increases significantly in incidence at this age group. However, < 5% of our entire cohort had renal impairment making it unlikely that this factor introduced significant bias into the analysis.

The SEER-Medicare database also does not provide data on performance status or lifestyle factors, which could have influenced clinicians' decisions to treat with specific therapeutic regimens. Finally, we did not have information on patients enrolled in health maintenance organizations (HMO) or fee-for-service plans since these data are not collected by Medicare. Treatment patterns, prognosis, and complications may differ between these alternative health care plans and Medicare enrollees, and this would be a productive area for additional evaluation.

6   Conclusions

This real-world analysis provides new information on treatment patterns and outcomes in an elderly, medically unfit, CLL patient population. Patients treated with R-mono and CLB were found to be older at diagnosis and had a higher comorbidity burden; while patients receiving R+IV Chemo were the youngest and had the lowest comorbidity burden at diagnosis. Adjusting for these differences in the survival analysis showed a non-significant mortality risk reduction with receipt of R-mono vs. CLB and a statistically significant mortality risk reduction with receipt of R+IV Chemo vs. IV Chemo-only. The survival benefit of R+IV Chemo vs. IV Chemo-only persisted in a subset of patients older than 75 years and in those with an NCI comorbidity score of 1. Altogether, these findings suggest that chemoimmunotherapy is more effective than chemotherapy in an elderly population with a high prevalence of comorbidity and this extends the conclusions from clinical trials in younger, medically fit patients.

Acknowledgements

Funding for this study was provided by Genentech, Inc. The authors acknowledge Faiyaz Momin, M.S. and Sridhar R. Guduru, M.S for programming support and Jia Li, Ph.D. for thoughtful review and comments. The authors also acknowledge the efforts of the Applied Research Program, NCI (Bethesda, MD), the Office of Information Services and the Office of Strategic Planning, Health Care Financing Administration (Baltimore, MD), Information Management Services, Inc. (Silver Spring, MD), and the Surveillance, Epidemiology, and End Results (SEER) Program tumor registries in the creation of the SEER–Medicare database. The interpretation and reporting of these data are the sole responsibility of the authors.

References

Binet, J. L., Auquier, A., Dighiero, G., Chastang, C., Piguet, H., Goasguen, J., . . . Gremy, F. (1981). A new prognostic classification of chronic lymphocytic leukemia derived from a multivariate survival analysis. Cancer, 48(1), 198–206.

Byrd, J. C., Murphy, T., Howard, R. S., Lucas, M. S., Goodrich, A., Park, K., . . . Flinn, I. W. (2001). Rituximab using a thrice weekly dosing schedule in B-cell chronic lymphocytic leukemia and small lymphocytic lymphoma demonstrates clinical activity and acceptable toxicity. J Clin Oncol, 19(8), 2153–2164.

Byrd, J. C., Rai, K., Peterson, B. L., Appelbaum, F. R., Morrison, V. A., Kolitz, J. E., . . . Larson, R. A. (2005). Addition of rituximab to fludarabine may prolong progression-free survival and overall survival in patients with previously untreated chronic lymphocytic leukemia: an updated retrospective comparative analysis of CALGB 9712 and CALGB 9011. Blood, 105(1), 49–53.

Carney, D. A., & Mulligan, S. P. (2009). Chronic lymphocytic leukaemia: current first-line therapy. Internal Medicine Journal, 39(1), 44–48.

Catovsky, D., Richards, S., Matutes, E., Oscier, D., Dyer, M. J., Bezares, R. F., . . . Group, N. C. L. L. W. (2007). Assessment of fludarabine plus cyclophosphamide for patients with chronic lymphocytic leukaemia (the LRF CLL4 Trial): a randomised controlled trial. Lancet, 370(9583), 230–239.

Charlson, M. E., Pompei, P., Ales, K. L., & MacKenzie, C. R. (1987). A new method of classifying prognostic comorbidity in longitudinal studies: development and validation. J Chronic Dis, 40(5), 373–383.

Danese, M. D., Griffiths, R. I., Gleeson, M., Satram-Hoang, S., Knopf, K., Mikhael, J., & Reyes, C. (2011). An observational study of outcomes after initial infused therapy in Medicare patients diagnosed with chronic lymphocytic leukemia. Blood, 117(13), 3505–3513.

de Groot, V., Beckerman, H., Lankhorst, G. J., & Bouter, L. M. (2003). How to measure comorbidity. a critical review of available methods. [Review]. J Clin Epidemiol, 56(3), 221–229.

Dighiero, G., & Hamblin, T. J. (2008). Chronic lymphocytic leukaemia. Lancet, 371(9617), 1017–1029.

Eichhorst, B., Busch, R., Hopfinger, G., Pasold, R., Hensel, M., Steinbrecher, C., . . . German, C. L. L. S. G. (2006). Fludarabine plus cyclophosphamide versus fludarabine alone in first-line therapy of younger patients with chronic lymphocytic leukemia. Blood, 107(3), 885–891.

Eichhorst, B., Goede, V., & Hallek, M. (2009). Treatment of elderly patients with chronic lymphocytic leukemia. Leuk Lymphoma, 50(2), 171–178.

Foon, K. A., Boyiadzis, M., Land, S. R., Marks, S., Raptis, A., Pietragallo, L., . . . Tarhini, A. (2009). Chemoimmunotherapy with low-dose fludarabine and cyclophosphamide and high dose rituximab in previously untreated patients with chronic lymphocytic leukemia. J Clin Oncol, 27(4), 498–503.

Forconi, F., Fabbri, A., Lenoci, M., Sozzi, E., Gozzetti, A., Tassi, M., . . . Lauria, F. (2008). Low-dose oral fludarabine plus cyclophosphamide in elderly patients with untreated and relapsed or refractory chronic lymphocytic Leukaemia. Hematol Oncol, 26(4), 247–251.

Goede, V., Fischer, K., Busch, R., Engelke, A., Eichhorst, B., Wendtner, C. M., . . . Hallek, M. (2014). Obinutuzumab plus Chlorambucil in Patients with CLL and Coexisting Conditions. N Engl J Med.

Greenland S, R. K. (1998). Modern Epidemiology (2nd ed.). Philadelphia, PA: Lippincott-Raven Publishers.

Gribben, J. G. (2010). Chronic lymphocytic leukemia: planning for an aging population. Expert Rev Anticancer Ther, 10(9), 1389–1394.

Hallek, M., Cheson, B. D., Catovsky, D., Caligaris-Cappio, F., Dighiero, G., Dohner, H., . . . International Workshop on Chronic Lymphocytic, L. (2008). Guidelines for the diagnosis and treatment of chronic lymphocytic leukemia: a report from the International Workshop on Chronic Lymphocytic Leukemia updating the National Cancer Institute-Working Group 1996 guidelines. Blood, 111(12), 5446–5456.

Hallek, M., Fischer, K., Fingerle-Rowson, G., Fink, A. M., Busch, R., Mayer, J., . . . German Chronic Lymphocytic Leukaemia Study, G. (2010). Addition of rituximab to fludarabine and cyclophosphamide in patients with chronic lymphocytic leukaemia: a randomised, open-label, phase 3 trial. Lancet, 376(9747), 1164–1174.

Han, T., Ezdinli, E. Z., Shimaoka, K., & Desai, D. V. (1973). Chlorambucil vs. combined chlorambucil-

corticosteroid therapy in chronic lymphocytic leukemia. Cancer, 31(3), 502–508.

Hines, R. B., Chatla, C., Bumpers, H. L., Waterbor, J. W., McGwin, G., Jr., Funkhouser, E., . . . Manne, U. (2009). Predictive capacity of three comorbidity indices in estimating mortality after surgery for colon cancer. J Clin Oncol, 27(26), 4339–4345.

Howlader N, N. A., Krapcho M, et al. (2011, October 10, 2012). SEER Cancer Statistics Review, 1975–2009 (Vintage 2009 Populations) Retrieved August 10, 2013, from http://seer.cancer.gov/csr/1975_2009_pops09/

Huhn, D., von Schilling, C., Wilhelm, M., Ho, A. D., Hallek, M., Kuse, R., . . . German Chronic Lymphocytic Leukemia Study, G. (2001). Rituximab therapy of patients with B-cell chronic lymphocytic leukemia. Blood, 98(5), 1326–1331.

Keating, M. J., O'Brien, S., Albitar, M., Lerner, S., Plunkett, W., Giles, F., . . . Kantarjian, H. (2005). Early results of a chemoimmunotherapy regimen of fludarabine, cyclophosphamide, and rituximab as initial therapy for chronic lymphocytic leukemia. J Clin Oncol, 23(18), 4079–4088.

Klabunde, C. N., Legler, J. M., Warren, J. L., Baldwin, L. M., & Schrag, D. (2007). A refined comorbidity measurement algorithm for claims-based studies of breast, prostate, colorectal, and lung cancer patients. Ann Epidemiol, 17(8), 584–590.

Knospe, W. H., Loeb, V., Jr., & Huguley, C. M., Jr. (1974). Proceedings: Bi-weekly chlorambucil treatment of chronic lymphocytic leukemia. Cancer, 33(2), 555–562.

Kurth, T., Walker, A. M., Glynn, R. J., Chan, K. A., Gaziano, J. M., Berger, K., & Robins, J. M. (2006). Results of multivariable logistic regression, propensity matching, propensity adjustment, and propensity-based weighting under conditions of nonuniform effect. Am J Epidemiol, 163(3), 262–270.

Lamanna, N., Kalaycio, M., Maslak, P., Jurcic, J. G., Heaney, M., Brentjens, R., . . . Weiss, M. A. (2006). Pentostatin, cyclophosphamide, and rituximab is an active, well-tolerated regimen for patients with previously treated chronic lymphocytic leukemia. J Clin Oncol, 24(10), 1575–1581.

Leporrier, M. (2004). Role of fludarabine as monotherapy in the treatment of chronic lymphocytic leukemia. Hematol J, 5 Suppl 1, S10–19.

Linn, B. S., Linn, M. W., & Gurel, L. (1968). Cumulative illness rating scale. J Am Geriatr Soc, 16(5), 622–626.

Lund, J. L., Sturmer, T., Harlan, L. C., Sanoff, H. K., Sandler, R. S., Brookhart, M. A., & Warren, J. L. (2013). Identifying Specific Chemotherapeutic Agents in Medicare Data: A Validation Study. Med Care, 51(5), e27–34.

National Cancer Institute. (2012). Number of Part D Enrollees (Publication no.). from National Cancer Institute   http://healthservices.cancer.gov/seermedicare/aboutdata/enrollees.html

Parmelee, P. A., Thuras, P. D., Katz, I. R., & Lawton, M. P. (1995). Validation of the Cumulative Illness Rating Scale in a geriatric residential population. J Am Geriatr Soc, 43(2), 130–137.

Potosky, A. L., Riley, G. F., Lubitz, J. D., Mentnech, R. M., & Kessler, L. G. (1993). Potential for cancer related health services research using a linked Medicare-tumor registry database. Med Care, 31(8), 732–748.

Rai, K. R., Sawitsky, A., Cronkite, E. P., Chanana, A. D., Levy, R. N., & Pasternack, B. S. (1975). Clinical staging of chronic lymphocytic leukemia. Blood, 46(2), 219–234.

Robak, T., Dmoszynska, A., Solal-Celigny, P., Warzocha, K., Loscertales, J., Catalano, J., . . . Moiseev, S. I. (2010). Rituximab plus fludarabine and cyclophosphamide prolongs progression-free survival *compared with fludarabine and cyclophosphamide alone in previously treated chronic lymphocytic leukemia. J Clin Oncol, 28(10), 1756–1765.*

Robak, T., Smolewski, P., Cebula, B., Szmigielska-Kaplon, A., Chojnowski, K., & Blonski, J. Z. (2006). *Rituximab combined with cladribine or with cladribine and cyclophosphamide in heavily pretreated patients with indolent lymphoprolife-rative disorders and mantle cell lymphoma. Cancer, 107(7), 1542–1550.*

Shavers, V. L., & Brown, M. L. (2002). *Racial and ethnic disparities in the receipt of cancer treatment. [Review]. J Natl Cancer Inst, 94(5), 334–357.*

Siegel, R., DeSantis, C., Virgo, K., Stein, K., Mariotto, A., Smith, T., . . . Ward, E. (2012). *Cancer treatment and survivorship statistics, 2012. CA Cancer J Clin, 62(4), 220–241.*

Smolej, L. (2010). *How I treat elderly or comorbid patients with chronic lymphocytic leukemia. Acta Medica (Hradec Kralove), 53(4), 213–220.*

Smolej, L. (2012). *Therapy of elderly/comorbid patients with chronic lymphocytic leukemia. Curr Pharm Des, 18(23), 3399–3405.*

Thurmes, P., Call, T., Slager, S., Zent, C., Jenkins, G., Schwager, S., . . . Shanafelt, T. (2008). *Comorbid conditions and survival in unselected, newly diagnosed patients with chronic lymphocytic leukemia. Leuk Lymphoma, 49(1), 49–56.*

Wang, M., Burau, K. D., Fang, S., Wang, H., & Du, X. L. (2008). *Ethnic variations in diagnosis, treatment, socioeconomic status, and survival in a large population-based cohort of elderly patients with non-Hodgkin lymphoma. Cancer, 113(11), 3231–3241.*

Warren, J. L., Harlan, L. C., Fahey, A., Virnig, B. A., Freeman, J. L., Klabunde, C. N., . . . Knopf, K. B. (2002). *Utility of the SEER-Medicare data to identify chemotherapy use. Med Care, 40(8 Suppl), IV-55–61.*

Warren, J. L., Klabunde, C. N., Schrag, D., Bach, P. B., & Riley, G. F. (2002). *Overview of the SEER-Medicare data: content, research applications, and generalizability to the United States elderly population. Med Care, 40(8 Suppl), IV–3–18.*

Wierda, W. G. (2006). *Current and investigational therapies for patients with CLL. [Review]. Hematology Am Soc Hematol Educ Program, 285–294.*

Yancik, R. (1997). *Epidemiology of cancer in the elderly. Current status and projections for the future. Rays, 22(1 Suppl), 3–9.*

Zent, C. (2010). *Chronic Lymphocytic Leukemia in the Elderly: Who Should Be Treated? 2010 Educational Book. Retrieved from http://www.asco.org/ascov2/Education+&+Training/Educational+Book?&vmview=edbk_detail_view&confID=74&abstractID=60*

Chapter 2

Immune Imbalance in Nasal Polyps of Caucasian Chronic Rhinosinusitis Patients

Michael Könnecke[1], Robert Böscke[1], Anja Waldmann[1],
Karl-Ludwig Bruchhage[1], Robert Linke[1], Ralph Pries[1],
Barbara Wollenberg[1]

1 Introduction

Chronic rhinosinusitis (CRS) affects about 5–15% of the population in Europe and the USA (Fokkens *et al.*, 2012) thus represents a popular health problem with significant medical costs (Hastan *et al.*, 2011). For many years, different medications did not offer a healing for every CRS patients and the effort of researchers to find a single treatment for CRS failed, because there is no general pathophysiology for CRS. CRS is just an umbrella term for many forms of chronic inflammation of the nose (Fokkens *et al.*, 2012). In current national and international guidelines, CRS is subdivided in chronic rhinosinusitis with nasal polyps (CRSwNP) and chronic rhinosinusitis without nasal polyps (CRSsNP) (Fokkens *et al.*, 2012; Stuck *et al.*, 2007). CRSwNP is characterized as a chronic inflammatory condition of the nasal and paranasal sinuses with nasal polyp growth and a prevalence about 1–4% of the general population (Fokkens *et al.*, 2012; Settipane *et al.*, 2013). Nasal polyps are characterized by grape-like structures in the upper nasal cavity and typical histological features of nasal polyps, like a dense inflammatory infiltrates and loose fibrous connective tissue with substantial tissue edema (Fokkens *et al.*, 2012; Stuck *et al.*, 2007). However, nasal polyps exhibit four histological patterns, in which the edematous, eosinophilic polyp is the most common form of nasal polyps with a probability of 65–90% (Couto *et al.*, 2008; Davidsson & Hellquist, 1993; Hellquist, 1996; Stuck

---

[1] Department of Otorhinolaryngology, University Hospital Schleswig-Holstein, Campus Lübeck, Lübeck, Germany

et al., 2007). Predominately eosiniphilic cellular infiltration and eosinophilic Th2 inflammation are the major phenotypic markers of CRSwNP, while the inflammatory process is characterized by interleukin (IL)-4, IL-5, eosinophil cationic protein (ECP) and eotaxin-1/-2/-3 expression (Fokkens *et al.*, 2012; Plager *et al.*, 2010; Van Zele *et al.*, 2006). During the last years, several T cell subsets were well characterized. Thus, for example CD4+ T cells are able to differentiate into T helper (Th)1, Th2, Th9, Th17, Th22 and T follicular helper (Tfh) effector cell subsets, but the balance between T helper subsets is essential (Annunziato & Romagnani, 2009; Zygmunt & Veldhoen, 2011). However, inflammation can destroy this balance and generate specific inflammatory pattern.

The innate immune system responds to inflammation with recruitment of eosinophils and other leukocytes from blood vessels into the site of inflammation. This process, called leukocyte adhesion cascade, is mediated by adhesion molecules and tightly regulated with multiple steps involving leukocyte adhesion, rolling along the surface of activated endothelial cells and transendothelial migration (Schmidt *et al.*, 2013; Tam *et al.*, 2011). The recruitment mainly appears in postcapillary blood vessels and starts with capturing of flowing leukocytes, followed by rolling along the blood vessel wall. Both, capture and rolling, are mediated by adhesions molecules called selectins, which interact with selectin ligands on leukocytes (Ley *et al.*, 2007). The selectin family consists of three members, L(eukocyte)-selectin, P(latelet)-selectin and E(ndothelial)-selectin. While L-selectin is expressed by most leukocytes, E-selectin and P-selectin are expressed by inflamed endothelial cells. P-selectin glycoprotein ligand 1 (PSGL1) has a dominant role as a ligand for all three selectins and is expressed on almost all leukocytes as well as endothelial cells (da Costa Martins *et al.*, 2007). Leukocyte arrest during rolling is triggered by chemokines and other chemoattractants like CC-chemokine ligand 5 (CCL5, also known as RANTES), CXC-chemokine ligand 4 (CXCL4) and CXCL5 (Ley *et al.*, 2007). This is mediated by binding of leukocyte integrins to immunoglobulin superfamily members, like intercellular adhesion molecule 1 (ICAM1) and vascular cell-adhesion molecule 1 (VCAM1), which were expressed by endothelial cells (Campbell *et al.*, 1998; Campbell *et al.*, 1996).

The pathogenesis of CRSwNP remains unclear, especially the ongoing chronic inflammation. The known role of the leukocyte adhesion cascade for the pathophysiology of inflammatory processes led us to investigate mRNA and protein expression profiles of leukocyte adhesion cascade related components in nasal polyps of chronic rhinosinusitis patients. Our results could represent a promising strategy in the future.

2   Results

Inflammation is an immune response of the organism to injury or tissue damage. During this process, native T-cells are activated and are able to differentiate into Th1-, Th2- or Th17-cells. Inflammation can affect the balance between these T-helper-cells and generate specific inflammatory pattern. Th1-cells primarily produce IL2, TNFα and INFγ, whereas Th2-cells predominantly produce IL4, IL5, IL10 and IL13. Th17- cells produce inter alia IL6, IL17 and TNFα. However it is possible that different cytokines are produced by more than one T-helper subgroup, like IL2, IL6 and TNFα. Chronic rhinosinusitis with nasal polyps is usually a Th2 related inflammatory disease and microarray analysis showed significantly ($p \leq 0.05$) increased expression of specific genes, which were involved in immune-regulatory and inflammatory processes. Detailed analysis revealed a significant up-regulation of Th-2 related genes in nasal polyps when compared to associated inferior turbinates (Figure 1). Scatterplots point out the increased expression of Th-2 related genes, like IL4 (3.44-fold), IL5 (14.75- fold), IL10 (1.73- fold) and IL13 (21.15- fold) while Th1 and Th17 specific genes were unregulated between nasal polyps and inferior turbinates (Figure 2), Quantitative real-time PCR confirmed the increased expression of IL4 (3.93-fold, $p \leq 0.05$), IL5 (24.35-fold, $p \leq 0.01$), IL10 (2.77-fold, $p \leq 0.01$) and IL13 (31.01-fold, $p \leq 0.01$) in nasal polyps (Figure 3).

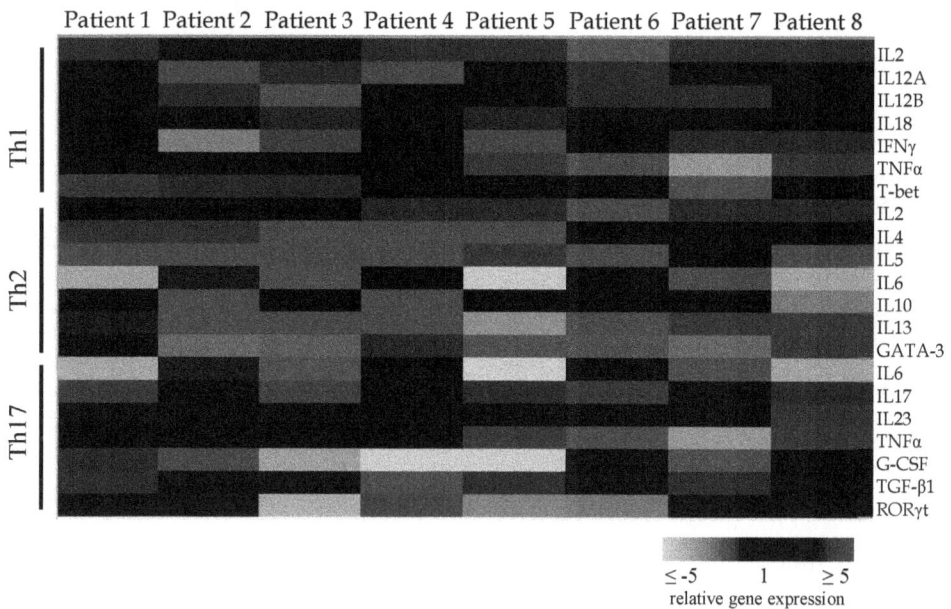

Figure 1: Gene expression of specific inflammatory patterns displayed as heat map. Expression of particular genes where assigned to specific T-helper sub-groups (Th1, Th2 and Th17). Gene expression alterations are color-coded as relative gene expression. Each line represents a gene and each column a tissue sample.

Further analysis of leukocyte adhesion cascade related components showed higher gene expression, P-selectin (1.62-fold, $n=7$), PSGL1 (1.74-fold, $n=7$) and VCAM1 (2.16-fold, $n=7$), while ICAM1 and CCL5 were unregulated. Surprisingly, E-selectin was strongly down-regulated in nasal polyps (0.32-fold, $n=7$) as well as CXCL4 (0.36-fold, $n=7$) and CXCL5 (0.12-fold, $n=7$) (Figure 4a). To confirm the data obtained by microarray analysis, we studied mRNA expression of adhesion molecules and chemokines.

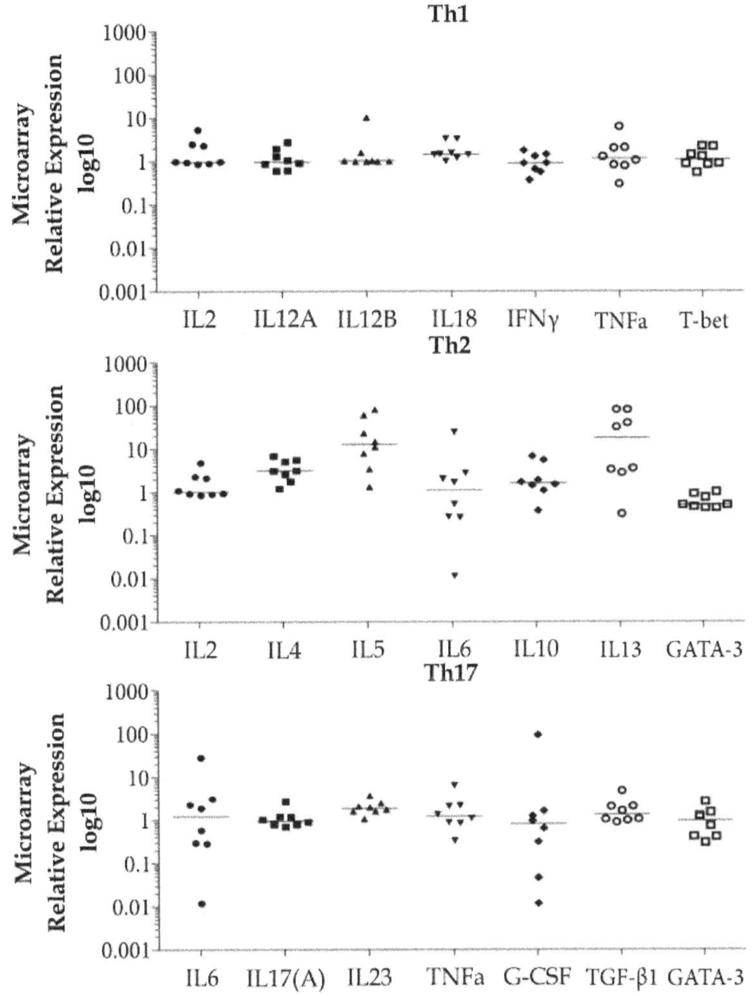

Figure 2: Detailed expression of Th1 (IL2, IL12A, IL18, IFNγ, TNFα, T-bet), Th2 (IL2, IL4, IL5, IL6, IL10, IL13, GATA-3) and Th17 (IL6, IL17(A), IL23, TNFα, G-CSF, TGF-β1, RORγt) related cytokines in nasal polyps compared to associated inferior turbinates by microarray analysis. Each single dot shows the relative expression of the target molecule in nasal polyps compared to associated inferior turbinates of one patient. Median is indicated as *horizontal bar*.

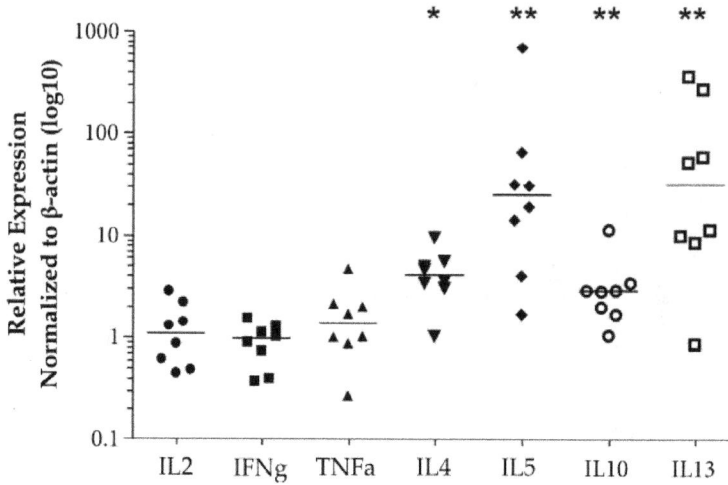

Figure 3: Expression of Th1 (IL2, IFNγ, TNFα) and Th2 (IL4, IL5, IL10, IL13) related cytokines in nasal polyps compared to associated inferior turbinates validated by quantitative real-time PCR. Each single dot shows the relative expression of the target molecule in nasal polyps compared to associated inferior turbinates of one patient. Median is indicated as *horizontal bar.*

The expression of E-selectin was significantly decreased (0.22-fold, $n=14$, $p \leq 0.01$) as well as CXCL4 (0.15-fold, $n=10$, $p \leq 0.05$) and CXCL5 (0.017-fold, $n=10$, $p \leq 0.05$), while P-selectin expression was significantly increased (2.37-fold, $n=15$, $p \leq 0.01$) in nasal polyps compared to associated inferior turbinates (Figure 4b). Expression levels of PSGL1, CCL5, ICAM1 and VCAM1 did not significantly differ between nasal polyps and inferior turbinates.

E-selectin, P-selectin, PSGL1, ICAM1 and VCAM1 are expressed by inflamed endothelial cells, due to this we determined the expression of CD31, a specific endothelial cell marker, in nasal polyps and inferior turbinates of seven patients. CD31 was not altered expressed (0.93-fold) in nasal polyps compared to inferior turbinates (Figure 5a). Additionally, we normalized our data to CD31 (Figure 5b) and alterations were insignificantly compared to the β-actin normalized data (Figure 5c, Table I). Most chemokines are known to be deposit by platelets onto the inflamed endothelium (Ley *et al.*, 2007). In this case, CCL5, CXCL4 and CXCL5 expression normalized to CD31 showed only insignificantly alterations when compared to the β-actin normalized data.

At the protein level, nasal polyps showed strongly decreased expression levels of E-selectin, while P-selectin was slightly up-regulated or equal expressed in nasal polyps when referenced to GAPDH and compared to inferior turbinates (Figure 6). After quantification and compared to inferior turbinates, protein expression of P-selectin was increased (145.8 % ± 30.3 %) and E-selectin was significantly decreased (62.6 % ± 6.96 %, $p=0.018$) in nasal polyps (Figure 7). Additional chemokine expression analysis revealed no significant altered availability of CCL5, CXCL4 and CXCL5 between nasal polyps and inferior turbinates (Figure 8).

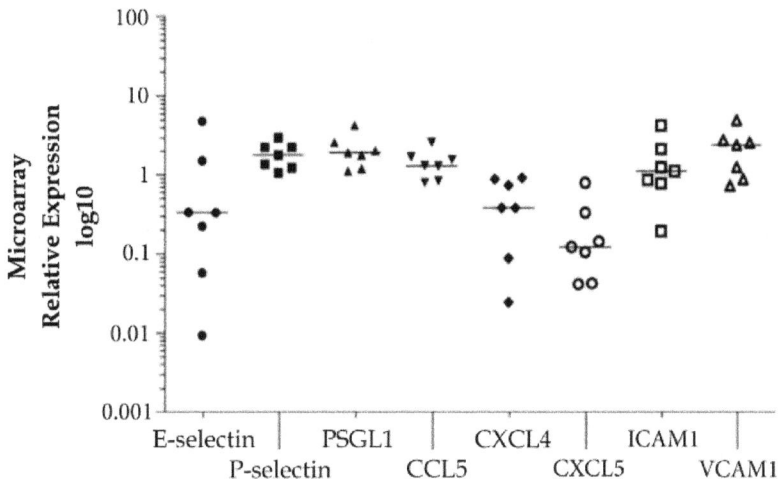

(a)

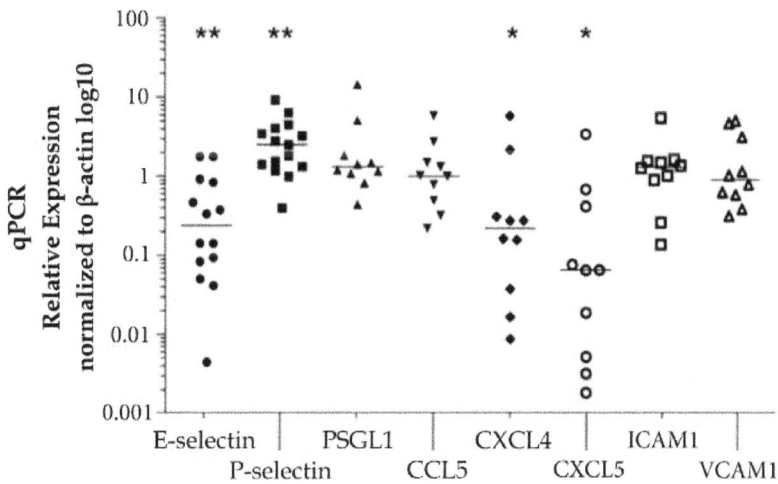

(b)

Figure 4: Expression of leukocyte adhesion cascade related components in nasal polyps compared to associated inferior turbinates using microarray (a) and validated by quantitative real-time PCR (b). Each single dot shows the relative expression of the target molecule in nasal polyps compared to associated inferior turbinates of one patient. Median is indicated as *horizontal bar*.

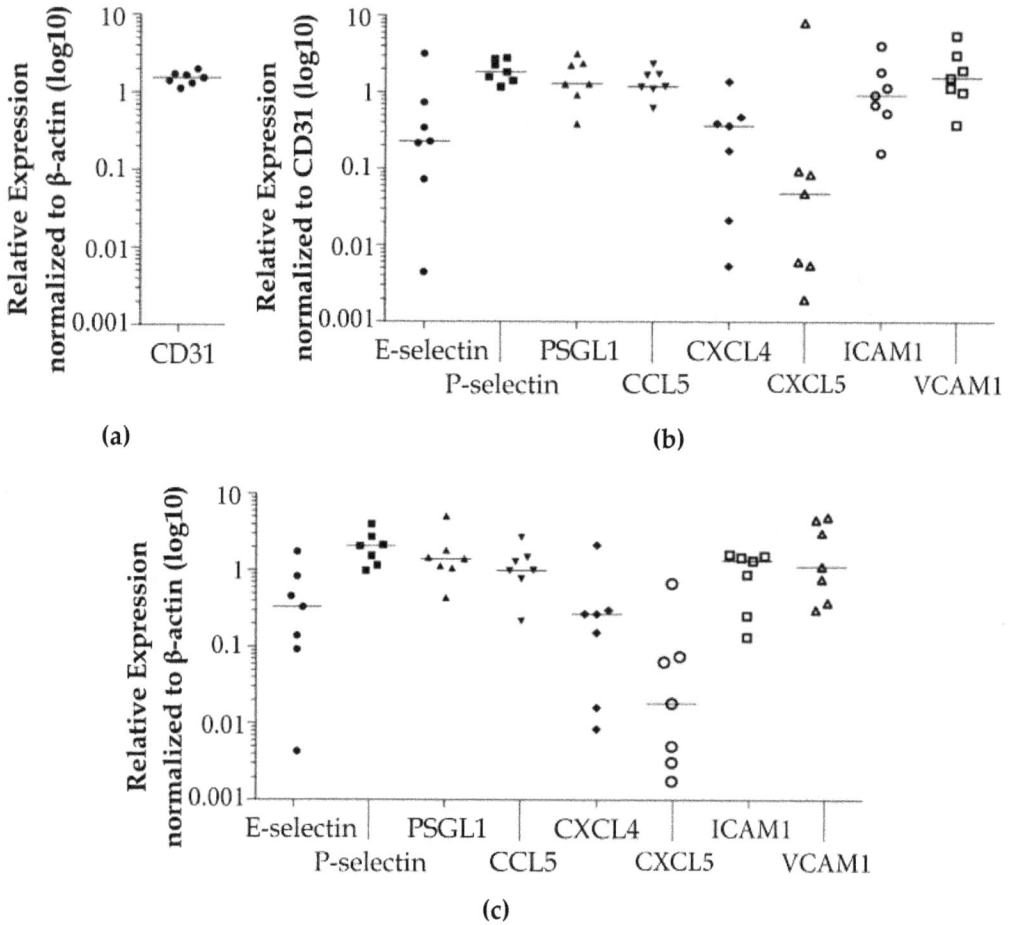

Figure 5: Expression of CD31 normalized to β-actin (a) and leukocyte adhesion cascade related components normalized to CD31 (b) and β-actin (c) in nasal polyps compared to associated inferior turbinates using quantitative real-time PCR. Each single dot shows the relative expression of the target molecule in nasal polyps compared to associated inferior turbinates of one patient. Median is indicated as *horizontal bar*.

Gene	Relative Expression	
	Normalized to CD31	Normalized to β-actin
E-selectin	0.22-fold	0.31-fold
P-selectin	1.82-fold	1.97-fold
PSGL1	1.29-fold	1.34-fold
ICAM1	0.93-fold	1.28-fold
VCAM1	1.56-fold	1.08-fold

Table 1: Comparison of CD31 and β-actin normalized qPCR data.

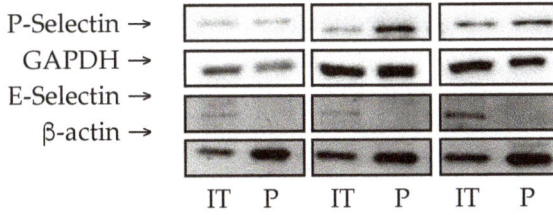

P-Selectin →
GAPDH →
E-Selectin →
β-actin →

IT P   IT P   IT P

Figure 6: Western blotting exhibited lower E-selectin expression in nasal polyps (P) than in the inferior turbinate (IT) of chronic rhinosinusitis patients (n=8). P-selectin was slightly up-regulated or equal expressed (n=8).

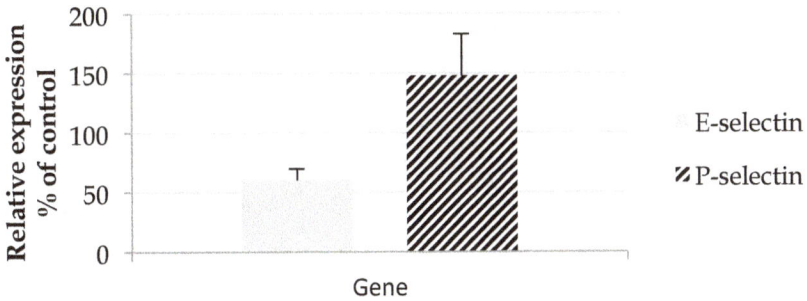

Figure 7: Quantification of E-selectin and P-selectin protein expression in nasal polyps referenced to endogenous control and compared to inferior turbinates (n=8).

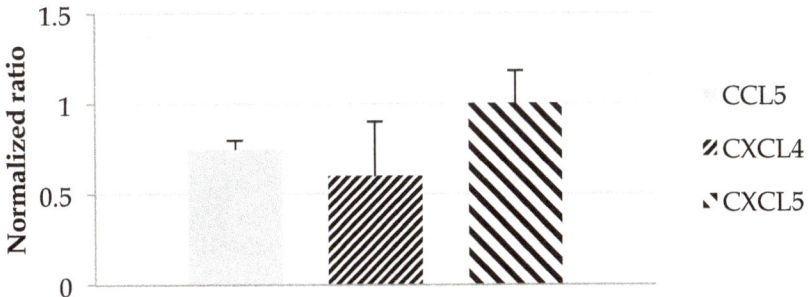

Figure 8: Availability of chemokines CCL5, CXCL4 and CXCL5 in nasal polyps compared to associated inferior turbinates (n=3).

Expression of E-selectin, P-selectin and ICAM1 was detected on the endothelium of nasal polyps and inferior turbinates (Figures 9, 10, 11). E-selectin was expressed at high levels in the inferior turbinates, whereas in nasal polyps E-selectin was irregularly expressed and always at a low level (Figure 9). P-selectin was expressed at high levels in the endothelium of all observed vessels in both inferior turbinates and nasal polyps (Figure 10). Additional staining of ICAM1 revealed similar high expression in both, nasal polyps and inferior turbinates (Figure 11).

Further examinations of stained sections revealed that eosinophil counts were significantly ($p \leq 0.01$) higher in nasal polyp tissues, and to a lesser extend in inferior turbinate tissues. Neutrophil counts did not significantly differ between nasal polyps and inferior turbinates (Figure 12). Strikingly, eosinophil and neutrophils counts significantly ($p \leq 0.01$) differ in nasal polyp tissues, whereas inferior turbinate tissues exhibited balanced counts of eosinophils and neutrophils. The mean values of eosinophils and neutrophils in nasal polyps and inferior turbinates are summarized in Table 2.

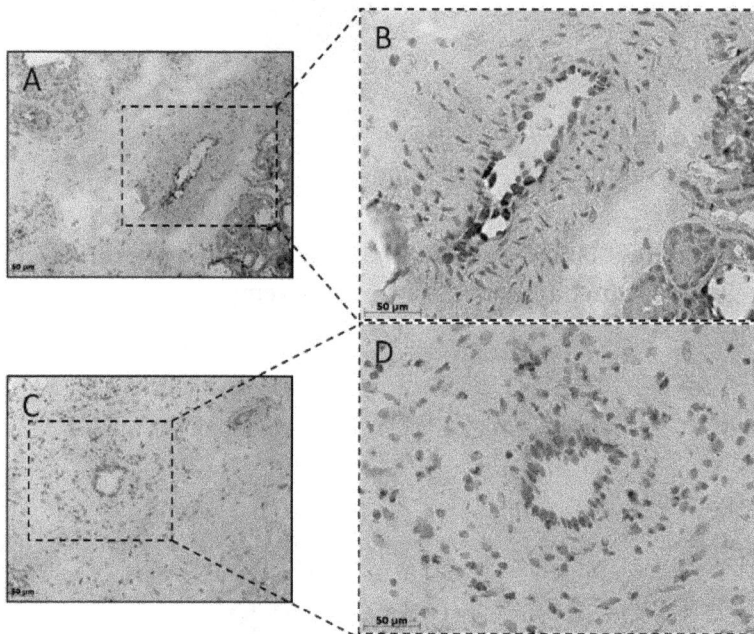

Figure 9: Expression and localization of E-selectin (n=10) in inferior turbinate (A/B) and nasal polyp (C/D) of chronic rhinosinusitis patients.

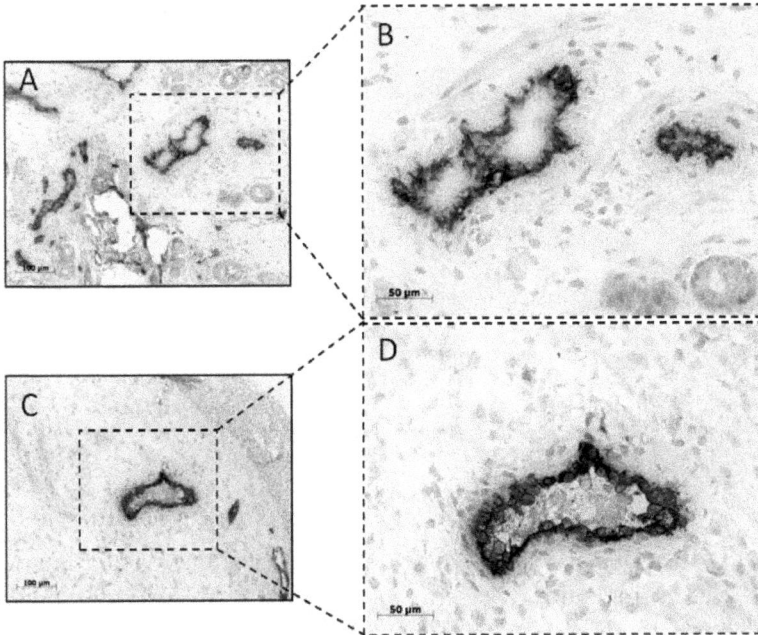

Figure 10: Expression and localization of P-selectin (*n*=10) in inferior turbinate (A/B) and nasal polyp (C/D) of chronic rhinosinusitis patients.

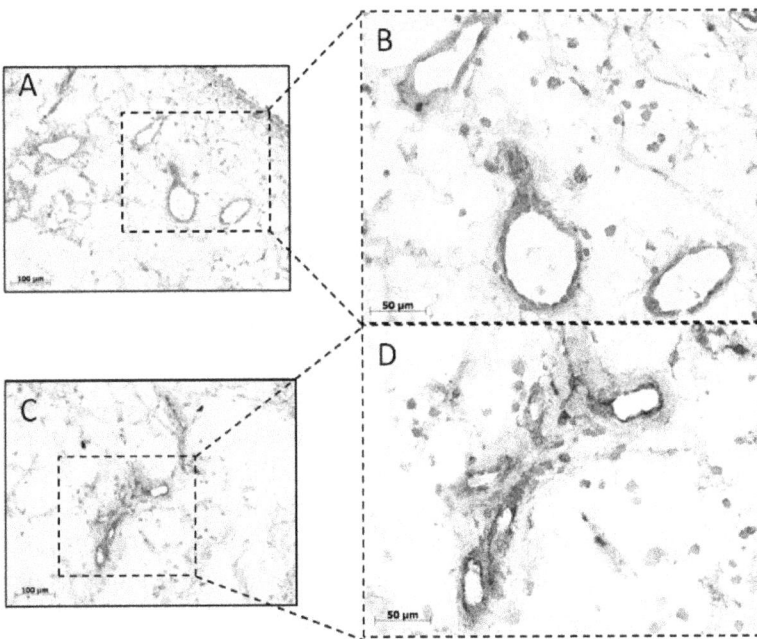

Figure 11: Expression and localization of ICAM1 (*n*=10) in inferior turbinate (A/B) and nasal polyp (C/D) of chronic rhinosinusitis patients.

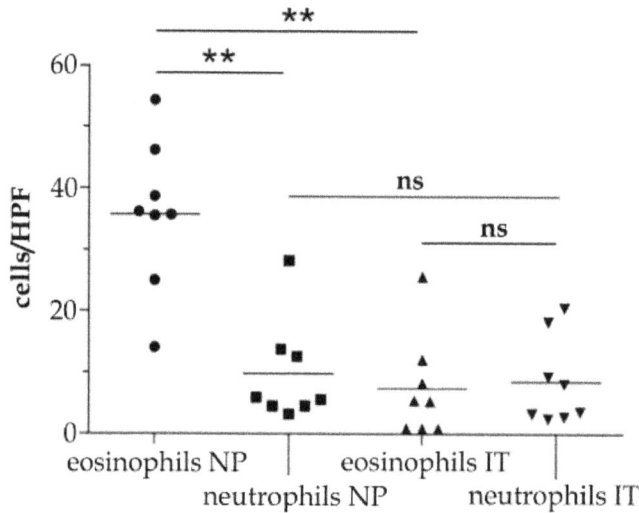

Figure 12: Eosinophils and neutrophils counts in nasal polyps and inferior turbinates ($n=8$). Each single dot represents the mean of 10 parts of high-power fields (HPF) at 400x magnification of one patient. Mean is indicated as *horizontal bar.*

Tissue	Eosinophils [cells/HPF]	Neutrophils [cells/HPF]
Nasal polyps	35.7±12.24	9.8±7.84
Inferior Turbinates	7.43±7.8	8.55±7.18

Table 2: Mean (±SD) values of eosinophils and neutrophils counts in nasal polyp and inferior turbinate tissues ($n=8$).

3 Discussion

Chronic rhinosinusitis is a multifunctional disease with several hypotheses that have been put forward regarding the pathogenesis of chronic rhinosinusitis with nasal polyps. However, there is a lack of detailed understanding of the basis of inflammation, especially the mechanisms responsible for recruitment and activation of leukocytes in nasal polyps. Inflammation in CRSsNP and CRSwNP are characterized by distinct inflammation patterns, showing a relatively Th1 biased inflammation pattern for CRSsNP, while CRSwNP portrays Th2-biased inflammation (Fokkens *et al.*, 2012). But this does not apply worldwide. While the clinical nature of nasal polyps persists equally between Caucasians and Asians, the inflammatory patterns differ between geographical areas. 65–95% of European nasal polyps are eosinophilic (Couto *et al.*, 2008; Stuck *et al.*, 2007), while the most of Asian nasal polyps are predominantly noneosinophilic and shows different immunopathologic features with Th1 and Th17 cytokine profiles (Bachert *et al.*, 2010; Cao *et al.*, 2009; Kim *et al.*, 2007; Zhang *et al.*, 2008), but the reason for this geographical differences remains unclear. In the current study we focused our examinations on Caucasian nasal polyps of chronic rhinosinusitis patients with the typical eosinophilic and Th2-biased inflammation. The recruitment of leukocytes from the blood into the sites of inflammation involves integrins, selectins and chemokines (Ley *et al.*, 2007). Several studies suggest a role of adhesion molecules for the pathogenesis of allergic, chronic and acute inflammatory diseases (Ciprandi *et al.*, 1993; Kyan-Aung *et al.*, 1991; Ley, 2003; Montefort *et al.*, 1992) as well as tumor growth and metastasis (Biancone *et al.*, 1996; Laubli & Borsig, 2010). E-selectin, ICAM1 and VCAM1 have been suggested to play a role in the pathophysiology of inflammatory airway diseases (Lukacs *et al.*, 2002). But also chemokines are thought to initiate and perpetuate the chronic inflammatory response in CRSwNP (Hulse *et al.*, 2014). For a better understanding of the mechanisms responsible for recruitment and activation of leukocytes in nasal polyps, we studied the expression profile of leukocyte adhesion cascade related components in nasal polyp and associated inferior turbinate tissue.

Selectins mediate the first adhesive contact of leukocytes to the endothelium under flow conditions (Schmidt *et al.*, 2013). P-selectin preferentially promotes the recruitment of eosinophils, because P-selectin is known to activate α4β1 integrin on eosinophils, resulting in adherence to VCAM1 on activated endothelial cells (Johansson & Mosher, 2011). In line with our results, others have reported that P-selectin is well expressed in nasal polyp tissue (Hamilos *et al.*, 1999; Symon *et al.*, 1994). However, the selective recruitment of eosinophils in nasal polyps cannot be explained by a strong expression of P-selectin, because P-selectin is also able to bind neutrophils. E-selectin primarily promotes the recruitment of neutrophils and can be considered as the counterpart of P-selectin, which primarily promotes the recruitment of eosinophils (Chase *et al.*, 2012), but E-selectin is also able to bind eosinophils. Accordingly, both, E-selectin and P-selectin, are able to support binding of both neutrophils and eosinophils, but E-selectin is most efficient at raising the affinity of CD18 integrins that support neutrophil deceleration and trafficking to sites of acute inflammation (Chase *et al.*, 2012). Eosinophils bind significantly less efficiently to E-selectin than neutrophils, because neutrophils express more of the ligands for E-selectin (sialyl Lewis X or sialyl dimeric Lewis X antigen) on their cell surface than eosinophils (Beck *et al.*, 1996; Bochner *et al.*, 1994; Jahnsen *et al.*, 1995). PSGL1 has a dominant role as a ligand for all three selectins in an inflammatory environment and is expressed on almost all leukocytes as well as endothelial cells (da Costa Martins *et al.*, 2007; Ley *et al.*, 2007). It is the best studied selectin ligand and important for neutrophil recruitment (Schmidt *et al.*, 2013). Our results revealed an equal expression of PSGL1 in nasal polyps and inferior turbinates. However, the current literature does not involve PSGL1 in the pathogenesis of CRSwNP, so far the role of PSGL1 in CRSwNP remains unclear. Between first adhesive contact of leukocyte and leukocyte arrest, chemokines are crucial for further conformational changes of leukocytes, which mediates leukocyte arrest (Ley, 2014). Several chemokines have been linked to the selective recruitment of inflammatory cells into the tissue and to chronic rhinosinusitis with nasal polyps (Fokkens *et al.*, 2012). Most of them are chemoattractants for eosinophils or are related to eosinophils. CCL5 was one of the first chemokines which was identified to be up-regulated in nasal polyps (Beck *et al.*, 1996; Davidsson *et al.*, 1996). CCL5 is a strong chemoattractant for eosinophils and T lymphocytes, but not for neutrophils. Recently, Cavallari et al. showed that CCL5 gene expression was up-regulated in eosinophilic nasal polyps compared to healthy controls (Cavallari et al., 2012). We used the inferior turbinate of the same patient as internal control due to the fact that it is not affected by nasal polyp growth and shares the same chronic inflammatory conditions as nasal polyps. However, we did not find a significantly altered expression of CCL5. Additionally, CXCL4 and CXCL5 gene expression was significantly down-regulated, but not at the protein level. CXCL4, a member of the CXC chemokine family, is produced by cells of the megakaryocytic lineage, but is also constitutionally produced by human monocytes (Lasagni et al., 2007; Schaffner et al., 2005). CXCL4 has many signaling functions and is immunomodulating, but most of the effects are on monocytes (Deuel et al., 1981; Fleischer et al., 2002; Gewirtz et al., 1989; Han et al., 1997; Horton et al., 1980; Marti et al., 2002). Furthermore, CXCL4 is a chemoattractant for monocytes, but also neutrophils, and prevent monocytes from apoptosis (Deuel et al., 1981; Flad et al., 1998). Additionally, in conjunction with IL4, monocytes differentiate into macrophages and antigenpresenting cells, like dendritic cells (Fricke et al., 2004; Scheuerer et al., 2000; Xia & Kao, 2003). CXCL5 is an epithelial cell-derived neutrophil-activating peptide, which mainly attracts neutrophils and is produced by a wide variety of cells, including macrophages, dendritic and epithelial cells, at sites of inflammation (Charo & Ransohoff, 2006; Middleton et al., 2002; Schwerk et al., 2013; Suzuki et al., 2002). Both, CXCL4 and CXCL5, are able to attract neutrophils and gene expression was down-regulated in nasal polyps of CRS patients, but not at the protein level. The current literature does not imply CXCL4 and CXCL5 expression in the pathophysiology of nasal polyps and needs to be further investigated. In this context and due to the fact that most chemokines are deposited by platelets onto the inflamed endothelium (Ley et al., 2007), platelets may also play an important role in the pathogenesis of CRSwNP, as already demonstrated in allergic diseases like asthma, or allergic rhinitis. Platelets have an important role in the recruitment of leucocytes into the inflamed tissue and it was indicated that platelets contribute inflammation by modulating processes involved in airway remodelling (Page & Pitchford, 2014).

The immunoglobulin superfamily members ICAM1 and VCAM1 convey the adhesion of different leukocytes. ICAM1 is known for a selective recruitment of eosinophils and neutrophils, whereas VCAM1 plays a favored role for eosinophil extravasation in chronic inflammatory conditions (Beck et al., 1996; Fokkens et al., 2012; Jahnsen et al., 1995). We did not find a significant alteration in VCAM1 and ICAM1 gene expression, but others reported an increased expression of VCAM1 in nasal polyps (Hamilos et al., 1999; Jahnsen et al., 1995). ICAM1 plays a dominant role in allergic rhinitis and asthma. It initiates and modulates different intercellular signaling events and cellular functions and is highly related to the proinflammatory infiltrate (Gorska-Ciebiada et al., 2006; Stanciu & Djukanovic, 1998). Nonetheless, ICAM1 is not specific for the lymphocyte response mainly of the Th2 type and its role was discussed controversially. On the one hand increased ICAM1 expression was found in nasal polyp tissue (Doner et al., 2004; Kong et al., 1999; Rogala et al., 2000; Zhou et al., 2004), on the other hand ICAM1 expression did not differ between nasal polyps and healthy controls (Bujia & Rasp, 1997;

Cavallari *et al.*, 2012; Corsi *et al.*, 2008; Jahnsen *et al.*, 1995). Several assumptions have been made to interpret this conflict, like different patient cohorts, differences in staining methods or preoperative corticosteroid medication. In our study we can exclude corticosteroid medication or associated diseases, which could affect the expression of several genes and proteins. Additionally, we used the inferior turbinate of the same patients as control, because it represents a good internal control due to the fact that it is not affected by nasal polyp growth and shares the same chronic inflammatory conditions as nasal polyps. However, we find a well expression of ICAM1, which did not significantly altered between nasal polyps and inferior turbinates. Further investigations are needed to clarify the role of ICAM1 in CRSwNP. When we put these results together, both P-selectin and VCAM1 predominantly recruit eosinophils and were up-regulated in nasal polyps. This could conceivably explain such selective recruitment of eosinophils, but not the high immune imbalance between eosinophils and neutrophils, because P-selectin as well as VCAM1 secondary recruit neutrophils.

However, a down-regulation of the neutrophil attracting chemokines CXCL4 and CXCL5 could contribute to this immune imbalance. Additionally, we found a down-regulation of E-selectin, which may be a crucial factor in the pathogenesis of nasal polyps, because E-selectin optimizes the mechanics and kinetics for the recognition of multiple ligands. The bond strength of E-selectin is more durable than that of P-selectin, because the membrane tethered with the substrate transmits force to the bonds with E-selectin ligands under shear forces of blood flow (Chase *et al.*, 2012). Once inhibited, E-selectin was not able to recruit neutrophils in a primate model, the influx of eosinophils was unaffected (Beck *et al.*, 1996; Symon *et al.*, 1994). In line with the down-regulation of E-selectin, we demonstrated a selective recruitment of eosinophils in nasal polyps and a final balance of eosinophils and neutrophils in inferior turbinates. The role of E-selectin in immune surveillance may be to amplify the sensitivity to locally activate neutrophil arrest and migratory function (Chase *et al.*, 2012). Neutrophils were suggested to play a significant role in the resolution of inflammation as well as for the pathology of the chronic inflammatory state (Mantovani *et al.*, 2011). Additionally, as it has been reported for bronchial biopsies and serum of asthmatic patients, we have expected increased expression of E-selectin in nasal polyps, following the concept of united airway disease (Bentley *et al.*, 1993; Gosset *et al.*, 1995; Kobayashi *et al.*, 1994; Yamashita *et al.*, 1997). However, we found a down-regulation of E-selectin in the endothelium of nasal polyps, like human squamous cell carcinomas of the skin, which down-regulated vascular E-selectin to evade the immune response (Clark *et al.*, 2008).

As mentioned above and consistently with our results, recent studies have demonstrated that CRSwNP is a T-helper-2 (Th2) disorder (Fokkens *et al.*, 2012), but this does not apply worldwide. In European countries 65-95% of nasal polyps are eosinophilic (Couto *et al.*, 2008; Stuck *et al.*, 2007) but nasal polyps in Asia show different immunopathologic features with Th1 and Th17 cytokine profiles and neutrophilic inflammation (Bachert *et al.*, 2010). E-selectin is responsible for the cellular influx of neutrophils and is down-regulated by the Th2 cytokine IL-4 (Raab *et al.*, 2002). Another study from China demonstrated an up-regulation of E-selectin in Asian nasal polyps (Kang *et al.*, 2006). So E-selectin may play an important role in the immune balance of eosinophils and neutrophils and so on in the pathophysiology of nasal polyps.

In summary, an imbalance between Th1 and Th2 responses leads to a chronic inflammatory answer and to establish the final balance between Th1 and Th2 may be essential for the enhancement or protection of disease (Delcenserie *et al.*, 2008; Nicolo *et al.*, 2006). Caucasian nasal polyps exhibit a Th2 inflammation and the inflammatory infiltrate is mostly dominated by eosinophils. Different therapeutic enhancements could represent a promising strategy in the future to reestablish the final balance between Th1 and Th2, and thus a balance between eosinophils and neutrophils. Investigations in platelet activation pathways could provide novel anti-inflammatory therapies without affecting haemostasis. This could, for example result in a better understanding in deposition of chemokines, and up- or down-regulation of specific chemokines could resolve inflammation. Anti-inflammatory therapies, like anti-IL5 or anti-IL13, were already tested in asthmatic patients (Hua *et al.*, 2015; Mukherjee *et al.*, 2014) and could be a promising strategy for Caucasian nasal polyps. An anti-IL5 therapy was already tested in patients with nasal polyps with a successful reduction of the size of nasal polyps (Gevaert *et al.*, 2006), but further examinations are necessary to evaluate the effectiveness of an anti-IL5 therapy. On the basis of our results, we suggest that an up-regulation of E-selectin and the associated influx of neutrophils may be essential to reestablish the immune balance in Caucasian nasal polyps, which are mostly dominated by eosinophils. On the other hand, a reduction of eosinophils is also a possible therapeutic therapy. P-selectin is able to activate $\alpha4\beta1$ integrin on eosinophils, which result in greater adherence to VCAM1 and influx into the inflamed tissue. A down-regulation of P-selectin could reduce the influx of eosinophils and reestablish the immune balance between eosinophils and neutrophils in Caucasian nasal polyps, like we detected in inferior turbinates. However, further studies are necessary to validate the best therapy in the pathogenesis of nasal polyps in CRS, and if so, whether its therapeutic effectiveness could represent a promising strategy in the future.

4   Materials and Methods

All patients were treated surgically at the Department of Otorhinolaryngology, University Hospital Schleswig-Holstein, Campus Lübeck, and have given their written informed consent. The study was approved by the local ethics committee of the University of Lübeck and conducted in accordance with the ethical principles for medical research formulated in the WMA Declaration of Helsinki. Nasal polyp tissue and associated inferior turbinate tissue, as internal control, were harvested from 34 Caucasian patients (28 males and 6 females, mean age 49.32 ± 14.10) who underwent functional endoscopic sinus surgery (FESS) or septoplasty with reduction of the inferior turbinates. Fresh tissue samples were flash frozen in liquid nitrogen immediately after resection, stored at -80 °C before RNA and protein extraction. All patients had a history of sinusitis of more than three months and did not respond to conservative therapy. Patients were skin tested for pollens, molds, dust mites, and pets using standardized extracts (Allergopharma Joachim Ganzer KG, Reinbek, Germany) within a time frame of four

weeks before surgery. Eosinophilic CRSwNP was determined by histopathologic examination and patients with mucoviscidosis or neutrophilic nasal polyps were not included in this study. All patients had been free of steroid medication for at least four weeks
before surgery and had no history of atopy, bronchial asthma or salicylate intoler-
ance/aspirin-exacerbated respiratory disease. Microarray, quantitative real-time PCR,
western blot and immunohistochemistry were performed as previously published
(Könnecke *et al.*, 2014). Additional material and methods are shown in Table 3, Table 4
and Section 4.1.

Gene Symbol	Assay ID	GeneBank	Length of Amplicon
CCL5	Hs00174575_m1	NM_002985.2	63 bp
CXCL4	Hs00236998_m1	NM_002619.2	86 bp
CXCL5	Hs00171085_m1	NM_002994.3	90 bp

Table 3: Additional TaqMan® Gene Expression Assays used for qPCR.

Antibody	Type	Concentration	Reference
P-selectin	rabbit polyclonal	1:400	Abcam PLC (Cambridge, MA)
ICAM1	mouse monoclonal	1:50	GeneTex (Irvine, Ca, USA)

Table 4: Additional antibodies used for western blot and immunohistochemistry.

4.1 Chemokine Detection

Chemokines were detected using the Proteome Profiler™ Human Chemokine Array Kit
(R&D Systems, Inc., NE, MN/USA, #ARY017) according to the manufacturer instructions. 200 μg of protein from nasal polyps and inferior turbinates were used for chemokine detection. For data analysis, pixel density of each spot was measured and average
signals calculated. The background was subtracted and the corresponding signals were
compared to determine the relative change in chemokine levels between nasal polyps
and inferior turbinates.

Acknowledgement

We are grateful to all the members of the Department of Otorhinolaryngology for helpful discussions and a stimulating atmosphere. This work was supported by the Cassella-
med GmbH & Co. KG, Köln, Germany, and the Rudolf Bartling-Stiftung, Hannover,
Germany.

References

Annunziato, F., & Romagnani, S. (2009). Heterogeneity of human effector CD4+ T cells. Arthritis Res Ther, 11(6), 257.

Bachert, C., Claeys, S. E., Tomassen, P., van Zele, T., & Zhang, N. (2010). Rhinosinusitis and asthma: a link for asthma severity. Curr Allergy Asthma Rep, 10(3), 194–201.

Beck, L. A., Stellato, C., Beall, L. D., Schall, T. J., Leopold, D., Bickel, C. A. et al. (1996). Detection of the chemokine RANTES and endothelial adhesion molecules in nasal polyps. J Allergy Clin Immunol, 98(4), 766–780.

Bentley, A. M., Durham, S. R., Robinson, D. S., Menz, G., Storz, C., Cromwell, O. et al. (1993). Expression of endothelial and leukocyte adhesion molecules interacellular adhesion molecule-1, E-selectin, and vascular cell adhesion molecule-1 in the bronchial mucosa in steady-state and allergen-induced asthma. J Allergy Clin Immunol, 92(6), 857–868.

Biancone, L., Araki, M., Araki, K., Vassalli, P., & Stamenkovic, I. (1996). Redirection of tumor metastasis by expression of E-selectin in vivo. J Exp Med, 183(2), 581–587.

Bochner, B. S., Sterbinsky, S. A., Bickel, C. A., Werfel, S., Wein, M., & Newman, W. (1994). Differences between human eosinophils and neutrophils in the function and expression of sialic acid-containing counterligands for E-selectin. J Immunol, 152(2), 774–782.

Bujia, J., & Rasp, G. (1997). [Determination of intercellular adhesion molecule-1 (ICAM-1) in nasal secretions of patients with rhinitis]. Acta Otorrinolaringol Esp, 48(1), 11–14.

Campbell, J. J., Hedrick, J., Zlotnik, A., Siani, M. A., Thompson, D. A., & Butcher, E. C. (1998). Chemokines and the arrest of lymphocytes rolling under flow conditions. Science, 279(5349), 381–384.

Campbell, J. J., Qin, S., Bacon, K. B., Mackay, C. R., & Butcher, E. C. (1996). Biology of chemokine and classical chemoattractant receptors: differential requirements for adhesion-triggering versus chemotactic responses in lymphoid cells. J Cell Biol, 134(1), 255–266.

Cao, P. P., Li, H. B., Wang, B. F., Wang, S. B., You, X. J., Cui, Y. H. et al. (2009). Distinct immunopathologic characteristics of various types of chronic rhinosinusitis in adult Chinese. J Allergy Clin Immunol, 124(3), 478–484, 484 e471–472.

Cavallari, F. E., Valera, F. C., Gallego, A. J., Malinsky, R. R., Kupper, D. S., Milanezi, C. et al. (2012). Expression of RANTES, eotaxin-2, ICAM-1, LFA-1 and CCR-3 in chronic rhinosinusitis patients with nasal polyposis. Acta Cir Bras, 27(9), 645–649.

Charo, I. F., & Ransohoff, R. M. (2006). The many roles of chemokines and chemokine receptors in inflammation. N Engl J Med, 354(6), 610–621.

Chase, S. D., Magnani, J. L., & Simon, S. I. (2012). E-selectin ligands as mechanosensitive receptors on neutrophils in health and disease. Ann Biomed Eng, 40(4), 849–859.

Ciprandi, G., Buscaglia, S., Pesce, G., Villaggio, B., Bagnasco, M., & Canonica, G. W. (1993). Allergic subjects express intercellular adhesion molecule--1 (ICAM-1 or CD54) on epithelial cells of conjunctiva after allergen challenge. J Allergy Clin Immunol, 91(3), 783–792.

Clark, R. A., Huang, S. J., Murphy, G. F., Mollet, I. G., Hijnen, D., Muthukuru, M. et al. (2008). Human squamous cell carcinomas evade the immune response by down-regulation of vascular E-selectin and recruitment of regulatory T cells. J Exp Med, 205(10), 2221–2234.

Corsi, M. M., Pagani, D., Dogliotti, G., Perona, F., Sambataro, G., & Pignataro, L. (2008). Protein biochip array of adhesion molecule expression in peripheral blood of patients with nasal polyposis. Int J Biol

Markers, 23(2), 115–120.

Couto, L. G., Fernades, A. M., Brandao, D. F., Santi Neto, D., Valera, F. C., & Anselmo-Lima, W. T. (2008). Histological aspects of rhinosinusal polyps. Braz J Otorhinolaryngol, 74(2), 207–212.

da Costa Martins, P., Garcia-Vallejo, J. J., van Thienen, J. V., Fernandez-Borja, M., van Gils, J. M., Beckers, C. et al. (2007). P-selectin glycoprotein ligand-1 is expressed on endothelial cells and mediates monocyte adhesion to activated endothelium. Arterioscler Thromb Vasc Biol, 27(5), 1023–1029.

Davidsson, A., Danielsen, A., Viale, G., Olofsson, J., Dell'Orto, P., Pellegrini, C. et al. (1996). Positive identification in situ of mRNA expression of IL-6, and IL-12, and the chemotactic cytokine RANTES in patients with chronic sinusitis and polypoid disease. Clinical relevance and relation to allergy. Acta Otolaryngol, 116(4), 604–610.

Davidsson, A., & Hellquist, H. B. (1993). The so-called 'allergic' nasal polyp. ORL J Otorhinolaryngol Relat Spec, 55(1), 30–35.

Delcenserie, V., Martel, D., Lamoureux, M., Amiot, J., Boutin, Y., & Roy, D. (2008). Immunomodulatory effects of probiotics in the intestinal tract. Curr Issues Mol Biol, 10(1–2), 37–54.

Deuel, T. F., Senior, R. M., Chang, D., Griffin, G. L., Heinrikson, R. L., & Kaiser, E. T. (1981). Platelet factor 4 is chemotactic for neutrophils and monocytes. Proc Natl Acad Sci U S A, 78(7), 4584–4587.

Doner, F., Sari, I., Yariktas, M., & Dogru, H. (2004). Intercellular adhesion molecule-1 expression in nasal polyps treated with corticosteroid. Am J Otolaryngol, 25(6), 407–410.

Flad, H. D., Grage-Griebenow, E., Scheuerer, B., Durrbaum-Landmann, I., Petersen, F., Brandt, E. et al. (1998). The role of cytokines in monocyte apoptosis. Res Immunol, 149(7–8), 733–736.

Fleischer, J., Grage-Griebenow, E., Kasper, B., Heine, H., Ernst, M., Brandt, E. et al. (2002). Platelet factor 4 inhibits proliferation and cytokine release of activated human T cells. J Immunol, 169(2), 770–777.

Fokkens, W. J., Lund, V. J., Mullol, J., Bachert, C., Alobid, I., Baroody, F. et al. (2012). European Position Paper on Rhinosinusitis and Nasal Polyps 2012. Rhinol Suppl(23), 3 p preceding table of contents, 1–298.

Fricke, I., Mitchell, D., Petersen, F., Bohle, A., Bulfone-Paus, S., & Brandau, S. (2004). Platelet factor 4 in conjunction with IL-4 directs differentiation of human monocytes into specialized antigen-presenting cells. FASEB J, 18(13), 1588–1590.

Gevaert, P., Lang-Loidolt, D., Lackner, A., Stammberger, H., Staudinger, H., Van Zele, T. et al. (2006). Nasal IL-5 levels determine the response to anti-IL-5 treatment in patients with nasal polyps. J Allergy Clin Immunol, 118(5), 1133–1141.

Gewirtz, A. M., Calabretta, B., Rucinski, B., Niewiarowski, S., & Xu, W. Y. (1989). Inhibition of human megakaryocytopoiesis in vitro by platelet factor 4 (PF4) and a synthetic COOH-terminal PF4 peptide. J Clin Invest, 83(5), 1477–1486.

Gorska-Ciebiada, M., Ciebiada, M., Gorska, M. M., Gorski, P., & Grzelewska-Rzymowska, I. (2006). Intercellular adhesion molecule 1 and tumor necrosis factor alpha in asthma and persistent allergic rhinitis: relationship with disease severity. Ann Allergy Asthma Immunol, 97(1), 66–72.

Gosset, P., Tillie-Leblond, I., Janin, A., Marquette, C. H., Copin, M. C., Wallaert, B. et al. (1995). Expression of E-selectin, ICAM-1 and VCAM-1 on bronchial biopsies from allergic and non-allergic asthmatic patients. Int Arch Allergy Immunol, 106(1), 69–77.

Hamilos, D. L., Thawley, S. E., Kramper, M. A., Kamil, A., & Hamid, Q. A. (1999). Effect of intranasal fluticasone on cellular infiltration, endothelial adhesion molecule expression, and proinflammatory cytokine mRNA in nasal polyp disease. J Allergy Clin Immunol, 103(1 Pt 1), 79–87.

Han, Z. C., Lu, M., Li, J., Defard, M., Boval, B., Schlegel, N. et al. (1997). *Platelet factor 4 and other CXC chemokines support the survival of normal hematopoietic cells and reduce the chemosensitivity of cells to cytotoxic agents. Blood, 89(7), 2328–2335.*

Hastan, D., Fokkens, W. J., Bachert, C., Newson, R. B., Bislimovska, J., Bockelbrink, A. et al. (2011). *Chronic rhinosinusitis in Europe–an underestimated disease. A GA(2)LEN study. Allergy, 66(9), 1216–1223.*

Hellquist, H. B. (1996). *Nasal polyps update. Histopathology. Allergy Asthma Proc, 17(5), 237–242.*

Horton, J. E., Harper, J., & Harper, E. (1980). *Platelet factor 4 regulates osteoclastic bone resorption in vitro. Biochim Biophys Acta, 630(3), 459–462.*

Hua, F., Ribbing, J., Reinisch, W., Cataldi, F., & Martin, S. (2015). *A pharmacokinetic comparison of anrukinzumab, an anti- IL-13 monoclonal antibody, among healthy volunteers, asthma and ulcerative colitis patients. Br J Clin Pharmacol, 80(1), 101–109.*

Hulse, K. E., Stevens, W. W., Tan, B. K., & Schleimer, R. P. (2014). *Pathogenesis of Nasal Polyposis. Clin Exp Allergy.*

Jahnsen, F. L., Haraldsen, G., Aanesen, J. P., Haye, R., & Brandtzaeg, P. (1995). *Eosinophil infiltration is related to increased expression of vascular cell adhesion molecule-1 in nasal polyps. Am J Respir Cell Mol Biol, 12(6), 624–632.*

Johansson, M. W., & Mosher, D. F. (2011). *Activation of beta1 integrins on blood eosinophils by P-selectin. Am J Respir Cell Mol Biol, 45(4), 889–897.*

Kang, H., Zhang, J., Tang, S., & Zhu, H. (2006). *[Secretion and expression of E-selectin in nasal polyps]. Lin Chuang Er Bi Yan Hou Ke Za Zhi, 20(5), 221–223.*

Kim, J. W., Hong, S. L., Kim, Y. K., Lee, C. H., Min, Y. G., & Rhee, C. S. (2007). *Histological and immunological features of non-eosinophilic nasal polyps. Otolaryngol Head Neck Surg, 137(6), 925–930.*

Kobayashi, T., Hashimoto, S., Imai, K., Amemiya, E., Yamaguchi, M., Yachi, A. et al. (1994). *Elevation of serum soluble intercellular adhesion molecule-1 (sICAM-1) and sE-selectin levels in bronchial asthma. Clin Exp Immunol, 96(1), 110–115.*

Kong, H., Dong, Z., Guo, Y., Yang, Z., & Bu, G. (1999). *Intercellular adhesion molecule-1 and accumulation of eosinophils in nasal polyp tissue. Chin Med J (Engl), 112(4), 366–368.*

Könnecke, M., Böscke, R., Waldmann, A., Bruchhage, K. L., Linke, R., Pries, R. et al. (2014). *Immune Imbalance in Nasal Polyps of Caucasian Chronic Rhinosinusitis Patients Is Associated with a Downregulation of E-Selectin. J Immunol Res, 2014, 959854.*

Kyan-Aung, U., Haskard, D. O., Poston, R. N., Thornhill, M. H., & Lee, T. H. (1991). *Endothelial leukocyte adhesion molecule-1 and intercellular adhesion molecule-1 mediate the adhesion of eosinophils to endothelial cells in vitro and are expressed by endothelium in allergic cutaneous inflammation in vivo. J Immunol, 146(2), 521–528.*

Lasagni, L., Grepin, R., Mazzinghi, B., Lazzeri, E., Meini, C., Sagrinati, C. et al. (2007). *PF-4/CXCL4 and CXCL4L1 exhibit distinct subcellular localization and a differentially regulated mechanism of secretion. Blood, 109(10), 4127–4134.*

Laubli, H., & Borsig, L. (2010). *Selectins promote tumor metastasis. Semin Cancer Biol, 20(3), 169–177.*

Ley, K. (2003). *The role of selectins in inflammation and disease. Trends Mol Med, 9(6), 263–268.*

Ley, K. (2014). *Arrest chemokines. Front Immunol, 5, 150.*

Ley, K., Laudanna, C., Cybulsky, M. I., & Nourshargh, S. (2007). *Getting to the site of inflammation: the leukocyte adhesion cascade updated.* Nat Rev Immunol, 7(9), 678–689.

Lukacs, N. W., John, A., Berlin, A., Bullard, D. C., Knibbs, R., & Stoolman, L. M. (2002). *E- and P-selectins are essential for the development of cockroach allergen-induced airway responses.* J Immunol, 169(4), 2120–2125.

Mantovani, A., Cassatella, M. A., Costantini, C., & Jaillon, S. (2011). *Neutrophils in the activation and regulation of innate and adaptive immunity.* Nat Rev Immunol, 11(8), 519–531.

Marti, F., Bertran, E., Llucia, M., Villen, E., Peiro, M., Garcia, J. et al. (2002). *Platelet factor 4 induces human natural killer cells to synthesize and release interleukin-8.* J Leukoc Biol, 72(3), 590–597.

Middleton, J., Patterson, A. M., Gardner, L., Schmutz, C., & Ashton, B. A. (2002). *Leukocyte extravasation: chemokine transport and presentation by the endothelium.* Blood, 100(12), 3853–3860.

Montefort, S., Feather, I. H., Wilson, S. J., Haskard, D. O., Lee, T. H., Holgate, S. T. et al. (1992). *The expression of leukocyte-endothelial adhesion molecules is increased in perennial allergic rhinitis.* Am J Respir Cell Mol Biol, 7(4), 393–398.

Mukherjee, M., Sehmi, R., & Nair, P. (2014). *Anti-IL5 therapy for asthma and beyond.* World Allergy Organ J, 7(1), 32.

Nicolo, C., Di Sante, G., Orsini, M., Rolla, S., Columba-Cabezas, S., Romano Spica, V. et al. (2006). *Mycobacterium tuberculosis in the adjuvant modulates the balance of Th immune response to self-antigen of the CNS without influencing a "core" repertoire of specific T cells.* Int Immunol, 18(2), 363–374.

Page, C., & Pitchford, S. (2014). *Platelets and allergic inflammation.* Clin Exp Allergy, 44(7), 901–913.

Plager, D. A., Kahl, J. C., Asmann, Y. W., Nilson, A. E., Pallanch, J. F., Friedman, O. et al. (2010). *Gene transcription changes in asthmatic chronic rhinosinusitis with nasal polyps and comparison to those in atopic dermatitis.* PLoS One, 5(7), e11450.

Raab, M., Daxecker, H., Markovic, S., Karimi, A., Griesmacher, A., & Mueller, M. M. (2002). *Variation of adhesion molecule expression on human umbilical vein endothelial cells upon multiple cytokine application.* Clin Chim Acta, 321(1–2), 11–16.

Rogala, B., Namyslowski, G., Mrowka-Kata, K., Gawlik, R., & Gabriel, A. (2000). *Concentration of s-ICAM-1 in nasal polyps tissue.* Med Sci Monit, 6(6), 1109–1112.

Schaffner, A., Rhyn, P., Schoedon, G., & Schaer, D. J. (2005). *Regulated expression of platelet factor 4 in human monocytes—role of PARs as a quantitatively important monocyte activation pathway.* J Leukoc Biol, 78(1), 202–209.

Scheuerer, B., Ernst, M., Durrbaum-Landmann, I., Fleischer, J., Grage-Griebenow, E., Brandt, E. et al. (2000). *The CXC-chemokine platelet factor 4 promotes monocyte survival and induces monocyte differentiation into macrophages.* Blood, 95(4), 1158–1166.

Schmidt, S., Moser, M., & Sperandio, M. (2013). *The molecular basis of leukocyte recruitment and its deficiencies.* Mol Immunol, 55(1), 49–58.

Schwerk, J., Koster, M., Hauser, H., Rohde, M., Fulde, M., Hornef, M. W. et al. (2013). *Generation of mouse small intestinal epithelial cell lines that allow the analysis of specific innate immune functions.* PLoS One, 8(8), e72700.

Settipane, R. A., Peters, A. T., & Chiu, A. G. (2013). *Chapter 6: Nasal polyps.* Am J Rhinol Allergy, 27 Suppl 1, S20–25.

Stanciu, L. A., & Djukanovic, R. (1998). The role of ICAM-1 on T-cells in the pathogenesis of asthma. Eur Respir J, 11(4), 949–957.

Stuck, B. A., Bachert, C., Federspil, P., Hosemann, W., Klimek, L., Mosges, R. et al. (2007). Rhinosinusitis guidelines of the German society for otorhinolaryngology, head and neck surgery. Hno, 55(10), 758–+.

Suzuki, S., Kobayashi, M., Chiba, K., Horiuchi, I., Wang, J., Kondoh, T. et al. (2002). Autocrine production of epithelial cell-derived neutrophil attractant-78 induced by granulocyte colony-stimulating factor in neutrophils. Blood, 99(5), 1863–1865.

Symon, F. A., Walsh, G. M., Watson, S. R., & Wardlaw, A. J. (1994). Eosinophil adhesion to nasal polyp endothelium is P-selectin-dependent. J Exp Med, 180(1), 371–376.

Tam, A., Wadsworth, S., Dorscheid, D., Man, S. F., & Sin, D. D. (2011). The airway epithelium: more than just a structural barrier. Ther Adv Respir Dis, 5(4), 255–273.

Van Zele, T., Claeys, S., Gevaert, P., Van Maele, G., Holtappels, G., Van Cauwenberge, P. et al. (2006). Differentiation of chronic sinus diseases by measurement of inflammatory mediators. Allergy, 61(11), 1280–1289.

Xia, C. Q., & Kao, K. J. (2003). Effect of CXC chemokine platelet factor 4 on differentiation and function of monocyte-derived dendritic cells. Int Immunol, 15(8), 1007–1015.

Yamashita, N., Kaneko, S., Kouro, O., Furue, M., Yamamoto, S., & Sakane, T. (1997). Soluble E-selectin as a marker of disease activity in atopic dermatitis. J Allergy Clin Immunol, 99(3), 410–416.

Zhang, N., Van Zele, T., Perez-Novo, C., Van Bruaene, N., Holtappels, G., DeRuyck, N. et al. (2008). Different types of T-effector cells orchestrate mucosal inflammation in chronic sinus disease. J Allergy Clin Immunol, 122(5), 961–968.

Zhou, B., Li, H., Han, D., & Liu, Z. (2004). [Role of ICAM-1 in eosinophilia and prognosis of nasal polyps]. Lin Chuang Er Bi Yan Hou Ke Za Zhi, 18(2), 72–73.

Zygmunt, B., & Veldhoen, M. (2011). T helper cell differentiation more than just cytokines. Adv Immunol, 109, 159–196.

Chapter 3

Synchronous DC/CIK and Thoracic Radiotherapy in Patients with Advanced NSCLC: An Open-label, Single-center, Phase II Study

Lu-Ping Zhang[1], Jian-Guo Sun[2], Yan-Mei Xu[3], Jie Shen[2,] Feng He[2],
Dan Zhang[2], Zheng-Tang Chen[2]

1 Introduction

Lung cancer is the most commonly diagnosed cancer worldwide (1.8 million, 13.0% of the total), and also the most common cause of cancer death (1.6 million, 19.4% of the total) (International Agency for Research on Cancer). Of the newly diagnosed lung cancer patients, more than 80% are diagnosed with non-small cell lung cancer (NSCLC) (Brodowicz et al., 2006). Chemotherapy, surgery and thoracic radiotherapy (TRT) are the three main therapies for lung cancer. Although much progress has been made in the last decade in lung cancer treatment, the survival rate has been improved only marginally; the overall 5 year survival rate is still less than 20% (Allemani et al., 2015). More efforts are needed to improve the prognosis of NSCLC.

TRT plays an irreplaceable role in treating NSCLC patients, especially those with medically inoperable or locally advanced unresectable NSCLC (Panakis et al., 2008). Accumulating evidence shows that TRT may stimulate the anti-tumor immune response (Apetoh et al., 2007; Liao et al., 2009; Gupta et al., 2012; Gameiro et al., 2014). Tumor cells killed by radiation can release tumor antigens and molecules that induce various im-

---

[1] Cancer Institute of PLA, Xinqiao Hospital, Chongqing, China

[2] Third Military Medical University, Chongqing, China

[3] Oncology Department, Leshan People's Hospital, Chongqing, China

mune modulatory effects (Friedman, 2002; Finkelstein *et al.*, 2011). Dendritic cells (DCs) are the major antigen-presenting cells, and play a central role in regulating and activating the immune response (Villadangos & Schnorrer, 2007; Steinman & Banchereau, 2007). Cytokine-induced killer cells (CIKs), which express the T-cell marker CD3+ and also the NK cell marker CD56+, have a strong anti-tumor activity (Sangiolo *et al.*, 2009). Immunotherapy with DCs and CIKs has been proven to have excellent clinical efficacy and be well tolerated in tumor patients (Toomey *et al.*, 2013; Cui *et al.*, 2013).

In this phase II trial from January 2012 to June 2014, we evaluated the efficacy, safety and immunologic effects of DC/CIK cytotherapy combined with TRT in patients with advanced NSCLC.

2   Patients and Methods

2.1   Study Design and Patients

This prospective open-label, single-center, phase II study was conducted at the Cancer Institute of PLA, Xinqiao Hospital, Third Military Medical University, Chongqing, China, from January 2012 to June 2014. This trial was registered at Chinese Clinical Trial Registry (ChiCTR-TRC-12002369, http://www.chictr.org/en/) and approved by the Ethics Committee of General Logistics Department of PLA, China.

Eligible patients were those who had been histologically or cytologically (excluding sputum cytology) diagnosed with unresectable stage III or IV advanced NSCLC (according to the 7th edition of the General Rule for Clinical and Pathological Record of Lung Cancer) (The Japan Lung Cancer Society, 2010). Other inclusion criteria included 18 years of age or older when signing consent form; a life expectancy of 3 months or longer at the registration; Eastern Cooperative Oncology Group (ECOG) performance status (PS) 0 – 2; adequate function of the liver, kidney, heart and hematopoietic system; two or more cycles of previous chemotherapy. No previous molecular targeted therapy or TRT was allowed. One or more measurable lesions are necessary for therapeutic evaluation based on Response Evaluation Criteria in Solid Tumors (RECIST 1.1) (Eisenhauer *et al.*, 2009).

Major exclusion criteria included an acute infection; any autoimmune disease; a history of severe allergic reaction; HIV-positivity; pregnancy or nursing.

Enrolled patients were randomly assigned to control group and treatment group (1:1) with a block randomization. Patients in control group received TRT alone, but the patients in treatment group received both TRT and DC/CIK cytotherapy starting from the 6th fraction of irradiation (Figure 1). The primary endpoint for this clinical trial was median progression-free survival (mPFS), and secondary endpoints were objective response rate (ORR), disease control rate (DCR), median overall survival (mOS), PS changes and side effects. Immunologic effects were to be explored. After TRT, enrolled patients would continue chemotherapy to reach a standard 6 cycles in total.

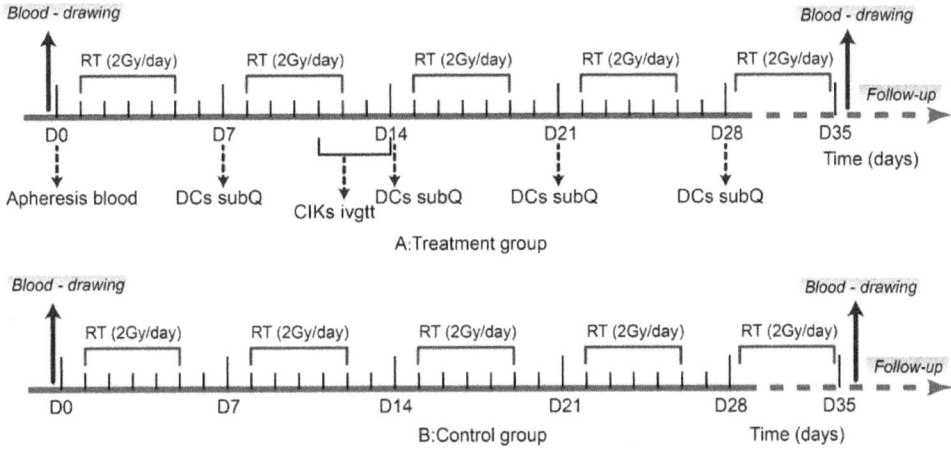

Figure 1: The study design of clinical trial.

2.2   Schedule of Cytotherapy

At the beginning of the study (day 0), we collected peripheral blood mononuclear cells (PBMCs) from the patients for culturing DCs and CIKs in vitro. Subsequently, more than 1×10^7 DCs were injected intradermally in the lymph node-rich regions (bilateral subaxillary or inguinal region) by multi-point injection on days 7, 14, 21, and 28. Over 1×10^9 CIKs in 100ml of normal saline (NS) 0.9%) were re-infused intravenously once a day for 4 successive days from day 11 (Figure 1).

2.3   Radiotherapy Regimens

Three dimensional conformal RT (3D-CRT) or intensity-modulated radiation therapy (IMRT) was adopted for the TRT. Contour delineation and therapeutic plan was designed and confirmed by the professional radiation oncologist. Briefly, TRT was performed at 2 Gy per fraction, 5 consecutive fractions per week to a total dose of 60–66 Gy in 6–7 weeks.

2.4   Preparation of Autologous DC Vaccines and CIKs

Autologous DCs and CIKs were prepared following the previous studies (Nicol *et al.*, 2011; Zhang *et al.*, 2011; Ma *et al.*, 2012; Kantoff *et al.*, 2010) (Figure 2). Briefly, PBMCs were isolated by Ficoll-Hypaque gradient density centrifugation, and then cultured in X-VIVO medium for 2h. The non-adherent cells were collected for culturing CIKs, and the adherent cells were collected for DCs in X-VIVO medium containing granulocyte macrophage colony-stimulating factor (GM-CSF) and interleukin-4 (IL-4). 5 days later, tumor necrosis factor-α (TNF-α) and peptide antigen (MUC-1 peptide: SAPDTRPAPGSTAPPAHGVT, GL Biochem, Shanghai, China) were added into DC culture for another 2 days. For preparing CIKs, non-adherent cells were cultured in X-

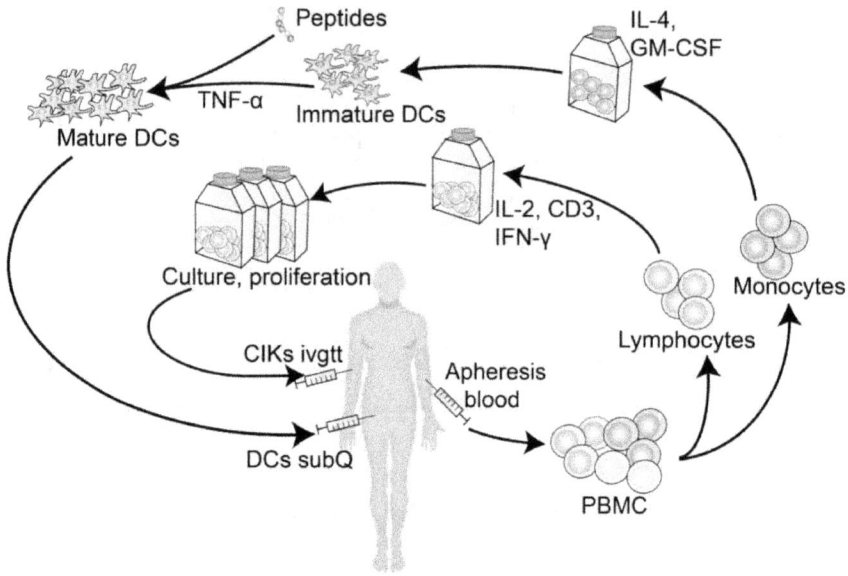

Figure 2: The schema of autologous infusion of DC vaccines and CIK cells.

VIVO medium containing interferon γ (IFN-γ), CD3 monoclonal antibody, and interleukin-2 (IL-2) for 10 days. The immune phenotype markers CD80, CD83, CD86, and HLA-DR for DCs and CD3, CD56 for CIKs were analyzed by flow cytometry. Levels of bacteria, fungi and endotoxin in all the cultured samples were detected during the course of cell culture.

2.5   Assessment of Clinic Effects and Follow-up

According to RECIST 1.1 (Eisenhauer *et al.*, 2009), the treatment efficacy was classified as complete response (CR), partial response (PR), stable disease (SD), and progression disease (PD). The ORR was defined as the percentage of patients with CR or PR, and DCR was defined as the percentage of patients with CR, or PR, or SD. Progression-free survival (PFS) was defined as the time scale from enrollment to disease progression while overall survival (OS) was the time scale from enrollment to death. The follow-up was performed at the 1st and 3rd month after TRT treatment, and then every 3 months for the one year, and thereafter every 6 months. Routine follow-up assessments included physical examinations, monitoring vital signs, computed tomographic (CT) scans and laboratory tests.

2.6   Assessment of Immunologic Effects

The serum levels of cytokines (IL-2, IFN-γ), T cell populations (CD3+, CD3+CD4+, CD3+CD8+ T lymphocytes) and CD3-CD56+ natural killer (NK) cells were monitored both before and after the TRT treatment. Blood-drawing from participants was performed on day 0 and within a week after TRT (Figure 1). 3 ml of peripheral blood in coagulant-promoting tube was collected for extracting serum. 3 ml of peripheral blood in EDTA anticoagulant tube was used for detecting T cell populations and NK cells by flow cytometry. Commercially available enzyme-linked immunosorbent assay (ELISA) kits (R&D Systems, MN, USA) were used to measure the levels of cytokines (IL-2, IFN-γ) following the manufacturer's instruction. For detecting the T cell populations and NK cells, 100 μl of fresh blood samples were stained with matched antibodies (anti-CD3+, anti-CD4+ combined with anti-CD8+ for T cell population, and anti-CD3+ combined with anti-CD56+ for NK cells, respectively) in darkness for 20 min. All the antibodies were purchased from BD Bioscience. Then, erythrocyte lysis buffer was added into the samples. After being vortexed for 15 seconds and incubated at room temperature for 5 min, the samples were centrifuged to remove the supernatant and washed with PBS. Next, after being re-suspended with staining buffer, the samples were analyzed on the BD Aria flow cytometer (BD Bioscience).

2.7   Qualities of Life (QOL) and Side Effects

Adverse effects, such as insomnia, anorexia, fever, skin rash, and joint pain, were monitored and were observed once a week during the therapy and once a month during the follow-up. PS was evaluated on day 0 of the study and within a week after the TRT.

2.8   Statistical Analysis

The data were analyzed using SPSS 18.0 statistical software (SPSS Inc., Chicago, IL, USA). The measurement data were expressed as means ± standard deviation ($\bar{x}$ ± s) and were compared with the independent Student's t-test. The enumeration data were analyzed using a χ^2 test. Kaplan-Meier curves with the log-rank test were used to estimate mPFS and mOS. Hazard ratio (HR) and 95% CI were also calculated by Cox proportional hazard regression models. A P value < 0.05 was considered to indicate statistical significance.

3   Results

3.1   Patient Characteristics

From January 2012 to June 2014, a total of 82 patients with advanced NSCLC were enrolled, with 21 in treatment group and 61 in control group (Figure 3). The mean follow-up time was 377 days (ranging from 60 – 685 days). Clinic-pathological characteristics such as age, gender, PS, clinical stage of tumor, previous chemotherapy, pathological type and PS in treatment and control groups were analyzed. None of these characteristics in the two groups showed significant differences (Table 1, P > 0.05), which meant a nearly identical baseline between the two groups. The number of patients with stage III NSCLC in the control group seems larger than that in treatment group. However, there was no statistically significant difference between these two groups.

```
                    ┌─────────────────────────────────────┐
                    │      82 assessed for eligibility     │
                    └─────────────────────────────────────┘
              ┌────────────────────────────┐   ┌────────────────────────────┐
              │  21 cases in treatment group│   │  61 cases in control group │
              └────────────────────────────┘   └────────────────────────────┘
```

| 21 cases received DC/CIK combined with RT
10 adverse events
21 cases had paired immunologic results before and after therapy | 61 cases received RT alone
27 adverse events
20 cases had paired immunologic results before and after therapy |

```
                    ┌─────────────────────────────────────┐
                    │        Post-study observation        │
                    └─────────────────────────────────────┘
```

| 21 cases with side effects assessment | 59 cases with side effects assessment
2 patients with incomplete follow-up data |

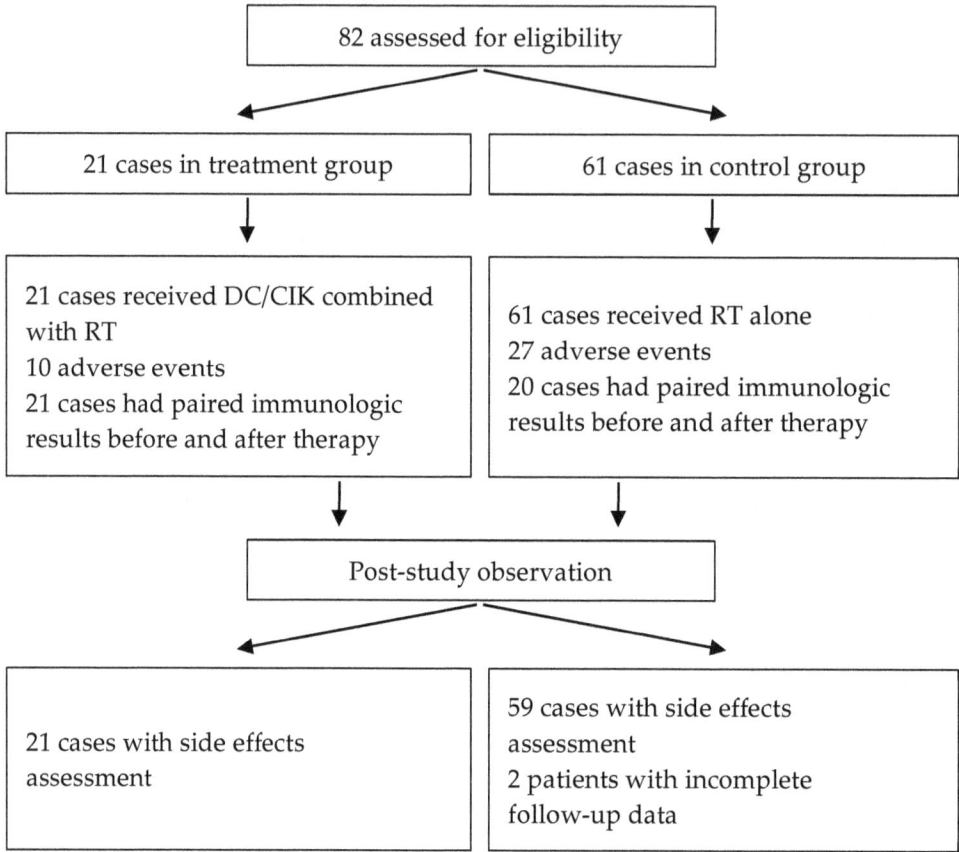

Figure 3: Trial profile.

Characteristics	Treatment Group	Control Group
Number	21	61
Age Mean (Range)	56.6 (32–74)	56.4 (31–74)
Gender: Male	19 (90.5%)	53 (86.9%)
Gender: Female	2 (9.5%)	8 (13.1%)
Stage Status: III	10 (47.6%)	37 (60.7%)
Stage Status: IV	11 (52.4%)	24 (39.3%)
Tumor Histology: Adenocarcinoma	8 (38.1%)	26 (42.6%)
Squamous carcinoma	13 (61.9%)	35 (57.4%)
Cycles of Previous Chemotherapy	2.9 ± 0.7	3.1 ± 0.8
PS score	0.4 ± 0.6	0.6 ± 0.7

Table 1: Baseline characteristics of two groups.

As for long-term evaluation, the mPFS of patients in treatment group (330 days) was significantly longer than that in control group (233 days) (HR 0.51, 95% CI 0.27–1.0, P=0.0483) (Figure 4A). However, there was no significant difference in mOS between treatment group (400 days) and control group (460 days) (HR 0.83, 95% CI 0.41–1.69, P=0.606) (Figure 4B).

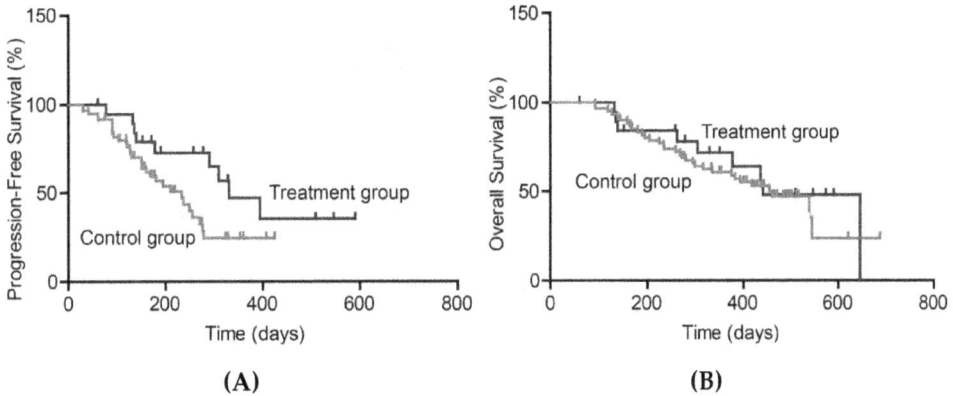

Figure 4: The long-term clinical effects of Kaplan-Meier curves. **(A)** Compared with control group, mPFS in treatment group is significantly longer (HR: 0.51, 95% CI: 0.27 – 1.0, P < 0.05). **(B)** No significant change in mOS between treatment group and control group (HR: 0.83, 95% CI: 0.41 – 1.69, P > 0.05).

3.2   Clinical Outcomes

The median follow-up time in treatment and control groups was 339 days (350.8 vs. 175.4) and 393 days (355.8 vs. 141.5), respectively. 0 CR, 10 PR, 9 SD and 2 PD were found in treatment group, and 0 CR, 15 PR, 39 SD and 7 PD were found in control group. ORR in treatment group is higher than that in control group (47.6% vs. 24.6%, P = 0.04) (Figure 5). However, no obvious difference in DCR was observed between treatment group and control group (90.5% vs. 88.5%, P = 0.767).

3.3   Immunologic Response

Among the 61 patients in control group, complete immunologic results were obtained in only 20 cases both before and after TRT treatment. There was a lack of some medical materials in the rest cases because of their refusal to draw blood and the delayed follow-up, and some other reasons. These 20 cases were analyzed by assessing the baseline (Table 2) and immunologic effects. The results of cytokines (IL-2, IFN-γ), T cell populations and NK cells were analyzed. The serum levels of IL-2 and IFN-γ did not differ significantly between the two groups both before and after the TRT (Table 3, P > 0.05). Moreover, there were also no obvious changes in the percentage of CD3+, CD3+CD4+, CD3+CD8+, CD3-CD56+ NK cells and CD4+/CD8+ T cell ratio before and after TRT in

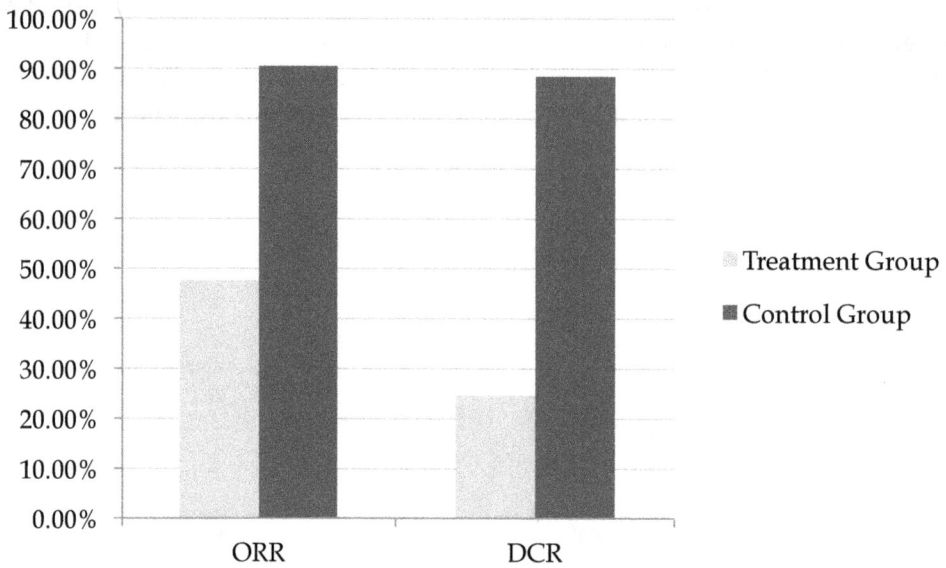

Group	Cases	ORR	DCR
Treatment Group	21	47.6% (10/21)*	90.5% (19/21)
Control Group	61	24.6% (15/61)	88.5% (54/61)

Figure 5: The short-term clinical effects. * = ORR is significantly higher than control group ($p < 0.05$).

Characteristics	Treatment Group	Control Group
Number	21	20
Age Mean (Range)	56.6 (32–74)	54.3 (39–68)
Gender: Male	19 (90.5%)	17 (85%)
Gender: Female	2 (9.5%)	3 (15%)
Stage Status: III	10 (47.6%)	10 (50%)
Stage Status: IV	11 (52.4%)	10 (50%)
Tumor Histology: Adenocarcinoma	8 (38.1%)	10 (50%)
Squamous carcinoma	13 (61.9%)	10 (50%)
Cycles of Previous Chemotherapy	2.9 ± 0.7	2.4 ± 0.5
PS score	0.4 ± 0.6	0.5 ± 0.6

Table 2: Baseline characteristics of treatment group and 20 cases in control group.

Group	CD3+ (%)	CD3+ CD4+ (%)	CD3+ CD8+ (%)	CD4+ / CD8+	CD3- CD56+ (%)	IL-2 (ng/L)	IFN-r (pg/mL)
Treatment group							
Pre-treatment	62.16 ±13.62	33.64 ±10.05	25.86 ±10.30	1.55 ±0.88	17.83 ±9.04	330.42 ±79.25	575.85 ±179.85
Post-treatment	66.34 ±13.65	34.63 ±13.28	29.73 ±11.14	1.45 ±0.97	17.31 ±9.50	330.94 ±66.12	567.12 ±151.64
P value	0.3	0.716	0.119	0.684	0.806	0.979	0.831
Control group							
Pre-treatment	68.70 ±15.48	39.48 ±12.76	27.30 ±8.79	1.57 ±0.67	10.25 ±6.12	358.37 ±49.00	491.19 ±60.00
Post-treatment	70.43 ±19.67	33.6471 ±18.02	33.65 ±17.19	1.27 ±0.96	8.52 ±6.52	376.09 ±44.44	507.32 ±59.87
P value	0.705	0.051	0.077	0.08	0.378	0.186	0.481

Table 3: Immunology response of patients ($\overline{x} \pm s$).

treatment group (P > 0.05). However, it should be noted that there was a decrease in CD4+/CD8+ T cell ratio after TRT in control group (Table 3, P = 0.08).

3.4   QOL and Side Effects

At the beginning of the study, the PS in the treatment and control groups was 0.4 ± 0.6 and 0.6 ± 0.7, respectively (Table 1). At the end of TRT, the PS in the treatment and control groups were 0.9 ± 0.8 and 1.4 ± 0.6, respectively. Little increase of PS was found in treatment group after TRT (0.48 ± 0.7). However, obvious increase of PS was observed in control group (0.9 ± 0.7). The PS in crease in treatment group was significantly lower than that in control group (P = 0.018, Table 4).

Side effects were assessed in all the 21 cases in treatment group, and 59 of 61 cases in control group with incomplete follow-up information in 2 cases. The functions of the liver, kidney and heart of all the participants remained normal at the end of the TRT treatment. The majority of side effects reported during the study were fever, anorexia, nausea, vomiting, myelosuppression, and radiation pneumonitis (Table 4). Most of them were at level I~II, except radiation pneumonitis. Grade 3 radiation pneumonitis was observed in 3 patients (14.3%) in treatment group, and 9 patients (15.3%) in control group. All the patients recovered after suitable treatment within 2 months. There were no cases with grade 4 radiation pneumonitis or treatment-related deaths.

Characteristics	Treatment group (n = 21)			Control group (n = 59)		
	Grade					
	1 – 2	3	4	1 – 2	3	4
Fever	5 (23.8%)	0	0	13 (22.0%)	0	0
Anorexia	3 (14.3%)	0	0	6 (10.2%)	0	0
Allergy	1 (4.8%)	0	0	0	0	0
Nausea, Vomiting	3 (14.3%)	0	0	9 (15.3%)	0	0
Heart Function	0	0	0	0	0	0
Liver Function	0	0	0	0	0	0
Renal Function	0	0	0	0	0	0
Myelosuppression	2 (9.5%)	0	0	8 (13.6%)	0	0
Radiation Pneumonitis	4 (19.0%)	3 (14.3%)	0	11 (18.6%)	9 (15.3%)	0
PS change after TRT	0.48 ± 0.7 *			0.9 ± 0.7		

Table 4: QOL and side effects. * = PS change is significantly better than control group (P < 0.05).

4   Discussion

Cancer cytotherapy is a novel therapeutic approach with great potential (Kantoff *et al.*, 2011; Mellman *et al.*, 2011; Szyszka-Barth *et al.*, 2014). Since the report of the first DCs-based cancer vaccine clinical trial in 1995 (Mukherji *et al.*, 1995), a lot of trials have been designed and conducted (Draube *et al.*, 2011; Engell-Noerregaard *et al.*, 2009). In 2010, Food and Drug Administration (FDA) approved the first DCs-based vaccine Provenge for the treatment of advanced prostate cancer (Mellman *et al.* 2011; Small *et al.*, 2000). Additionally, the cytotoxic and regulatory anti-tumor effects of CIKs are also attractive and promising. The combined use of DCs and CIKs is a viable adoptive cellular immunotherapy with a strong anti-tumor effect (Rosenberg *et al.*, 2008; Wang *et al.*, 2014). It has been shown that irradiation enhanced MHC I expression, and changed the tumor microenvironment to promote greater infiltration of immune-effector cells (Chakraborty *et al.*, 2008; Garnett *et al.*, 2004; Lugade *et al.*, 2005). Tumor cells killed by irradiation release tumor antigens (Finkelstein *et al.*, 2011) which are presented by ectopic DCs. Both preclinical and clinical researches demonstrated that radiotherapy combined with cytotherapy elicited greater anti-tumor response (Hodge *et al.*, 2012; Kwilas *et al.*, 2014).

In the present study, we aimed to analyze the efficacy of combining DC/CIK with TRT in patients with locally advanced or metastatic NSCLC. All the patients were identified with stage III or IV NSCLC with more than 2 cycles of systemic chemotherapy. We know the standard treatment of stage III NSCLC is concurrent chemo-radiotherapy. However, quite a part of patients with stage III NSCLC couldn't tolerate concurrent chemo-radiotherapy because of huge primary tumors, potential risk of heart failure and respiratory dysfunction, etc. Therefore, some patients preferred sequential chemotherapy/radiotherapy to concurrent chemo-radiotherapy. Moreover, some patients had received several cycles of chemotherapy alone in other hospitals prior to admission to our oncology department. These patients with stage III NSCLC were eligible to be enrolled in the present clinical trial.

The interval between chemotherapy and this study was no less than 14 days. After several cycles of chemotherapy, TRT should be the standard treatment according to NCCN guideline for patients with locally advanced or metastatic NSCLC. Thus we designated TRT alone, instead of DC/CIK alone, as control group. A block randomization was designed at the beginning of the study. However, it was very difficult to recruit patients because of the high medical cost of DC/CIK cytotherapy which was excluded from medical insurance in China. Consequently, it would take a very long period to finish the enrollment. In this condition, therefore, we made some adjustments. Using the same inclusion criteria for treatment group and control group, we assigned eligible patients who accepted both DC/CIK and TRT to treatment group.

As for the clinical outcomes of our study, a longer mPFS was observed in treatment groupthan in control group (330 days vs. 233 days, P < 0.05), and ORR was higher in treatment group (47.6% vs. 24.6%, P < 0.05). Although there was no significant difference in DCR and OS between the two groups (P > 0.05), the positive results in mPFS and ORR were still encouraging. Better clinical outcomes were observed in patients treated with DC/CIK combined with TRT. Our results confirmed the hypothesis that tumor antigens released by TRT enhance tumor-specific killing via ectopic DC/CIK cytotherapy.

Cancer patients often suffer from immune deficiency, including a decrease of CD4+/CD8+T cell ratio, especially during a long period of systemic chemotherapy (Zhong *et al.*, 2012). In the present study, we found a tendency of decrease in CD4+/CD8+ T cell ratio after TRT in control group (P = 0.08) but not in treatment group (Table 3). Thus, a reasonable explanation could be that radical TRT with conventional fractionation caused immune suppression in control group, while DC/CIK cytotherapy partially rescued immune suppression induced by TRT in treatment group. However, the sample size is not big enough. The inference that DC/CIK cytotherapy partially rescued immune suppression induced by TRT, thus, needs further investigation in the future.

Meanwhile, we examined other cytokines in the current study, such as IL-2 and IFN-γ in peripheral blood, which were supposed to play critical roles in specific immunological effects and promoting innate and adaptive immune responses (Yang *et al.*, 2003). The serum levels of IL-2 and IFN-γ did not change significantly after TRT in both groups (P > 0.05). Since the immune response is very complex in DC/CIK combined with TRT, further researches are needed to reveal cytokine activity in the future.

In addition, we found a significant PS increase after TRT in control group (P < 0.05). Nevertheless, PS did not increase so much in treatment group (P > 0.05). Taken together, these results suggest that combined cytotherapy improved the QOL for patients with advanced NSCLC receiving TRT. During the treatment with DC/CIK combined with TRT, a majority of side effects were mild and could be tolerated and no treatment-related deaths occurred.

Given that irradiation-mediated immune responses alter the tumor microenvironment, more and more researches have explored that local radiation combined with CTLA-4 blockade (Demaria *et al.*, 2005) or PD-L1 blockade (Deng *et al.*, 2014) could promote anti-tumor immunity. Our results also suggest that the combination of DC/CIK cytotherapy with TRT has a great potential in application. It achieves better clinical outcomes and a good tolerance, and boosts the immunity to some extent. However, further studies with a larger number of cases are still needed. In addition, it is necessary to perform a phase III multicenter clinical trial to confirm the conclusion. Standardized treatment schedule and detailed mechanism of DC/CIK cytotherapy combined with TRT need to be elucidated in the ongoing research.

5   Conclusions

Our study confirms the efficiency and safety of the combination of DC/CIK cytotherapy with TRT in advanced NSCLC. Indeed, this novel strategy enhances immunity, improves ORR, prolongs PFS, and improves QOL, with no severe treatment-related adverse effects. It is therefore a potentially viable option for patients with advanced NSCLC.

Acknowledgements

This work was supported by the National Natural Science Foundation of China (No. 81272496), Chongqing Natural Science Foundation (No. cstc2012jjB0003, cstc2012jjA10096), Clinical Research Fund of Third Military Medical University (No. 2011XLC38). We also appreciate the English editing by Department of Medical English, Third Military Medical University.

Competing Interests

The authors declare that they have no competing interests.

References

Apetoh L, Ghiringhelli F, Tesniere A, Obeid M, Ortiz C, Criollo A, Mignot G, Maiuri MC, Ullrich E, Saulnier P, Yang H, Amigorena S, Ryffel B, Barrat FJ, Saftig P, Levi F, Lidereau R, Nogues C, Mira JP, Chompret A, Joulin V, Clavel-Chapelon F, Bourhis J, Andre F, Delaloge S, Tursz T, Kroemer G, Zitvogel L. Toll-like receptor 4-dependent contribution of the immune system to anticancer chemotherapy and radiotherapy. NAT MED. 2007, 13(9). 1050–1059.

Brodowicz T, Krzakowski M, Zwitter M, et al. Cisplatin and gemcitabine first-line chemotherapy followed by maintenance gemcitabine or best supportive care in advanced non-small cell lung cancer: a phase III trial. Lung Cancer. 2006, 52(2): 155–163.

Chakraborty M, Wansley EK, Carrasquillo JA, Yu S, Paik CH, Camphausen K, Becker MD, Goeckeler WF, Schlom J, Hodge JW. The use of chelated radionuclide (samarium-153-ethylenediaminetetra-

methylenephosphonate) to modulate phenotype of tumor cells and enhance T cell-mediated killing. CLIN CANCER RES. 2008, 14(13). 4241–4249.

Claudia Allemani, Hannah K Weir, Helena Carreira, et al. Global surveillance of cancer survival 1995–2009: analysis of individual data for 25676887 patients from 279 population-based registries in 67 countries. Lancet. 2015, 385(9972): 977–1010.

Cui Y, Yang X, Zhu W, Li J, Wu X, Pang Y. Immune response, clinical outcome and safety of dendritic cell vaccine in combination with cytokine-induced killer cell therapy in cancer patients. ONCOL LETT. 2013, 6(2). 537–541.

Demaria S, Kawashima N, Yang AM, Devitt ML, Babb JS, Allison JP, Formenti SC. Immune-mediated inhibition of metastases after treatment with local radiation and CTLA-4 blockade in a mouse model of breast cancer. Clin Cancer Res. 2005, 11(2 Pt 1).728–734.

Deng L, Liang H, Burnette B, Beckett M, Darga T, Weichselbaum RR, Fu YX. Irradiation and anti-PD-L1 treatment synergistically promote antitumor immunity in mice. J Clin Invest. 2014, 124(2).687–695.

Draube A, Klein-Gonzalez N, Mattheus S, Brillant C, Hellmich M, Engert A, von BM. Dendritic cell based tumor vaccination in prostate and renal cell cancer: a systematic review and meta-analysis. PLOS ONE. 2011, 6(4). e18801.

Eisenhauer EA, Therasse P, Bogaerts J, Schwartz LH, Sargent D, Ford R, Dancey J, Arbuck S, Gwyther S, Mooney M, Rubinstein L, Shankar L, Dodd L, Kaplan R, Lacombe D, Verweij J. New response evaluation criteria in solid tumours: revised RECIST guideline (version 1.1). EUR J CANCER. 2009, 45(2). 228–247.

Engell-Noerregaard L, Hansen TH, Andersen MH, Thor SP, Svane IM. Review of clinical studies on dendritic cell-based vaccination of patients with malignant melanoma: assessment of correlation between clinical response and vaccine parameters. CANCER IMMUNOL IMMUN. 2009, 58(1). 1–14.

Finkelstein SE, Timmerman R, McBride WH, Schaue D, Hoffe SE, Mantz CA, Wilson GD. The confluence of stereotactic ablative radiotherapy and tumor immunology. CLIN DEV IMMUNOL. 2011, 2011.

Friedman EJ. Immune modulation by ionizing radiation and its implications for cancer immunotherapy. CURR PHARM DESIGN. 2002, 8(19). 1765–1780.

Gameiro SR, Jammeh ML, Wattenberg MM, Tsang KY, Ferrone S, Hodge JW. Radiation-induced immunogenic modulation of tumor enhances antigen processing and calreticulin exposure, resulting in enhanced T-cell killing. ONCOTARGET. 2014, 5(2). 403–416.

Garnett CT, Palena C, Chakraborty M, Tsang KY, Schlom J, Hodge JW. Sublethal irradiation of human tumor cells modulates phenotype resulting in enhanced killing by cytotoxic T lymphocytes. CANCER RES. 2004, 64(21). 7985–7994.

Gupta A, Probst HC, Vuong V, Landshammer A, Muth S, Yagita H, Schwendener R, Pruschy M, Knuth A, van den Broek M. Radiotherapy promotes tumor-specific effector CD8+ T cells via dendritic cell activation. J IMMUNOL. 2012, 189(2). 558–566.

Hodge JW, Sharp HJ, Gameiro SR. Abscopal regression of antigen disparate tumors by antigen cascade after systemic tumor vaccination in combination with local tumor radiation. CANCER BIOTHER RADIO. 2012, 27(1). 12–22.

International Agency for Research on Cancer. Latest World Cancer Statistics Global Cancer Burden Rises to 14.1 Million New Cases in 2012: Marked Increase in Breast Cancers must be Addressed. World Health Organization, 2013 (223): 1–3.

Kantoff PW, Higano CS, Shore ND, Berger ER, Small EJ, Penson DF, Redfern CH, Ferrari AC, Dreicer R, Sims RB, Xu Y, Frohlich MW, Schellhammer PF. Sipuleucel-T immunotherapy for castration-resistant prostate cancer. NEW ENGL J MED. 2010, 363(5). 411–422.

Kwilas AR, Donahue RN, Bernstein MB, Hodge JW. In the field: exploiting the untapped potential of immunogenic modulation by radiation in combination with immunotherapy for the treatment of cancer. Front Oncol. 2012, 2:104.

Liao YP, Wang CC, Schaue D, Iwamoto KS, McBride WH. Local irradiation of murine melanoma affects the development of tumour-specific immunity. IMMUNOLOGY. 2009, 128(1 Suppl). e797–804.

Lugade AA, Moran JP, Gerber SA, Rose RC, Frelinger JG, Lord EM. Local radiation therapy of B16 melanoma tumors increases the generation of tumor antigen-specific effector cells that traffic to the tumor. J IMMUNOL. 2005, 174(12). 7516–7523.

Ma Y, Zhang Z, Tang L, Xu YC, Xie ZM, Gu XF, Wang HX. Cytokine-induced killer cells in the treatment of patients with solid carcinomas: a systematic review and pooled analysis. CYTOTHERAPY. 2012, 14(4). 483–493.

Mellman I, Coukos G, Dranoff G. Cancer immunotherapy comes of age. NATURE. 2011, 480(7378). 480–489.

Mukherji B, Chakraborty NG, Yamasaki S, Okino T, Yamase H, Sporn JR, Kurtzman SK, Ergin MT, Ozols J, Meehan J, et a. Induction of antigen-specific cytolytic T cells in situ in human melanoma by immunization with synthetic peptide-pulsed autologous antigen presenting cells. P NATL ACAD SCI USA. 1995, 92(17). 8078–8082.

Nicol AJ, Tazbirkova A, Nieda M. Comparison of clinical and immunological effects of intravenous and intradermal administration of alpha-galactosylceramide (KRN7000)-pulsed dendritic cells. CLIN CANCER RES. 2011, 17(15). 5140–5151.

Panakis N, McNair HA, Christian JA, Mendes R, Symonds-Tayler JR, Knowles C, Evans PM, Bedford J, Brada M. Defining the margins in the radical radiotherapy of non-small cell lung cancer (NSCLC) with active breathing control (ABC) and the effect on physical lung parameters. RADIOTHER ONCOL. 2008, 87(1). 65–73.

Rosenberg SA, Restifo NP, Yang JC, Morgan RA, Dudley ME. Adoptive cell transfer: a clinical path to effective cancer immunotherapy. NAT REV CANCER. 2008, 8(4). 299–308.

Sangiolo D, Mesiano G, Carnevale-Schianca F, Piacibello W, Aglietta M, Cignetti A. Cytokine induced killer cells as adoptive immunotherapy strategy to augment graft versus tumor after hematopoietic cell transplantation. EXPERT OPIN BIOL TH. 2009, 9(7). 831–840.

Small EJ, Fratesi P, Reese DM, Strang G, Laus R, Peshwa MV, Valone FH. Immunotherapy of hormone-refractory prostate cancer with antigen-loaded dendritic cells. J CLIN ONCOL. 2000, 18(23). 3894–3903.

Steinman RM, Banchereau J. Taking dendritic cells into medicine. NATURE. 2007, 449(7161). 419–426.

Szyszka-Barth K, Ramlau K, Gozdzik-Spychalska J, Spychalski L, Bryl M, Golda-Gocka I, Kopczynska A, Barinow-Wojewodzki A, Ramlau R. Actual status of therapeutic vaccination in non-small cell lung cancer. Contemp Oncol (Pozn). 2014, 18(2). 77–84.

The Japan Lung Cancer Society. General Rule for Clinical and Pathological Record of Lung Cancer, 7th edn. Tokyo: Kanehara Press, 2010.

Toomey PG, Vohra NA, Ghansah T, Sarnaik AA, Pilon-Thomas SA. Immunotherapy for gastrointestinal malignancies. CANCER CONTROL. 2013, 20(1). 32–42.

Villadangos JA, Schnorrer P. Intrinsic and cooperative antigen-presenting functions of dendritic-cell subsets in vivo. NAT REV IMMUNOL. 2007, 7(7). 543–555.

Wang D, Zhang B, Gao H, Ding G, Wu Q, Zhang J, Liao L, Chen H. Clinical research of genetically modified dendritic cells in combination with cytokine-induced killer cell treatment in advanced renal cancer. BMC CANCER. 2014, 14(1). 251.

Yang L, Ng KY, Lillehei KO. Cell-mediated immunotherapy: a new approach to the treatment of malignant glioma. CANCER CONTROL. 2003, 10(2). 138–147.

Zhang SN, Choi IK, Huang JH, Yoo JY, Choi KJ, Yun CO. Optimizing DC vaccination by combination with oncolytic adenovirus coexpressing IL-12 and GM-CSF. MOL THER. 2011, 19(8). 1558–1568.

Zhong GC, Yan B, Sun Y, Zhang XY, Chen J, Su Y, Sun HP, Zhu B. Clinical efficacy of immunotherapy of dendritic cell and cytokine-induced killer cell combined with chemotherapy for treatment of multiple myeloma. Zhonghua xueyexue zazhi. 2012, 33(12). 1000–1003.

Chapter 4

Understanding the Roles of the Immune System in Cow's Milk Allergy

Juandy Jo[1], Johan Garssen[2,3], Leon M.J. Knippels[2,3], Elena Sandalova[1,3]

1 Introduction

Cow's milk allergy (CMA) is one of the most commonly reported food allergies in infancy (Prescott *et al.* 2013). Incidence of CMA peaks during early childhood and tends to recede later, with the reported prevalence to be 0.6–2.5% in pre-schoolers, 0.3% in older children and teens, and less than 0.5% in adults (Fiocchi *et al.* 2010). A recent study performed in Europe supports these findings by demonstrating the overall incidence of challenge-proven CMA of 0.54% (Schoemaker *et al.* 2015). The self-perceived prevalence is unfortunately higher: 1–17.5% in pre-schoolers, 1–13.5% in older children and teens, and 1–4% in adults (Fiocchi *et al.* 2010; Jarvenpaa *et al.* 2014). This imposes dietary restriction on the CMA-suspected subjects, impairing the quality of life of both children and family, impeding children's growth and causing unnecessary health care cost (Koletzko *et al.* 2012). The repetitive exposure to cow's milk proteins in patients with persistent CMA could result in chronic allergic inflammation accompanied along with anatomical and physiological defects, such as eosinophilic gastroenteropathies (Galli *et al.* 2008; Leung *et al.* 2013). Of note is the phenomenon of atopic march, in which CMA patients (particularly the persistent cases) are having substantial risk to suffer from respiratory allergies, such as asthma, in their later life (Sprikkelman *et al.* 2000; Sampaio *et al.* 2005). It is therefore important to understand the CMA pathogenesis in order to correctly diagnose and to effectively prevent and manage the disease and its later life

[1] Program of Immunology, Nutricia Research, Singapore

[2] Department of Immunology, Nutricia Research, Utrecht, the Netherlands

[3] Division of Pharmacology, Utrecht Institute for Pharmaceutical Sciences, Utrecht University, the Netherlands

consequences, such as the atopic march (van den Hoogen *et al.* 2014).

By definition, CMA is a repeated, immune-mediated aberrant reaction to certain proteins within cow's milk. These proteins, which are harmless food ingredients, comprise of αS1-casein (Bos d 9), β-lactoglobulin (Bos d 5) and others (Table 1). CMA can be mechanis-tically classified into: 1) the "acute onset" immunoglobulin E (IgE)-mediated; 2) the "delayed onset" non-IgE, cell-mediated; or 3) the mixed type-mediated allergy. The proper CMA diagnosis, thus its management, is complicated by the variation of onsets and clinical manifestations of these different clusters (Fiocchi *et al.* 2010). Therefore, the reference standard to diagnose CMA is an oral, preferably placebo-controlled and double-blind cow's milk challenge in suspected subjects after a successful elimination diet (Fiocchi *et al.* 2011; Savilahti and Savilahti 2013). However, it is resource intensive and not easily to be conducted or interpreted. The oral challenge also carries a substantial risk of anaphylaxis (Fiocchi *et al.* 2010), thus many clinicians prefer to utilize less hazardous techniques for diagnosing CMA. The IgE-mediated CMA can be diagnosed by performing skin prick test against cow's milk proteins and measuring cow's milk-specific IgE levels (Fiocchi *et al.* 2010). In contrast to the non-IgE-mediated CMA, the IgE-mediated CMA typically persists to school age and seemed to be a risk factor for the atopic march (Saarinen *et al.* 2005; Schoemaker *et al.* 2015).

Fraction (Proportion)	Allergen Name [*Protein*]	Size (kDalton)	Concentration (g/L)	Prevalence (patients %)
Casein (80%)	Bos d 9 [*αS1-casein*]	23.6	12–15	65–100
	Bos d 10 [*αS2-Casein*]	25.2	3–4	no data
	Bos d 11 [*β-Casein*]	24	9–11	35–44
	Bos d 12 [*κ-Casein*]	19	3–4	35–41
Whey (20%)	Bos d 4 [*α-Lactalbumin*]	14.2	1–1.5	0–67
	Bos d 5 [*β-lactoglobulin*]	18.3	3–4	13–62
	Bos d 6 [*Bovine Serum Albumin*]	66.3	0.1–0.4	0–76
	Bos d 7 [*Immunoglobulins*]	160	0.6–10	12–36
	Bos d Lactoferrin [*Lactoferrin*]	80	0.09	0–35

Table 1: Main allergens in cow's milk. This table is adapted from (Hochwallner *et al.* 2014).

Immune responses consist of both humoral and cellular components. A close and complex interaction occurs between humoral and cellular immunities. While the availability of pro-allergic soluble factors is crucially dependent on immune-cell activities, the allergen-induced cross-linking of surface-bound IgEs provoke pro-allergic immune cells to unleash inflammatory mediators, causing allergy reactions. There is a growing data to address the roles of both humoral and cellular immunities in allergy and upon its tolerance induction and maintenance. This chapter focuses on the roles of both immune components in the IgE-mediated CMA in order to enhance our understanding of the CMA immunopathogenesis. Therapeutic strategies for inducing immune tolerance against cow's milk are also discussed. In addition, mechanistic interactions between CMA and other inflammatory diseases are also proposed and discussed.

2   The Roles of Immune System during CMA Pathogenesis

2.1   Humoral Immunity

Due to the significant overlap between inflammatory mechanisms due to helminth infections and allergy, the humoral aspect of CMA immunopathogenesis has been extensively studied. It is known that helminth infections incite $T_{Helper}2$ (T_H2)-polarized immune responses, hence elevated IgE levels in order to eliminate the parasites (Fallon and Mangan 2007). IgE is the Ig isotype with the lowest abundance *in vivo* (~50–200 ng/mL of blood in healthy humans compared with ~1–10 mg/mL of blood for other Ig isotypes), the Ig isotype with the shortest serum half-life (~2 days compared with ~20 days for IgG in humans) and the Ig isotype with a tight regulation of its concentration (Dullaers *et al.* 2012; Wu and Zarrin 2014). IgE binds to its receptors (the high affinity FcεRI and the low-affinity FcεRII/CD23) expressed by immune cells, including mast cells, basophils, dendritic cells, macrophages and B cells (Dullaers *et al.* 2012; Wu and Zarrin 2014). The facts that IgE half-life is significantly prolonged until weeks or months upon binding to its receptors (Achatz *et al.* 2010) and that most IgEs are retained in tissues (Dullaers *et al.* 2012) suggest that IgE plays an important role in local immunity. The *in vivo* production site of IgE is intriguing. While plasma cells ('Ig-producing B cells') could secrete IgE into the blood circulation and subsequently IgEs diffuse into the inflamed sites, growing evidences indicate that the IgE synthesis could occur as well at the sites of allergic inflammation in response to persistent allergen exposure (Gould *et al.* 2006; Wu and Zarrin 2014). With this possibility, it is pertinent to be aware that local IgE production might not be reflected as high levels of circulating allergen-specific IgE (Gould *et al.* 2006). Of note, the IgE production can occur via two main pathways of Ig class switching: 1) a direct pathway from the IgM to the IgE; or 2) a sequential pathway from IgM to an IgG1 intermediate then to IgE (Wu and Zarrin 2014). It is elusive of whether the direct class switching pathway is more dominant in humans (Wu and Zarrin 2014) or of how to activate a certain pathway of IgE production. It has been suggested that, at least in the murine model, the sequential class switching produces high-affinity IgE antibodies, whereas the direct class switching may generate lower affinity IgE antibodies (Xiong *et al.* 2012). Of note, among the IgE-mediated CMA patients, the early-phase of CMA clinical manifestations are due to the cross-linking of surface-bound allergen-specific IgEs by allergens that subsequently activate mast cells and basophils to release biologically active substances, such as histamine, interleukin-4 (IL-4), serine proteases, TNF-α and platelet-activating factor (Galli *et al.* 2008). These factors contribute to the progression of allergic reactions as well as the tissue inflammation.

It is debatable whether other Ig isotypes also play a pro-allergic role. It is important to remember that any Ig isotype is primarily secreted as a part of physiological immune responses following exposure to any foreign antigen, including food allergen. Hence besides IgE, the existence of other isotype of allergen-specific Ig (e.g., IgM or IgG) perhaps merely indicates an exposition to allergen without any obvious pro-allergic role. Nonetheless, despite one study reported that there was no association between the allergic manifestations and cow's milk-specific IgG within CMA subjects (Hidvegi *et al.* 2002), several other studies suggested that CMA subjects had slightly elevated levels of cow's milk-specific total IgG or IgG subtypes (Ruiter *et al.* 2007; Scott-Taylor *et al.* 2010). By referring to the sequential pathway of IgE production via IgG1 as an intermediate (Wu and Zarrin 2014), it is possible that the current existence of cow's milk-specific IgG1 suggests the subsequent existence of cow's milk-specific IgE. To rephrase it, allergen-specific IgG1 could be an indicator of present allergen sensitization and thus subsequent allergic reaction (Kukkonen *et al.* 2011; Orivuori *et al.* 2014).

As a more obscure Ig isotype, functionality of secreted IgD is elusive despite it is known as a transmembrane antigen receptor for mature B cells before antigenic stimulation (Chen and Cerutti 2011). Nevertheless, an interesting study using human upper respiratory mucosal samples demonstrated that IgD could bind to basophils and mast cells; subsequently, cross-linking of surface-bound IgDs induced basophil to produce BAFF (a mandatory B cell survival factor) and pro-inflammatory cytokines, including IL-4 and IL-13 (Chen *et al.* 2009). Taken together, this suggests that IgD may exert a pro-allergic role as well. Nonetheless, further study focusing on CMA subject is definitely required to confirm this hypothesis.

Immunoglobulin-free light chains (Ig-fLCs) are proposed to be a pro-allergic soluble mediator as well. Free κ or λ light chains were shown to be able to induce murine mast-cell degranulation, causing immediate allergic inflammation (Redegeld *et al.* 2002). Ig-fLC blockade indeed strongly reduced the allergic skin responses in murine models of contact hypersensitivity (van Houwelingen *et al.* 2007) and CMA (Schouten *et al.* 2010). Interestingly, one study demonstrated that in its cohort, serum levels of Ig-fLCs in CMA patients were significantly elevated as compared to the ones observed in non-allergic subjects (Schouten *et al.* 2010), suggesting the pro-allergic role of Ig-fLCs. It is elusive whether in humans, Ig-fLCs exert the pro-allergic role in the presence of allergen-specific IgE ('complementing the IgE role') or whether Ig-fLCs could replace allergen-specific IgE in mediating the allergic inflammation ('substituting IgE in the non-IgE-mediated allergy'). This latter role is possible since it has been reported that the depletion of CD4+CD25+ T cells in whey-allergic mice switched the pathogenesis of allergic inflammation from an IgE-mediated to an Ig-fLC-mediated reactions (van Esch *et al.* 2010). Of note, elevated levels of Ig-fLCs have been associated with numerous chronic diseases as well, e.g., chronic obstructive pulmonary disease, non-allergic rhinitis with eosinophilia syndrome, rheumatoid arthritis, systemic lupus erythematosus, multiple sclerosis and breast cancer (Redegeld and Nijkamp 2003; Powe *et al.* 2010; Braber *et al.* 2012; Groot Kormelink *et al.* 2014), suggesting that this potential humoral arm of allergic reaction can also mediate other types of chronic inflammatory diseases.

2.2   Cellular Immunity

It is important to remember that innate and adaptive immune cells influence each other extensively, which contribute to the occurrence of allergy and its clinical characteristics. Nonetheless, for the sake of simplicity, cellular components of innate and adaptive immunity are discussed separately. A key feature is that most allergens, including cow's milk proteins, are sampled, processed and presented by antigen-presenting cells (APCs), in particular dendritic cells (DCs), in order to initiate the cascade of cellular and humoral immune reactions leading to allergic inflammation (Figure 1). It is also worthy to mention that type 2 innate lymphoid cells (type 2 ILCs or ILC2s) could respond to the epithelial-derived cytokines in order to initiate or mediate allergic inflammation as well.

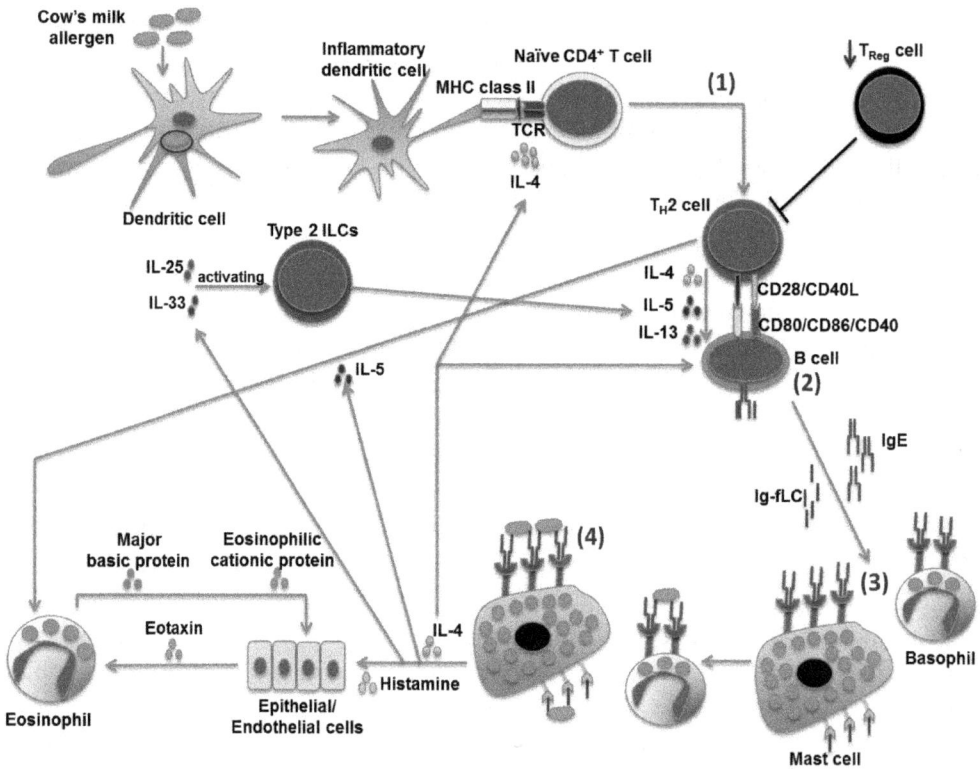

Figure 1: The intricate cascade of allergic inflammation. Allergen's exposure to inflammatory dendritic cells (DCs) allows these cells to process and to present allergen-derived peptides to naïve CD4+ T cells. In the early presence of IL-4 (from an unidentified source, probably basophils and mast cells), naïve CD4+ T cells differentiate into pro-allergic TH2 cells.

In Figure 1: **(1)** Activated type 2 innate lymphoid cells (type 2 ILCs) also contribute the allergy reaction by releasing pro-allergic cytokines, such as IL-4, IL-5 and IL-13. Of note, type 2 ILCs are activated by cytokines IL-25 and IL-33, probably released by mast cells. Concurrently, it appears that there is an impairment of T_{Reg}-cell frequency and/or activity, hence no/minimum suppression is exerted on $T_{H}2$-cell activity. Subsequently, $T_{H}2$ cells will drive B cells ('plasma cells'), via cell-contact as well as IL-4, IL-5 and IL-13, to undergo immunoglobulin class switching recombination, in which they eventually produce IgE; **(2)** Along with the antibody production, plasma cells also secrete significant amount of κ and λ Ig-free light chains (Ig-fLCs). IgE and/or Ig-fLCs will then bind to mast cells and basophils, causing sensitization; **(3)** Following subsequent exposure to allergen, cross-linking of surface-bound antibodies occurs, causing mast cells and basophils to degranulate and release their biologically active substances, including histamine, IL-4 and IL-5; **(4)** Released L-4 amplifies the differentiation of $T_{H}2$ and IgE-producing plasma cells, while released IL-5 (also secreted by type 2 ILCs and $T_{H}2$ cells) induces accumulation and activation of eosinophils in the affected tissues. Similarly, histamine activates epithelial or endothelial cells to release eotaxin that also attracts eosinophils into the tissues. Activated eosinophils release active substances, including major basic and eosinophilic cationic proteins that are toxic to the surrounding cells, contributing to further inflammation. Please notice that this figure only enlists major pro-allergic cytokines. This figure is adapted from (Jo *et al.* 2014).

2.2.1 Innate Components

The principal effector cells upon allergen exposure are subsets of innate immune cells, including tissue mast cells, basophils and eosinophils. Due to their surface expression of high-affinity receptors for IgE (FcεRI) and their ability to secrete mediators of allergic inflammation following IgE cross-linking by the specific allergens, tissue mast cells and basophils play pivotal roles in the IgE-mediated allergic inflammation (Schouten *et al.* 2010; MacGlashan 2013). These subsets contribute to the early- (immediate) and late-phase reactions of allergy (2–6 hours after exposure) (Galli *et al.* 2008). In addition, several studies have demonstrated that murine mast cells can be activated by Ig-fLCs to release pro-allergic mediators as well (Redegeld *et al.* 2002; Schouten *et al.* 2010).

Routine assessment assays on mast-cell and basophil activation in humans and mice have been developed and extensively used. Mast-cell activity in humans can be indirectly measured by the size of the induced wheal after skin prick test (SPT) with milk extract (Ford *et al.* 2013). In mice, mast-cell activity can be measured either by the size of cow's milk protein-induced ear-skin swelling or by the elevation of serum levels of murine mast cell β-chymase or mMCP-1, a specific marker for mucosal mast-cell degranulation (Caughey 2007; Schouten *et al.* 2008). Basophil activation in humans and mice can be assessed through the measurement of released mediators (e.g., histamine or IL-4) or the up-regulation of degranulation-associated cell-surface proteins, e.g., CD203c or CD63 (MacGlashan 2013). As indicated by the key roles of mast cells and basophils in allergy, wheal diameter as well as expression levels of CD203c and CD63 on milk protein-activated basophils were indeed much more pronounced in patients with more severe CMA (Ford *et al.* 2013).

Mediators released upon mast-cell degranulation, particularly histamine, could stimulate endothelial or epithelial cells to release a potent eosinophil chemoattractant, i.e., eotaxin (Menzies-Gow *et al.* 2004). This causes the infiltration of eosinophils, along with basophils, into inflamed tissues (Menzies-Gow *et al.* 2002). In addition, mast cells, type 2 ILCs and TH2 cells also release IL-5 that attracts eosinophils, prolongs their survival, increases adhesion to endothelial cells and enhances their effector function (Galli *et al.* 2008; Takatsu and Nakajima 2008; Diefenbach *et al.* 2014). The tissue-infiltrating eosinophils subsequently release highly basic and cytotoxic granule proteins, including major basic protein and eosinophil cationic protein, which are toxic to epithelial and endothelial cells (Gleich *et al.* 1979; Kita 2013), contributing to the late-phase reaction of allergy (Galli *et al.* 2008). This tissue inflammation eventually results in eosinophilic gastroenteropathies (Hogan *et al.* 2001).

It is worthy to briefly mention the pro-allergic roles of type 2 ILCs as well. These are a recently identified subset of innate lymphocytes that do not express rearranged receptors and play important roles in innate immunity and tissue remodelling. Three subsets of ILCs are identified currently: type 1 (ILC1s), type 2 (ILC2s) and type 3 ILCs (ILC3s) (Diefenbach *et al.* 2014; Hazenberg and Spits 2014). Type 2 ILCs are activated by epithelial-derived cytokines IL-25 and IL-33 in order to produce TH2-cytokines, such as IL-4, IL-5 and IL-13 (Moro *et al.* 2010; Neill *et al.* 2010; Price *et al.* 2010; Saenz *et al.* 2010). Due the production of these cytokines, type 2 ILCs are highly suggested to play important roles in immune responses against helminth infections as well as allergens (Barlow and McKenzie 2014). Of note, activated mast cells, among other cells, could produce IL-25 (Ikeda *et al.* 2003) and IL-33 (Hsu *et al.* 2010), suggesting the very intricate cross-talks among cellular components during allergic inflammation. Importantly, it has been reported that ILC2s existed in human skin and were enriched in patients with atopic dermatitis. These cells were activated by IL-25 and IL-33, but could be inhibited by the E-cadherin ligation on human ILC2s (Salimi *et al.* 2013). Following this notion, it is also possible that type 2 ILCs play an important role in initiating or even mediating CMA immunopathogenesis.

Roles of other innate immune subsets including neutrophils, monocytes, NK, γδ and NK T cells during allergic reaction to cow's milk are elusive yet. Despite accumulation of neutrophils, γδ and NK T cells in the chronically inflamed digestive tissues of CMA patients (Turunen *et al.* 2004; Semeniuk *et al.* 2009; Jyonouchi *et al.* 2014), actual roles of these innate cells within allergic reaction are unknown. It is possible that these cells are accumulated in the inflamed sites due to the high levels of inflammatory chemokines during chronic allergic reaction. These cells can be indirectly activated by the circulating inflammatory cytokines as well, further contributing to the chronic inflammatory reactions (Galli *et al.* 2008). Nonetheless, several murine studies suggest that these cells could play key roles during allergy. Neutrophils have been proposed to be important in both sensitization and induction of allergic skin inflammatory reactions as well as mediating alternative mechanisms of anaphylactic reaction (Mocsai 2013; Orivuori *et al.* 2014). In addition, murine tissue γδ and invariant NK T cells were suggested to exert regulatory roles to suppress food allergy (Bol-Schoenmakers *et al.* 2011; Schouten *et al.* 2012). Human studies are definitely required to clarify these murine findings. The different cellular elements between human and murine immune systems further complicate the extrapolation of murine data to the human setting. For example, several studies (Treiner and Lantz 2006; Tang *et al.* 2013) have demonstrated that while CD1d-restricted invariant NK T cells are abundant in mice but low in human, MR1-restricted mucosal-associated invariant T (MAIT) cells are instead abundant in human but low in mice. Pertaining to CMA, it will be more relevant to study a particular immune cell subset that is enriched in humans, such as MAIT instead of NK T cells.

As a part of professional APCs, DCs are crucial in order to sample, process and display antigens to naïve T cells, either to initiate immune responses or to induce immune tolerance (Steinman *et al.* 2003). Pertaining to food-derived antigens, DCs in the intestine and associated lymphoid tissues are of particular interest, partly due to facts that these cells can pick-up antigens directly from the intestinal lumen or antigens that have been transported across the intestinal epithelial cells (IECs) (Coombes and Powrie 2008). Importantly in the healthy gastrointestinal tract, commensal bacteria and their products modulate intestinal DCs to be hyporesponsive or tolerant via interaction with the pattern recognition receptors of DCs (Coombes and Powrie 2008; de Kivit *et al.* 2014). In addition, non-inflamed healthy IECs are also able to suppress activity of inflammatory DCs while inducing tolerogenic DCs (de Kivit *et al.* 2014). Taken together, an interaction between gut microbiota, IECs and intestinal DCs under homeostatic conditions contributes to immune tolerance in the healthy gastrointestinal tract. Of particular interest is the existence of tolerogenic CD103$^+$ DCs in murine intestines and mesenteric lymph nodes because they were able to convert naïve CD4$^+$ T into FOXP3$^+$ T$_{Regulatory}$ (T$_{Reg}$) cells via TGF-β and retinoic acid (Coombes *et al.* 2007). T$_{Reg}$ cells are proposed able to suppress allergic sensitization. A recent study shows a functional homology between murine CD103$^+$ DCs and human CD141^{high} DCs in cross-presenting antigens to CD8$^+$ T cells (Haniffa *et al.* 2012), hence eliciting a query of whether human intestinal CD141^{high} DCs can also serve as tolerogenic DCs. Notably in a murine model of peanut allergy, oral sensitization with peanut extract was accompanied by a shift in intestinal DC subsets, i.e., less tolerogenic CD103$^+$ DCs but more inflammatory CD11b$^+$ DCs (Smit *et al.* 2011). DC-recognition of allergens can be mediated by their C-type lectin receptors, such as DC-SIGN and mannose receptor (Salazar and Ghaemmaghami 2013). Subsequently in the early presence of IL-4 (potentially released by activated pro-allergic innate immune cells, including basophils and mast cells), allergen-presenting DCs polarize naïve CD4$^+$ T cells into T$_H$2 cells, which in turn differentiate Ig-producing B cells ('plasma cells') to produce IgE (Galli *et al.* 2008). Of note, the important role of DCs for mediating allergic reaction against cow's milk proteins is supported by a finding from the adoptive transfer study of DCs from cow's milk-allergic mice into naïve recipients. This DC transfer induced spontaneous production of cow's milk-specific IgE in the naïve mice in the absence of antigen challenge (Chambers *et al.* 2004). In summary, inflammatory DCs initiate the allergic reaction by sampling and processing cow's milk allergens, then presenting allergen-derived peptides to CD4$^+$ T cells to become T$_H$2 cells. Type 2 ILCs could also be activated by specific cytokines to release T$_H$2-cytokines during allergy. These events are followed by the IgE class switching and the activation of pro-allergic effectors including tissue mast cells, basophils and eosinophils.

2.2.2   Adaptive Components

CD4$^+$ T cells serve an important role as the master regulator of adaptive immune responses. CD4$^+$ T cells crucially influence the outcome of inflammatory reactions via their plasticity to differentiate into at least pro-inflammatory T$_H$1-T$_H$2-T$_H$17 or anti-inflammatory T$_{Reg}$ cells (Zhu et al. 2010), either resulting as a resolved reaction or a persistent inflammation. While T$_H$1 and T$_H$17 cells are physiologically important to eliminate intracellular and extracellular pathogens respectively, T$_H$2 cells are important for eradicating helminth infections. T$_H$2 cells also contribute to the pathogenesis of allergy through secretion of T$_H$2-cytokines (Galli et al. 2008; Zhu et al. 2010). CMA patients indeed exhibited cow's milk protein-specific T$_H$2-polarized immune responses in their peripheral blood, i.e., high levels of IL-4, IL-5 and IL-13, with low production of T$_H$1-cytokine IFN-γ (Andre et al. 1996; Campbell et al. 1998; Schade et al. 2000; Tiemessen et al. 2004; Vocca et al. 2011; Michaud et al. 2014). This T$_H$2-cytokine profile was importantly also displayed by duodenum-infiltrating T cells derived from CMA patients upon stimulation with cow's milk proteins (Beyer et al. 2002). In addition, cow's milk-specific T$_H$2-immune responses were observed in murine models of CMA as well (Li et al. 1999; Adel-Patient et al. 2005). Of note, partly due to many potential allergens within cow's milk, it is still elusive whether there is any difference of T-cell epitopes recognized by CMA patients who developed tolerance and by the ones who developed persistent allergy (Schade et al. 2003). Taken together, CMA partially occurs due to persistent uncontrolled T$_H$2-polarized immune responses.

It is important to elucidate whether there is any regulatory mechanism exists against allergy. One possible mechanism is partly attributed to the suppressive role of T$_{Reg}$ cells. These cells can be further classified as thymus-derived, peripherally derived, or in vitro-induced T$_{Reg}$ cells (Abbas et al. 2013). However in order to simplify the nomenclature used in this review, various T$_{Reg}$ cells are grouped as one entity. Their suppressive functions can occur through either secretion of inhibitory cytokines (e.g., IL-10 and TGF-β), cytolysis, metabolic disruption, or attenuation of DC maturation and/or functionality (Vignali et al. 2008). It has been demonstrated that a fine balance between T$_{Reg}$ and pro-allergic T$_H$2 cells, including cell frequency and functionality, determines the development of allergy (Akdis et al. 2004). Noteworthy, a supporting evidence of a T$_{Reg}$–cell suppressive role in allergy came from clinical studies of patients with IPEX ('Immune dysregulation, Polyendocrinopathy, Enteropathy, X-linked') syndrome caused by a deletion in a noncoding region of the FOXP3 gene, the central gene for T$_{Reg}$ differentiation (Bennett et al. 2001). These patients had defects in T$_{Reg}$ frequency as well as functionality and more importantly exhibited severe food allergic phenotype particularly against cow's milk proteins (Torgerson et al. 2007). IPEX patients also suffer from autoimmune diabetes and/or thyroiditis (Cheng and Anderson 2012), indicating that the impairment of T$_{Reg}$ cells loosens the brakes for many types of inflammation to occur. Indeed, CMA patients who had a higher frequency of circulating cow's milk protein-specific TReg cells exhibited a milder symptom and a favourable prognosis (Shreffler *et al.* 2009). In addition, lower frequencies of TGF-β-producing T cells were observed in the duodenal mucosa of children with food allergy as compared to non-allergic subjects (Perez-Machado *et al.* 2003; Westerholm-Ormio *et al.* 2010). To summarize, defects in TReg-cell frequency and functionality partly contribute to CMA pathogenesis.

Of note, several studies demonstrated the existence of regulatory B (BReg) cells that were associated with the suppression of excessive inflammation in mice and humans (Mauri and Bosma 2012). This subset of lymphocytes potentially supports the immunological tolerance via the production of anti-inflammatory cytokines IL-10, IL-35 and TGF-β (Rosser and Mauri 2015). Furthermore, BReg cells are required for the development and maintenance of TReg cells as well (Sun *et al.* 2008; Carter *et al.* 2011; Tadmor *et al.* 2011; Flores-Borja *et al.* 2013), thus can also indirectly regulate the immune responses. It is therefore of interest to elucidate BReg-cell role within CMA patients. However, it is difficult to study this subset of cells due the rarity in its frequency, the heterogeneity of its phenotypes and the lack of a unique transcription factor unlike TReg cells (Rosser and Mauri 2015; Tedder 2015). The last notion can be partially interpreted that BReg cells are not a lineage-specific B cell, but rather are expanded in response to inflammation (Rosser and Mauri 2015). In addition, BReg cells can differentiate into the Ig-producing plasma cells after the resolution of inflammatory responses (Maseda *et al.* 2012; Rosser and Mauri 2015), aggravating the difficulty to study this subset of cells. Nonetheless, a few *in vitro* studies suggested the presence of BReg cells in milk-tolerant subjects based on the IL-10 or TGF-β production upon casein stimulation (Lee *et al.* 2010; Noh *et al.* 2010; Lee *et al.* 2011). Whether these cells actively mediate immune tolerance against cow's milk allergens *in vivo*, it remains inconclusive.

Despite exogenous antigens, including cow's milk proteins, can be cross-presented by DCs to initiate CD8+ T-cell responses (Joffre *et al.* 2012), it is elusive whether CD8+ T cells play any role within CMA immunopathogenesis. It was even reported that upon unspecific stimulation, there was a significant difference in the frequency of IFN-γ-expressing CD4+, but not of CD8+ T cells, between CMA infants and healthy controls (Osterlund and Suomalainen 2002). On contrary, it is obvious that differentiated Ig-producing B cells ('plasma cells') serve an important pathogenic role during allergy. The presence of IL-4 and IL-13 released by TH2 cells promote immunoglobulin class switching recombination, inducing plasma cells to secrete IgE (Galli *et al.* 2008). Taken together, CMA pathogenesis is attributed to the pro-allergic activity of cellular components of innate (DCs, tissue mast cells, basophils, eosinophils and type 2 ILCs) and adaptive immunity (TH2 and IgE-producing plasma cells along with the impaired TReg-cell activity), as summarized in Table 2.

Type	Cell	Role in Allergy

Innate Cells	Tissue Mast cells	**Key effectors** during allergy.
		Upon Ig-E cross-linking (perhaps Ig-fLCs as well) with allergen, 3 classes of biologically active product are secreted (Caughey 2007):
		(1) Pre-stored cytoplasmic granules:
		  a) biogenic amines (e.g., histamine);
		  b) serglycin proteoglycans (e.g., heparin and chondroitin sulphate);
		  c) serine proteases (tryptases, chymases and carbozypeptida-ses); and
		  d) some cytokines (e.g., TNF-α and VEGFA).
		(2) Lipid-derived mediators (prostaglandins, leukotriene B4, cyste-inyl leukotrienes and platelet-activating factors).
		(3) Newly synthesized factors (cytokines, chemokines and growth factors).

	Basophils	**Key effectors** during allergy. Similar to mast cells, upon cross-linkage of IgE, 3 type of mediators can be released (MacGlashan 2013): (1) Preformed, immediately released (e.g., histamine); (2) Newly synthesized, immediately released (phospholipid meta-bolites including leukotriene C4); and (3) Newly synthesized, slowly released (cytokines including IL-4).
	Eosinophils	**Key effectors** during allergy. Upon activation with cytokine (e.g., IL-5), highly basic and cyto-toxic granule proteins are secreted (Kita 2013): (1) Major basic protein/MBP and MBP2; (2) Eosinophilic cationic protein/ECP; (3) Eosinophilic peroxidase/EPX; and (4) Eosinophil-derived neurotoxin/EDN.
	Inflammatory Dendritic cells/DCs	**Initiators of T$_H$2-cell response** during allergy (Galli *et al.* 2008). Inflammatory DCs uptake and process allergens, subsequently presenting allergen-derived peptides to naïve CD4+ T cells. In the presence of IL-4, DCs polarizing naïve CD4+ T becomes T$_H$2 cells.

Continues on next page…

...Continued from previous page

	Type 2 Innate Lymphoid Cells (ILC2s)	Probably act as **the initial drivers** of allergic inflammation by secreting T$_H$2-cytokines (Barlow and McKenzie 2014; Diefenbach *et al.* 2014; Hazenberg and Spits 2014).
	Other innate cells (Neutrophils, NK, MAIT and $\gamma\delta$ T cells)	Unknown roles.
Adaptive Cells	CD4$^+$ T$_H$2 cells	**Drivers** of allergic inflammation. Through cell-contact and cytokines (IL-4 and IL-13), T$_H$2 cells promote immunoglobulin class-switch recombination in B cells to drive the IgE production (Galli *et al.* 2008).
	CD4$^+$ T$_{Reg}$ cells	**Suppressors** of allergic inflammation, via (Akdis 2012): (1) Suppression of tissue mast cells, basophils and eosinophils; (2) Suppression of inflammatory DCs and induction of tolerogenic DCs; (3) Suppression of allergen-specific T$_H$2 cells; and (4) Early induction of IgG4 and late decrease in IgE.
	Ig-producing B cells (Plasma cells)	**Co-drivers** of allergic inflammation along with T$_H$2 cells by secret-ing IgE and Ig-fLCs (Galli *et al.* 2008).
	Other B- and T-cell subsets	Unknown roles.

Table 2: The roles of cellular immunity in allergy. This table is adapted from (Jo *et al.* 2014).

3   The Roles of Immune System upon Tolerance to Cow's Milk Proteins

The majority of infants with CMA spontaneously develop clinical tolerance to cow's milk proteins or outgrow the allergic disorder to cow's milk proteins by school age (Savilahti and Savilahti 2013). However, it has been shown that infants with the IgE-mediated CMA recovered later than those with the non-IgE-mediated allergy (Host *et al.* 2002; Vanto *et al.* 2004; Schoemaker *et al.* 2015). Hence, the dire consequences due to the dietary restriction before these children outgrow their allergic reactions, the tissue damage due to chronic allergic inflammation, as well as the potential atopic march in later life serve as an important reminder that CMA need to be properly diagnosed and managed early on. A proper understanding of immunity upon tolerance induction to cow's milk is crucial for diagnosing and managing CMA effectively.

3.1   Humoral Ommunity

A few studies had demonstrated an association among the IgE-mediated CMA subjects who later develop tolerance with the reduction of allergen-specific IgE and with the increment of allergen-specific IgG4 levels (Ruiter *et al.* 2007; Savilahti and Savilahti 2013). This alteration is apparently mediated by IL-10 secreted by T$_{Reg}$ cells (Akdis 2012). IgG4, which is normally found at very low concentrations, is unique because it is the only IgG subtype unable to form any immune complex as well unable to activate complement (Tao *et al.* 1993; van der Neut Kolfschoten *et al.* 2007; Aalberse *et al.* 2009; Jackson *et al.* 2014). It is postulated that IgG4 acts as a blocking antibody via competition with allergens for binding to IgE on the Fcε receptors (James *et al.* 2011) and as an anti-inflammatory factor due to its dynamic Fab arm exchange resulting as a bi-specific antibody with a substantially decreased capacity for cross-linking (van der Neut Kolfschoten *et al.* 2007). Therefore it is considered to have an anti-inflammation (hence anti-allergic) role. However, it is prudent to be cautious on generalizing anti-allergic role of IgG4 since not all allergy studies observed a correlation between elevated levels of IgG4 and anti-allergic effects (Williams *et al.* 2012). It remains possible that since IL-10 exerts anti-inflammatory role and since IL-10 promotes class switching of IgG1 to IgG4 instead to IgE, IgG4 does not directly induce immune tolerance (Williams *et al.* 2012; Jackson *et al.* 2014).

Several groups have also studied role of antigen-specific IgA (either in blood or as a secretory form) upon tolerance induction. An association was reported between cow's milk avoidance by breast-feeding mothers with low levels of cow's milk-specific IgA in their breast milk and in their infants' sera and with the development of CMA, suggesting high levels of cow's milk specific-IgA, in particular secretory IgA (such as in the breast milk), might have a protective effect against cow's milk allergens (Jarvinen *et al.* 2014). In addition, several recent studies suggesting an association of elevated levels of cow's milk-specific IgA with the development of tolerance against cow's milk (Savilahti *et al.* 2010; Jarvinen *et al.* 2014; Savilahti *et al.* 2014). Whether the IgA-induced immune tolerance is achieved by simply removing food allergens before they are absorbed by the gastrointestinal tract (Silbart and Keren 1989) or by a more intricate mechanism (Corthesy 2013), it remains to be elucidated.

Infants who received non-digestible carbohydrates ('prebiotics') during the first six months of age had a lower incidence of atopic dermatitis, which was linearly associated with lower levels of Ig-fLCs (Schouten *et al.* 2011). Hence this suggests that the decreasing levels of Ig-fLCs might be associated with an anti-allergic role. Taken together, the decreasing levels of allergen-specific specific IgE (probably Ig-fLCs too) as well as the increasing levels of allergen-specific IgG4 and/or allergen-specific secretory IgA partly contribute to the development of immune tolerance (Table 3).

3.2   Cellular Immunity

With regard to the cellular immunity, the tolerance mechanism is essentially contributed by two primary mechanisms: 1) the suppression of pro-allergic innate effectors and type 2 ILCs; and 2) the up-regulation of T$_{Reg}$-cell regulatory activity.

Isotype	Role in Allergy
Allergen-specific IgE	**Key effector** during allergy. Cross-linkage of surface-bound IgEs induce tissue mast cells and basophils to degranulate and release allergic mediators (Galli *et al.* 2008).
Allergen-specific IgG	Not-well defined for allergen-specific IgG1-IgG2-IgG3. Allergen-specific IgG4 probably exerts an **anti-allergic** role (van der Neut Kolfschoten *et al.* 2007).
Allergen-specific IgM	Unknown role.
Allergen-specific IgA	Not-well defined; secretory IgA probably exerts an **anti-allergic** role (Jarvinen *et al.* 2014; Savilahti *et al.* 2014).
Allergen-specific IgD	Not-well defined; probably exerts a **pro-allergic** role (Chen and Cerutti 2011).
Ig-fLCs	Probably exert a **pro-allergic** role (Redegeld *et al.* 2002).

Table 3: The roles of secreted immunoglobulins and immunoglobulin-free light chains (Ig-fLCs) in allergy.

Arguably, the latter mechanism is the principal way to induce and maintain tolerance to allergens because it partially affects the former mechanism in the disease progression. Moreover, activity of functional T_{Reg} cells could contribute to T-cell anergy, i.e., a tolerance mechanism in which the lymphocyte is intrinsically functionally inactivated following an antigen encounter, but remains alive (Schwartz 2003). Immunologic findings of spontaneously and treatment-induced tolerance against cow's milk allergens are discussed together because both approaches, arguably, follow similar immune mechanisms.

3.2.1   Inhibition of Pro-allergic Innate Effector Cells and Type 2 ILCs

During tolerance development, pro-allergic innate effectors could undergo rapid desensit-ization against allergens, causing them to be less likely to release inflammatory factors (Akdis 2012). One probable mechanism is due to the presence of allergen-specific IgG4, as mentioned briefly above. It has been demonstrated that basophils from CMA children who developed clinical tolerance were significantly less responsive to the allergen (Wanich *et al.* 2009; Ford *et al.* 2013). Interestingly, the reduced responsiveness of basophils was partially due to an inhibitory factor present in serum probably allergen-specific IgG4 (Wanich *et al.* 2009). Furthermore, it is also known that the secreted anti-inflammatory IL-10 cytokine reduced the release of pro-inflammatory cytokines by mast cells (Marshall *et al.* 1996) and suppressed activity of eosinophils (Takanaski *et al.* 1994). Of note, due to the ability to respond to epithelial-derived cytokines IL-25 and IL-33, type 2 ILCs could secrete T_H2-cytokines to mediate allergic reactions (Barlow and McKenzie 2014). Thus, it is possible that the immune tolerance against allergens is partly contributed by the activation blockade of type 2 ILCs. Supporting evidences for this notion indeed come from a few studies which demonstrated the existence of natural factors that inhibited the activation of type 2 ILCs, such as lipoxin A4 (Barnig *et al.* 2013) or soluble excretory/secretory products of parasitic nematode *Heligmosomoides polygyrus*, e.g., IL-1β (Zaiss *et al.* 2013; McSorley *et al.* 2014). Taken together, these findings suggest that tolerance to cow's milk allergens is associated with suppressed activities of innate type 2 ILCs and pro-allergic innate effectors.

3.2.2. Up-regulation of T_{Reg}-cell Activity

Up-regulated T_{Reg} cells can attenuate allergic responses through 1) suppression of mast cells, basophils and eosinophils; 2) suppression of inflammatory DCs and induction of tolerogenic DCs; 3) suppression of allergen-specific T_H2 cells, hence contributing to T-cell anergy; and 4) early induction of IgG4 and late reduction of IgE production (Akdis 2012). All of these mechanisms can be mediated through secretion of IL-10 and TGF-β or through cell contact-dependent suppression (Akdis 2012). By treating a CMA murine model with various kind of treatments, including dietary long-chain n-3 polyunsaturated fatty acids, prebiotics, *Bifidobacterium breve* M-16V strain ('probiotics'), synbiotics ('prebiotics + probiotics'), or cow's milk protein-derived peptides, a linear correlation of T_{Reg}-cell frequency and activity with the CMA suppression were observed (Schouten *et al.* 2009; Schouten *et al.* 2012; Meulenbroek *et al.* 2013; van den Elsen *et al.* 2013; van den Elsen *et al.* 2013). Furthermore, several human studies also demonstrated the association between the increment of frequency and *in vitro* suppressive capacity of T_{Reg} cells with the clinical tolerance in children who outgrown CMA (Karlsson *et al.* 2004; Shreffler *et al.* 2009). Collectively, these findings indicate that the up-regulation of T_{Reg}-cell functionality would partly contribute to the tolerance to cow's milk allergens.

4   Therapeutic Strategies to Induce Immune Tolerance

As mentioned, there is no established method to cure CMA to date. The only available approach to date is to apply strict avoidance of cow's milk proteins, either by 1) perform maternal elimination diet of cow's milk for breast-fed infants; 2) use partial or extensively hydrolysed milk formula for formula-fed children less than 2 years of age; or 3) switch to a milk-free diet for children more than 2 years of age (Fiocchi *et al.* 2010). This strict dietary avoidance should be accompanied with ready access to self-injectable epinephrine (Muraro *et al.* 2014). Drawbacks of this approach include impairment of the quality of life of both child and family, restricted children's growth and higher health care cost (Koletzko *et al.* 2012). Therefore, novel therapeutic strategies are currently being developed for preventing and curing allergy in general and food allergy in particular. Hereby we review two promising approaches (Table 4).

Biological Immune Response Modifiers	Allergen-Specific Immunotherapy
Targeting (Akdis 2012): (a) IgE or its receptor, or (b) pro-allergic cytokines.	Consisting the whole antigen or a part of it, e.g., peptide (Kostadinova *et al.* 2013).

	Administered via (Akdis 2012; Narisety and Keet 2012):
	1) Skin:
	    (a) Subcutaneous immunotherapy (SCIT), or
	    (b) Epicutaneous immunotherapy (EPIT).
	2) Gastrointestinal tract:
	    (a) Sublingual immunotherapy (SLIT), or
	    (b) Oral immunotherapy (OIT).

Table 4: Therapeutic strategies for treating the allergic inflammation.

4.1   Biological Immune Response Modifiers

The first strategy is to develop biological immune response modifiers to suppress pathological immune responses (Akdis 2012). The immune modifiers are developed to suppress pro-allergic soluble mediators, including IgE and cytokines (e.g., IL-4, IL-5, IL-13, IL-25 or IL-33). IgE, the pro-allergic Ig isotype, is the most obvious target for this approach. Several humanized monoclonal antibodies (mAbs) targeting the Fc portion of IgE have been developed and tested (Akdis 2012). One of the anti-IgE mAbs, omalizumab, has been suggested to be effective in a few clinical trials on patients with poorly controlled, moderate to severe respiratory allergic reactions (Casale *et al.* 2001; Lin *et al.* 2004; Busse *et al.* 2011). Omalizumab acts by decreasing the free IgE levels in serum and the expression of FcεRI on various immune cells (Lin *et al.* 2004). However, the clinical application of anti-IgE mAbs is very limited due to a few reasons: 1) high doses of anti-IgE mAbs are required to successfully neutralize IgE; 2) low cost effectiveness of using anti-IgE mAbs; and 3) unexpected efficacy without any reasonable explanation in some cases (Oba and Salzman 2004; Akdis 2012). Therefore an alternative approach is developed to replace mAbs, i.e., by using designed ankyrin repeat proteins ('DARPins'). DARPins represent a promising scaffold due to high specificity and low concentration binding to the respected target. A few studies have demonstrated that DARPins can effectively bind to the Fc portion of IgE as well as the alpha chain of FcεRI, hence preventing the release of pro-inflammatory mediators (Eggel *et al.* 2009; Baumann *et al.* 2010). These exciting findings indicate that the DARPins technology is promising to be utilized to create allergy-attenuating candidate molecules.

Immune modifiers are also developed to target pro-allergic cytokines because these cytokines coordinate the inflammatory processes upon allergy. Cytokine inhibitors have been developed and tested for, at least, IL-4, IL-5, IL-13 or TNF-α. However, the low efficacy (due to the intricate cytokine network, hence targeting a single cytokine only may not induce any significant improvement) and/or the unfavourable risk-benefit ratio of using cytokine inhibitors become a big hurdle in order to bring forward this therapeutic option to the clinical settings (Akdis 2012).

4.2   Allergen-Specific Immunotherapy (Allergen SIT)

The ultimate goal in allergology is to discover a long-term cure for allergic diseases. This goal potentially can be achieved by using allergen SIT, since its primary mode of action is to induce desensitization and subsequently immune tolerance to the allergens, by administering repeated, increased doses of the allergens (Akdis 2012). Desensitization means an increment in threshold of exposed/ingested harmless antigen needed to cause allergic symptoms (Jones *et al.* 2009). Immune tolerance refers to the state of immunologic hyporesponsiveness to harmless antigen (Kostadinova *et al.* 2013). Despite allergen SIT actually has been performed for several allergic reactions in the clinic, the current strategy of administering allergen SIT has limited efficacy, high side effects, low patient adherence and high cost due to long duration of the treatment (Akdis 2012; Kostadinova *et al.* 2013). This indicates that an improved/novel strategy is crucially required.

With regard to food allergy, allergen SIT requires thorough evaluation in two aspects. The first aspect is to properly choose the most optimum route of administering allergen SIT. The classical way to administer allergen SIT is through the subcutaneous route (SCIT), i.e., injecting soluble allergen under the skin. It is employed frequently for respiratory and bee venom allergies due to its safety and effectiveness (Kostadinova *et al.* 2013). The only food allergen that has been tested via SCIT thus far is peanut allergen. Unfortunately, despite the promising efficacy rate of SCIT, the rate of systemic adverse reactions, including anaphylactic shock, was high when using peanut allergen (Oppenheimer *et al.* 1992; Nelson *et al.* 1997). Hence this finding discourages the SCIT utilization in its current form for treating food allergy (Kostadinova *et al.* 2013). A modified method for SCIT is the epicutaneous immunotherapy (EPIT), i.e., administering soluble allergen via skin patch into the stratum corneum, the outer layer of the skin. Due to the non-invasive nature of EPIT, it is possibly a safer method for treating food allergy (Kostadinova *et al.* 2013). Interestingly, a pilot study of using EPIT to treat the IgE-mediated CMA-diagnosed children in France demonstrated that this method is safe and acceptable (Dupont *et al.* 2010). Further clinical trials will definitely be required in order to determine the efficacy of EPIT in treating CMA, similar to the ones that have been initiated for peanut allergy (Senti *et al.* 2014).

Besides the cutaneous route, allergen SIT can be administered via the enteral route, including sublingual immunotherapy (SLIT) and oral immunotherapy (OIT). For SLIT, concentrated liquid allergen extract is administered under the tongue for 2 minutes and subsequently discarded or swallowed. For OIT, the powder form or mixture of culprit food with a vehicle (e.g., apple sauce) is directly ingested (Narisety and Keet 2012; Kostadinova *et al.* 2013). Due to the difference of used forms, allergen quantity in the OIT can be increased from milligram amounts to several grams, while the one in the SLIT can only be increased from microgram amounts to maximum milligram amounts. Nonetheless, SLIT has other advantages, i.e., allowing the food proteins to bypass gastric digestion and potentially enhancing tolerance induction because the oral mucosa supposedly contains many tolerogenic APCs but fewer effector cells responsible for the allergic reactions (Narisety and Keet 2012). The safety profile of SLIT for treating CMA has been tested in a few clinical studies. Indeed, it has been shown that the SLIT for CMA has an encouraging safety profile (de Boissieu and Dupont 2006; Keet *et al.* 2012). However, it has been demonstrated that for desensitizing CMA-diagnosed patients, the efficacy of SLIT was much lower than the one belongs to OIT (Keet *et al.* 2012). Thus far, OIT is the most actively studied form of allergen SIT for primary food allergies including CMA, partially due to the ability to use allergen at high doses reaching the actual amount of ingested food (Narisety and Keet 2012). Several clinical studies performed in Europe and North America demonstrated that OIT with cow's milk could induce desensitization, as reflected by ability to consume larger amount of cow's milk without exhibiting any adverse effect, reduction of sensitivity on skin prick test, reduction of cow's milk-specific IgE levels and/or elevation of cow's milk-specific IgG4 levels (Patriarca *et al.* 2003; Meglio *et al.* 2004; Staden *et al.* 2007; Longo *et al.* 2008; Skripak *et al.* 2008; Narisety *et al.* 2009; Pajno *et al.* 2010; Martorell *et al.* 2011; Salmivesi *et al.* 2013; Savilahti *et al.* 2014). The subsequent question is of course whether OIT could induce immune tolerance for long term or even permanently. Interestingly, a few clinical studies have demonstrated the OIT efficacy to induce oral tolerance against cow's milk for a long period, even for more than 3 years of follow-up (Staden *et al.* 2007; Martorell *et al.* 2011; Salmivesi *et al.* 2013). It is important to notice that OIT has been tested in children with severe cases of CMA as well, resulting as 36% of tested subjects were able to tolerate at least 150 mL of cow's milk (Longo *et al.* 2008). Taken together, cow's milk OIT is potential to induce desensitization and immune tolerance that can persist in the long term. However, higher dose of cow's milk allergen used in OIT (than SLIT) is also associated with a higher risk to develop adverse effects (Keet *et al.* 2012). Therefore, it is mandatory to exert cautions while administering OIT in its current form.

The second aspect of evaluation is related to how to minimize the high rates of adverse effects in OIT by reducing the size and structure of administered food protein. A way to do this is by using peptides ('peptide immunotherapy'), as they consist T-cell epitopes (hence, potentially retain their therapeutic benefit) but less likely to induce side effects due to peptides' inability to cross-link surface-bound IgE on effector immune cells. Theoretically, since the distance between two FcεRI molecules is ranging from 8 to 24 nm, using peptides shorter than 30 amino acids should not cross-link surface-bound IgEs, but shall retain T-cell epitopes (Knipping *et al.* 2012) . This strategy of peptide immunotherapy has been more actively studied for respiratory allergies, in particular of allergy to cat and bee venom (Larche 2005; Moldaver and Larche 2011). Several clinical studies focusing on both allergens had been performed. Indeed, allergen-specific hyporesponsiveness can be induced via down-regulation of T-cell allergic responses (skewing to the regulatory phenotype) as well as of pro-allergic cytokine (e.g., IL-4 and IL-13) and IgE production (Larche 2005; Verhoef *et al.* 2005; Moldaver and Larche 2011). Furthermore, exposure of tolerogenic peptide induces early apoptotic deletion in naïve CD4+ T cells (Kearney *et al.* 1994; Hochweller and Anderton 2005; Hochweller *et al.*

2006). It was also demonstrated that the peptide immunotherapy could reduce allergic responses if the allergy was driven by effector memory CD4$^+$ T (T$_{EM}$), but not by central memory T (T$_{CM}$) cells (Mackenzie *et al.* 2014). Interestingly, a study demonstrated that follow-ing at least two rounds of peptide exposure, reactivated memory CD4$^+$ T cells failed to survive (marked by low expression of the antiapoptotic molecule Bcl2 and high expression of activated caspase molecules), hence fewer pro-allergic T cells existed to sustain subsequent hyper-sensitivity response (David *et al.* 2014). Furthermore, the peptide immunotherapy is associated with a phenomenon called 'linked epitope suppression', i.e., a treatment with selected epitopes form a single allergen can suppress responses to other epitopes from the same allergen, probably through the action of IL-10 (Campbell *et al.* 2009). Of note, the peptide immunotherapy was generally well tolerated, although a few adverse effects were observed in some studies, including delayed symptoms of asthma or erythema with palm pruritus, hence it is still of concern (Larche 2005; Moldaver and Larche 2011). Taken together, these findings support the concept to utilize selected peptides in order to prevent inflammatory responses against an allergen; however, the clinical efficacy of the peptide immunotherapy potentially will be varied among different allergies and individuals.

Pertaining to CMA, peptide immunotherapy has been mainly investigated in murine models. Several groups demonstrated that prior treatment with αS1-casein- or β-lactoglobulin-derived peptide(s) rendered mice to be immune tolerant to cow's milk protein (Hirahara *et al.* 1995; Pecquet *et al.* 2000). In a recent study, particular β-lactoglobulin-derived tolerogenic peptides were identified, in which these peptides were able to reduce acute allergic response in a murine model of CMA. The allergic reduction, as manifested as a reduction in ear swelling, was importantly associated with decreasing levels of cow's milk-specific IgE and increasing frequencies of T$_{Reg}$ cells (Meulenbroek *et al.* 2013). Collectively, this alternative approach is promising to prevent or treat CMA, although further clinical studies are required to assess its clinical efficacy and safety.

5   Possible Mechanistic Interaction between CMA and Other Inflammatory Reactions

The allergic reactions are characterised by the T$_H$2-polarized immune responses, by the activation of pro-allergic innate effectors and by the impairment of T$_{Reg}$ cells. As mentioned above, CD4$^+$ T cells are heterogeneous due to their ability to differentiate into T$_H$1, T$_H$2, T$_H$9, T$_H$17, T$_H$22, T$_{follicular\ helper}$ (T$_{fh}$) or T$_{Reg}$ cells, hallmarked by different lineage-specifying transcription factors and different signature cytokines (O'Shea and Paul 2010). For example, T$_H$1 cells express T-bet and secrete IFN-γ, T$_H$2 cells express GATA3 and secrete IL-4, T$_H$17 cells express RORγt and secrete IL-17, while T$_{Reg}$ cells express Foxp3 and secrete IL-10 and TGF-β. It was originally proposed that each subset of CD4$^+$ T cells permanently retain their differentiated identity, resulting as non-overlapping distinct subsets (O'Shea and Paul 2010). However, it is clear now that the differentiation process is dynamic instead, particularly during chronic inflammation *in vivo* (Hirahara *et al.* 2013). This allows a particular differentiated subset of CD4$^+$ T cells to secrete signature cytokines that belong to other subsets or even to further convert into another subset. For example, it has been shown that T cells derived from chronic allergic asthma patients co-expressed and co-produced both T$_H$2- and T$_H$17-transcription factors and cytokines (Wang *et al.* 2010). In addition, atopic dermatitis patients predominantly displayed T$_H$2-immune responses with a T$_H$17 component at the acute phase of the disease, which often converted into T$_H$1-immune responses at the chronic stage (Oyoshi *et al.* 2009). Thus, it incites a speculation of whether T$_H$2-polarized immune responses in CMA could also exhibit or even convert to T$_H$1- or T$_H$17-immune responses in minority group of patients who never outgrow their CMA.

The consensus of food allergy occurs due to the imbalance between T$_H$2- and T$_{Reg}$-polarized immune responses indeed incites a speculation of whether inflammation of CMA affects other type of inflammatory reactions (infection as well as other chronic inflammatory non-communicable diseases or NCDs) and vice versa. The published data does not allow a definite conclusion to be constructed; nonetheless it provides some hints that permit various speculations. First, despite there is no prospective study following children with food allergy to determine whether they have a lower predilection to suffer from helminth infection, CMA infants with the elevated T$_H$2-polarized immune responses should be more protected against helminths. A supporting finding came from a population study in Cameroon who demonstrated that subjects with elevated IL-5 and IL-13 cytokines indeed had reduced reinfection rates with *Ascaris lumbricoides* and *Trichiuris trichiura* (Jackson *et al.* 2004), supporting the importance of T$_H$2-immune responses against helminths. On the other hand, helminth infections is associated with T$_H$2-polarized immune responses, hence theoretically it could increase the susceptibility of infected hosts to develop allergic reactions. However, it appears not to be the case. A study on infants living in areas endemic for helminth infections suggested that despite potent T$_H$2-responses were observed early in life, it did not translate into a higher SPT reactivity to various allergens at 4 years of age (Djuardi *et al.* 2013). A supporting finding came from a study on mice chronically infected with *Heligmosomoides polygyrus bakeri* suggested that the helminths induced IL-1β secretion in small intestines that acts to suppress the production of IL-25 and IL-33, thus resulting in suboptimal T$_H$2-immune responses and hence chronic helminth infection (Zaiss *et al.* 2013). Helminth infections could also induce activation of T$_{Reg}$ cells, resulting in IL-10 and IgG4 production, hence attenuating the T$_H$2-immune responses (Fallon and Mangan 2007). A murine study indeed demonstrated that infection with intestinal helminths (*Heligmosomoides polygyrus*) prior to the sensitization and challenge with peanut extract *per oral* indeed significantly reduced peanut-specific IgE levels and diminished systemic anaphylactic symptoms via IL-10 production (Bashir *et al.* 2002). More importantly, several clinical studies demonstrated associations between human infections with *Schistosoma haematobium* or *Schistosoma mansoni* and lowered allergic responses, probably through the action of IL-10 (Araujo *et al.* 2000; van den Biggelaar *et al.* 2000; Medeiros *et al.* 2003). Therefore, prior exposures to helminths might reduce allergy incidence to cow's milk proteins.

Second, the activation of T$_H$1-polarized immune responses is required for the control and elimination of intracellular pathogens. Due to the suppression of IFN-γ gene transcription by IL-4, i.e., T$_H$2 cytokine suppresses T$_H$1-functionality (Nakamura *et al.* 1997), it is plausible to assume that allergic infants might be more susceptible to be infected with intracellular pathogens. Interestingly, a prospective birth cohort study in the Netherlands, PIAMA (*n*=4,146), demonstrated an association between children having risk factors for allergy (i.e., having allergic parents and attending child care or having older siblings) with a higher risk of suffering low respiratory tract infections in the first year of life (Koopman *et al.* 2001). However, it is elusive whether CMA infants are more susceptible than healthy infants to develop infections in the gastrointestinal tract, respiratory tract or skin. Next, gastrointestinal infection with intracellular pathogens can cause enteral inflammation along with the disruption of the healthy intestinal flora. This perturbs homeostasis among host immunity, host gut microbiota and gut antigens, which may represent the critical determinant in the development of food allergy, including CMA (Macdonald and Monteleone 2005). Indeed, there is a case report demonstrating a Japanese infant who developed CMA associated with enterotoxigenic *Escherichia coli* and methicillin-resistant *Staphylococcus aureus* infections (Omata *et al.* 2008). In addition, another study of Japanese newborns who underwent small intestine surgery and received antibiotics due to symptoms resembling postoperative infection showed that 9 out of 30 subjects subsequently developed CMA (Ezaki *et al.* 2012). Importantly, within a subset of patients who received prophylactic probiotics, most of the patients (~98%) did not suffer from CMA (Ezaki *et al.* 2012), suggesting that restoration and maintenance of gastrointestinal immune tolerance is imperative in order to prevent food allergy. Arguably, gastrointestinal infections that incite enteral inflammation may represent an important risk factor to develop CMA.

Third, consistent with the fact that allergy is the most common and earliest-onset of inflammatory NCDs (Prescott 2013), it is important to understand how the immune mechanisms underlying food allergy interact with the ones constituting other NCDs, including other types of allergy, metabolic diseases, autoimmunity and cancer. It is noteworthy to mention that there are common risk factors for most NCDs, i.e., diet patterns, microbial patterns, behaviour and environmental pollutants (Prescott 2013). These common risks may initiate similar alterations within the immune system to cause many NCDs, arguably through the impairment of T$_{Reg}$ cells. T$_{Reg}$-cell defect causes uncontrolled inflammation (Vignali *et al.* 2008), contributing to the pathogenesis of many NCDs (Prescott 2013). Indeed, the reduction of T$_{Reg}$ cells has been linked to the dysregulated inflammation of other NCDs, such as obesity and insulin resistance (Priceman *et al.* 2013). Furthermore, a prospective mother-child study conducted in Germany, LINA (*n*=629), demonstrated a clear correlation between history of maternal exposure to tobacco smoke, lower T$_{Reg}$-cell frequencies in maternal and cord blood, as well as a higher risk for those children to develop atopic dermatitis within the first 3 years of life (Herberth *et al.* 2013). It is arguably that the common defect of immune regulation may cause several NCDs to occur concurrently, though the responsible mechanism still needs to be confirmed. Nonetheless, it is of interest to quote a recent data from the National Health and Nutrition Examination Survey, demonstrating that US children and adolescents who were obese indeed had higher levels of total IgE and

C-reactive protein levels as well as higher incidences of food allergy (Visness *et al.* 2009). Taken together, similar impairment in the immune mechanism that causes inflammation may mediate occurrence of many NCDs.

As allergic inflammation still remains a big mystery of the immune system, it is worthy to view allergy from a different perspective in order to understand it better. The current belief is that allergy is an adverse effect of an aberrant or misdirected immune response that evolved to provide immunity to macroparasites, e.g., helminths (Fallon and Mangan 2007; Galli *et al.* 2008). However, this view does not reconcile issues of 1) why many allergens do not have any relationship with helminth antigens as well as why many allergens do not share any common characteristic (e.g., peanut and penicillin); and 2) why many allergic responses occur very fast despite helminths are slowly replicating relatively to bacteria or viruses (Palm *et al.* 2012). In order to reconcile this issue, Medzhitov's group proposed that allergic inflammation actually provide an important defence mechanism against various noxious environmental factors, including 1) macroparasites; 2) noxious xenobiotics; 3) venoms and haematophagous fluids; and 4) environmental irritants (Palm *et al.* 2012). The induced allergic reactions reduce exposure and promote expulsion of noxious factors as well as ensure avoidance of unfavourable environments (Palm *et al.* 2012). Despite it is an interesting concept, this hypothesis could not explain why certain innocuous antigens, such as cow's milk or peanut, induce allergic inflammation and why the induced allergic inflammation only occurs in certain groups of people. It will be extremely important to analyse allergic reactions as well as specific allergens from various perspectives in order to elucidate our understanding of allergic inflammation.

6   Conclusion

Immune system, comprising both the innate and adaptive components, mediates allergic reactions as well as immune tolerance toward cow's milk proteins. The CMA pathogenesis is mediated by the activation of pro-allergic innate (inflammatory DCs, tissue mast cells, basophils, eosinophils and type 2 ILCs) and adaptive effectors (T_H2 and IgE-producing plasma cells), by the suppression of T_{Reg} cells as well by the production of cow's milk-specific IgE. The immune tolerance against cow's milk proteins is contributed by the activation of T_{Reg} cells and by the suppression of T_H2-polarized immune responses as well as pro-allergic effectors. Possible therapeutic strategies to induce immune tolerance against CMA have been discussed, including the usage of the biological immune response modifiers or the allergen-specific immunotherapy. One of the promising methods of the allergen-specific immunotherapy is the utilization of peptide immunotherapy. Finally, due to the significant overlapping between the inflammatory reaction of CMA and of infection or other NCDs, the proper management of CMA may positively contribute to a better control of systemic inflammation.

References

Aalberse, R. C., S. O. Stapel, et al. (2009). *Immunoglobulin G4: an odd antibody. Clin Exp Allergy 39(4): 469–477.*

Abbas, A. K., C. Benoist, et al. (2013). *Regulatory T cells: recommendations to simplify the nomenclature. Nat Immunol 14(4): 307–308.*

Achatz, G., G. Achatz-Straussberger, et al. (2010). *The Biology of IgE: Molecular Mechanism Restraining Potentially Dangerous High Serum IgE Titres In Vivo. Cancer and IgE: Introducing the Concept of AllergoOncology. M. L. Penichet and E. Jensen-Jarolim, Humana Press: 13–36.*

Adel-Patient, K., H. Bernard, et al. (2005). *Peanut- and cow's milk-specific IgE, Th2 cells and local anaphylactic reaction are induced in Balb/c mice orally sensitized with cholera toxin. Allergy 60(5): 658–664.*

Akdis, C. A. (2012). *Therapies for allergic inflammation: refining strategies to induce tolerance. Nat Med 18(5): 736–749.*

Akdis, M., J. Verhagen, et al. (2004). *Immune responses in healthy and allergic individuals are characterized by a fine balance between allergen-specific T regulatory 1 and T helper 2 cells. J Exp Med 199(11): 1567–1575.*

Andre, F., J. Pene, et al. (1996). *Interleukin-4 and interferon-gamma production by peripheral blood mononuclear cells from food-allergic patients. Allergy 51(5): 350–355.*

Araujo, M. I., A. A. Lopes, et al. (2000). *Inverse association between skin response to aeroallergens and Schistosoma mansoni infection. Int Arch Allergy Immunol 123(2): 145–148.*

Barlow, J. L. and A. N. McKenzie (2014). *Type-2 innate lymphoid cells in human allergic disease. Curr Opin Allergy Clin Immunol 14(5): 397–403.*

Barnig, C., M. Cernadas, et al. (2013). *Lipoxin A4 regulates natural killer cell and type 2 innate lymphoid cell activation in asthma. Sci Transl Med 5(174): 174ra126.*

Bashir, M. E., P. Andersen, et al. (2002). *An enteric helminth infection protects against an allergic response to dietary antigen. J Immunol 169(6): 3284–3292.*

Baumann, M. J., A. Eggel, et al. (2010). *DARPins against a functional IgE epitope. Immunol Lett 133(2): 78–84.*

Bennett, C. L., J. Christie, et al. (2001). *The immune dysregulation, polyendocrinopathy, enteropathy, X-linked syndrome (IPEX) is caused by mutations of FOXP3. Nat Genet 27(1): 20–21.*

Beyer, K., R. Castro, et al. (2002). *Human milk-specific mucosal lymphocytes of the gastrointestinal tract display a TH2 cytokine profile. J Allergy Clin Immunol 109(4): 707–713.*

Bol-Schoenmakers, M., M. Marcondes Rezende, et al. (2011). *Regulation by intestinal gammadelta T cells during establishment of food allergic sensitization in mice. Allergy 66(3): 331–340.*

Braber, S., M. Thio, et al. (2012). *An association between neutrophils and immunoglobulin free light chains in the pathogenesis of chronic obstructive pulmonary disease. Am J Respir Crit Care Med 185(8): 817–824.*

Busse, W. W., W. J. Morgan, et al. (2011). *Randomized trial of omalizumab (anti-IgE) for asthma in inner-city children. N Engl J Med 364(11): 1005–1015.*

Campbell, D. E., D. J. Hill, et al. (1998). *Enhanced IL-4 but normal interferon-gamma production in children with isolated IgE mediated food hypersensitivity. Pediatr Allergy Immunol 9(2): 68–72.*

Campbell, J. D., K. F. Buckland, et al. (2009). Peptide immunotherapy in allergic asthma generates IL-10-dependent immunological tolerance associated with linked epitope suppression. J Exp Med 206(7): 1535–1547.

Carter, N. A., R. Vasconcellos, et al. (2011). Mice lacking endogenous IL-10-producing regulatory B cells develop exacerbated disease and present with an increased frequency of Th1/Th17 but a decrease in regulatory T cells. J Immunol 186(10): 5569–5579.

Casale, T. B., J. Condemi, et al. (2001). Effect of omalizumab on symptoms of seasonal allergic rhinitis: a randomized controlled trial. JAMA 286(23): 2956–2967.

Caughey, G. H. (2007). Mast cell tryptases and chymases in inflammation and host defense. Immunol Rev 217: 141–154.

Chambers, S. J., E. Bertelli, et al. (2004). Adoptive transfer of dendritic cells from allergic mice induces specific immunoglobulin E antibody in naive recipients in absence of antigen challenge without altering the T helper 1/T helper 2 balance. Immunology 112(1): 72–79.

Chen, K. and A. Cerutti (2011). The function and regulation of immunoglobulin D. Curr Opin Immunol 23(3): 345–352.

Chen, K., W. Xu, et al. (2009). Immunoglobulin D enhances immune surveillance by activating antimicrobial, proinflammatory and B cell-stimulating programs in basophils. Nat Immunol 10(8): 889–898.

Cheng, M. H. and M. S. Anderson (2012). Monogenic autoimmunity. Annu Rev Immunol 30: 393–427.

Coombes, J. L. and F. Powrie (2008). Dendritic cells in intestinal immune regulation. Nat Rev Immunol 8(6): 435–446.

Coombes, J. L., K. R. Siddiqui, et al. (2007). A functionally specialized population of mucosal CD103+ DCs induces Foxp3+ regulatory T cells via a TGF-beta and retinoic acid-dependent mechanism. J Exp Med 204(8): 1757–1764.

Corthesy, B. (2013). Multi-faceted functions of secretory IgA at mucosal surfaces. Front Immunol 4: 185.

David, A., F. Crawford, et al. (2014). Tolerance induction in memory CD4 T cells requires two rounds of antigen-specific activation. Proc Natl Acad Sci U S A 111(21): 7735–7740.

de Boissieu, D. and C. Dupont (2006). Sublingual immunotherapy for cow's milk protein allergy: a preliminary report. Allergy 61(10): 1238–1239.

de Kivit, S., M. C. Tobin, et al. (2014). Regulation of Intestinal Immune Responses through TLR Activation: Implications for Pro- and Prebiotics. Front Immunol 5: 60.

Diefenbach, A., M. Colonna, et al. (2014). Development, differentiation, and diversity of innate lymphoid cells. Immunity 41(3): 354–365.

Djuardi, Y., T. Supali, et al. (2013). The development of TH2 responses from infancy to 4 years of age and atopic sensitization in areas endemic for helminth infections. Allergy Asthma Clin Immunol 9(1): 13.

Dullaers, M., R. De Bruyne, et al. (2012). The who, where, and when of IgE in allergic airway disease. J Allergy Clin Immunol 129(3): 635–645.

Dupont, C., N. Kalach, et al. (2010). Cow's milk epicutaneous immunotherapy in children: a pilot trial of safety, acceptability, and impact on allergic reactivity. J Allergy Clin Immunol 125(5): 1165–1167.

Eggel, A., M. J. Baumann, et al. (2009). DARPins as bispecific receptor antagonists analyzed for immunoglobulin E receptor blockage. J Mol Biol 393(3): 598–607.

Ezaki, S., K. Itoh, et al. (2012). Prophylactic probiotics reduce cow's milk protein intolerance in neonates after small intestine surgery and antibiotic treatment presenting symptoms that mimics postoperative infection. Allergol Int 61(1): 107–113.

Fallon, P. G. and N. E. Mangan (2007). Suppression of TH2-type allergic reactions by helminth infection. Nat Rev Immunol 7(3): 220–230.

Fiocchi, A., G. R. Bouygue, et al. (2011). Molecular diagnosis of cow's milk allergy. Curr Opin Allergy Clin Immunol 11(3): 216–221.

Fiocchi, A., H. J. Schunemann, et al. (2010). Diagnosis and Rationale for Action Against Cow's Milk Allergy (DRACMA): a summary report. J Allergy Clin Immunol 126(6): 1119–1128 e1112.

Flores-Borja, F., A. Bosma, et al. (2013). CD19+CD24hiCD38hi B cells maintain regulatory T cells while limiting TH1 and TH17 differentiation. Sci Transl Med 5(173): 173ra123.

Ford, L. S., K. A. Bloom, et al. (2013). Basophil reactivity, wheal size, and immunoglobulin levels distinguish degrees of cow's milk tolerance. J Allergy Clin Immunol 131(1): 180-186 e181–183.

Galli, S. J., M. Tsai, et al. (2008). The development of allergic inflammation. Nature 454(7203): 445–454.

Gleich, G. J., E. Frigas, et al. (1979). Cytotoxic properties of the eosinophil major basic protein. J Immunol 123(6): 2925–2927.

Gould, H. J., P. Takhar, et al. (2006). Germinal-centre reactions in allergic inflammation. Trends Immunol 27(10): 446–452.

Groot Kormelink, T., D. G. Powe, et al. (2014). Immunoglobulin free light chains are biomarkers of poor prognosis in basal-like breast cancer and are potential targets in tumor-associated inflammation. Oncotarget 5(10): 3159–3167.

Haniffa, M., A. Shin, et al. (2012). Human tissues contain CD141hi cross-presenting dendritic cells with functional homology to mouse CD103+ nonlymphoid dendritic cells. Immunity 37(1): 60–73.

Hazenberg, M. D. and H. Spits (2014). Human innate lymphoid cells. Blood 124(5): 700–709.

Herberth, G., M. Bauer, et al. (2013). Maternal and cord blood miR-223 expression associates with prenatal tobacco smoke exposure and low regulatory T–cell numbers. J Allergy Clin Immunol.

Hidvegi, E., E. Cserhati, et al. (2002). Serum immunoglobulin E, IgA, and IgG antibodies to different cow's milk proteins in children with cow's milk allergy: association with prognosis and clinical manifestations. Pediatr Allergy Immunol 13(4): 255–261.

Hirahara, K., T. Hisatsune, et al. (1995). Profound immunological tolerance in the antibody response against bovine alpha s1-casein induced by intradermal administration of a dominant T cell determinant. Clin Immunol Immunopathol 76(1 Pt 1): 12–18.

Hirahara, K., A. Poholek, et al. (2013). Mechanisms underlying helper T-cell plasticity: implications for immune-mediated disease. J Allergy Clin Immunol 131(5): 1276–1287.

Hochwallner, H., U. Schulmeister, et al. (2014). Cow's milk allergy: from allergens to new forms of diagnosis, therapy and prevention. Methods 66(1): 22–33.

Hochweller, K. and S. M. Anderton (2005). Kinetics of costimulatory molecule expression by T cells and dendritic cells during the induction of tolerance versus immunity in vivo. Eur J Immunol 35(4): 1086–1096.

Hochweller, K., C. H. Sweenie, et al. (2006). Circumventing tolerance at the T cell or the antigen-presenting cell surface: antibodies that ligate CD40 and OX40 have different effects. Eur J Immunol 36(2): 389–396.

Hogan, S. P., A. Mishra, et al. (2001). A pathological function for eotaxin and eosinophils in eosinophilic gastrointestinal inflammation. Nat Immunol 2(4): 353–360.

Host, A., S. Halken, et al. (2002). Clinical course of cow's milk protein allergy/intolerance and atopic diseases in childhood. Pediatr Allergy Immunol 13 Suppl 15: 23–28.

Hsu, C. L., C. V. Neilsen, et al. (2010). IL-33 is produced by mast cells and regulates IgE-dependent inflammation. PLoS One 5(8): e11944.

Ikeda, K., H. Nakajima, et al. (2003). Mast cells produce interleukin-25 upon Fc epsilon RI-mediated activation. Blood 101(9): 3594–3596.

Jackson, J. A., J. D. Turner, et al. (2004). T helper cell type 2 responsiveness predicts future susceptibility to gastrointestinal nematodes in humans. J Infect Dis 190(10): 1804–1811.

Jackson, K. J., Y. Wang, et al. (2014). Human immunoglobulin classes and subclasses show variability in VDJ gene mutation levels. Immunol Cell Biol 92(8): 729–733.

James, L. K., M. H. Shamji, et al. (2011). Long-term tolerance after allergen immunotherapy is accompanied by selective persistence of blocking antibodies. J Allergy Clin Immunol 127(2): 509–516 e501–505.

Jarvenpaa, J., M. Paassilta, et al. (2014). Stability of parent-reported food allergy in six and 7-year-old children: the first 5 years of the Finnish allergy programme. Acta Paediatr 103(12): 1297–1300.

Jarvinen, K. M., J. E. Westfall, et al. (2014). Role of maternal elimination diets and human milk IgA in the development of cow's milk allergy in the infants. Clin Exp Allergy 44(1): 69–78.

Jo, J., J. Garssen, et al. (2014). Role of cellular immunity in cow's milk allergy: pathogenesis, tolerance induction, and beyond. Mediators Inflamm 2014: 249784.

Joffre, O. P., E. Segura, et al. (2012). Cross-presentation by dendritic cells. Nat Rev Immunol 12(8): 557–569.

Jones, S. M., L. Pons, et al. (2009). Clinical efficacy and immune regulation with peanut oral immunotherapy. J Allergy Clin Immunol 124(2): 292–300, 300 e291–297.

Jyonouchi, S., C. L. Smith, et al. (2014). Invariant natural killer T cells in children with eosinophilic esophagitis. Clin Exp Allergy 44(1): 58–68.

Karlsson, M. R., J. Rugtveit, et al. (2004). Allergen-responsive CD4+CD25+ regulatory T cells in children who have outgrown cow's milk allergy. J Exp Med 199(12): 1679–1688.

Kearney, E. R., K. A. Pape, et al. (1994). Visualization of peptide-specific T cell immunity and peripheral tolerance induction in vivo. Immunity 1(4): 327–339.

Keet, C. A., P. A. Frischmeyer-Guerrerio, et al. (2012). The safety and efficacy of sublingual and oral immunotherapy for milk allergy. J Allergy Clin Immunol 129(2): 448–455, 455 e441–445.

Kita, H. (2013). Eosinophils: multifunctional and distinctive properties. Int Arch Allergy Immunol 161 Suppl 2: 3–9.

Knipping, K., B. C. van Esch, et al. (2012). Enzymatic treatment of whey proteins in cow's milk results in differential inhibition of IgE-mediated mast cell activation compared to T-cell activation. Int Arch Allergy Immunol 159(3): 263–270.

Koletzko, S., B. Niggemann, et al. (2012). Diagnostic approach and management of cow's-milk protein allergy in infants and children: ESPGHAN GI Committee practical guidelines. J Pediatr Gastroenterol Nutr 55(2): 221–229.

Koopman, L. P., H. A. Smit, et al. (2001). Respiratory infections in infants: interaction of parental allergy, child care, and siblings — The PIAMA study. Pediatrics 108(4): 943–948.

Kostadinova, A. I., L. E. Willemsen, et al. (2013). Immunotherapy — risk/benefit in food allergy. Pediatr Allergy Immunol 24(7): 633–644.

Kukkonen, A. K., E. M. Savilahti, et al. (2011). Ovalbumin-specific immunoglobulins A and G levels at age 2 years are associated with the occurrence of atopic disorders. Clin Exp Allergy 41(10): 1414–1421.

Larche, M. (2005). Peptide therapy for allergic diseases: basic mechanisms and new clinical approaches. Pharmacol Ther 108(3): 353–361.

Lee, J. H., J. Noh, et al. (2011). Allergen-specific transforming growth factor-beta-producing CD19+CD5+ regulatory B-cell (Br3) responses in human late eczematous allergic reactions to cow's milk. J Interferon Cytokine Res 31(5): 441–449.

Lee, J. H., J. Noh, et al. (2010). Allergen-specific B cell subset responses in cow's milk allergy of late eczematous reactions in atopic dermatitis. Cell Immunol 262(1): 44–51.

Leung, J., N. V. Hundal, et al. (2013). Tolerance of baked milk in patients with cow's milk-mediated eosinophilic esophagitis. J Allergy Clin Immunol 132(5): 1215–1216 e1211.

Li, X. M., B. H. Schofield, et al. (1999). A murine model of IgE-mediated cow's milk hypersensitivity. J Allergy Clin Immunol 103(2 Pt 1): 206–214.

Lin, H., K. M. Boesel, et al. (2004). Omalizumab rapidly decreases nasal allergic response and FcepsilonRI on basophils. J Allergy Clin Immunol 113(2): 297–302.

Longo, G., E. Barbi, et al. (2008). Specific oral tolerance induction in children with very severe cow's milk-induced reactions. J Allergy Clin Immunol 121(2): 343–347.

Macdonald, T. T. and G. Monteleone (2005). Immunity, inflammation, and allergy in the gut. Science 307(5717): 1920–1925.

MacGlashan, D. W., Jr. (2013). Basophil activation testing. J Allergy Clin Immunol 132(4): 777–787.

Mackenzie, K. J., D. J. Nowakowska, et al. (2014). Effector and central memory T helper 2 cells respond differently to peptide immunotherapy. Proc Natl Acad Sci U S A 111(8): E784–793.

Marshall, J. S., I. Leal-Berumen, et al. (1996). Interleukin (IL)-10 inhibits long-term IL-6 production but not preformed mediator release from rat peritoneal mast cells. J Clin Invest 97(4): 1122–1128.

Martorell, A., B. De la Hoz, et al. (2011). Oral desensitization as a useful treatment in 2-year-old children with cow's milk allergy. Clin Exp Allergy 41(9): 1297–1304.

Maseda, D., S. H. Smith, et al. (2012). Regulatory B10 cells differentiate into antibody-secreting cells after transient IL-10 production in vivo. J Immunol 188(3): 1036–1048.

Mauri, C. and A. Bosma (2012). Immune regulatory function of B cells. Annu Rev Immunol 30: 221–241.

McSorley, H. J., N. F. Blair, et al. (2014). Blockade of IL-33 release and suppression of type 2 innate lymphoid cell responses by helminth secreted products in airway allergy. Mucosal Immunol 7(5): 1068–1078.

Medeiros, M., Jr., J. P. Figueiredo, et al. (2003). Schistosoma mansoni infection is associated with a reduced course of asthma. J Allergy Clin Immunol 111(5): 947–951.

Meglio, P., E. Bartone, et al. (2004). A protocol for oral desensitization in children with IgE-mediated cow's milk allergy. Allergy 59(9): 980–987.

Menzies-Gow, A., S. Ying, et al. (2004). Interactions between eotaxin, histamine and mast cells in early microvascular events associated with eosinophil recruitment to the site of allergic skin reactions in humans. *Clin Exp Allergy* 34(8): 1276–1282.

Menzies-Gow, A., S. Ying, et al. (2002). Eotaxin (CCL11) and eotaxin-2 (CCL24) induce recruitment of eosinophils, basophils, neutrophils, and macrophages as well as features of early- and late-phase allergic reactions following cutaneous injection in human atopic and nonatopic volunteers. *J Immunol* 169(5): 2712–2718.

Meulenbroek, L. A., B. C. van Esch, et al. (2013). Oral treatment with beta-lactoglobulin peptides prevents clinical symptoms in a mouse model for cow's milk allergy. *Pediatr Allergy Immunol* 24(7): 656–664.

Michaud, B., J. Aroulandom, et al. (2014). Casein-specific IL-4- and IL-13-secreting T cells: a tool to implement diagnosis of cow's milk allergy. *Allergy* 69(11): 1473–1480.

Mocsai, A. (2013). Diverse novel functions of neutrophils in immunity, inflammation, and beyond. *J Exp Med* 210(7): 1283–1299.

Moldaver, D. and M. Larche (2011). Immunotherapy with peptides. *Allergy* 66(6): 784–791.

Moro, K., T. Yamada, et al. (2010). Innate production of T(H)2 cytokines by adipose tissue-associated c-Kit(+)Sca-1(+) lymphoid cells. *Nature* 463(7280): 540–544.

Muraro, A., G. Roberts, et al. (2014). Anaphylaxis: guidelines from the European Academy of Allergy and Clinical Immunology. *Allergy* 69(8): 1026–1045.

Nakamura, T., Y. Kamogawa, et al. (1997). Polarization of IL-4- and IFN-gamma-producing CD4+ T cells following activation of naive CD4+ T cells. *J Immunol* 158(3): 1085–1094.

Narisety, S. D. and C. A. Keet (2012). Sublingual vs oral immunotherapy for food allergy: identifying the right approach. *Drugs* 72(15): 1977–1989.

Narisety, S. D., J. M. Skripak, et al. (2009). Open-label maintenance after milk oral immunotherapy for IgE-mediated cow's milk allergy. *J Allergy Clin Immunol* 124(3): 610–612.

Neill, D. R., S. H. Wong, et al. (2010). Nuocytes represent a new innate effector leukocyte that mediates type-2 immunity. *Nature* 464(7293): 1367–1370.

Nelson, H. S., J. Lahr, et al. (1997). Treatment of anaphylactic sensitivity to peanuts by immunotherapy with injections of aqueous peanut extract. *J Allergy Clin Immunol* 99(6 Pt 1): 744–751.

Noh, J., J. H. Lee, et al. (2010). Characterisation of allergen-specific responses of IL-10-producing regulatory B cells (Br1) in Cow Milk Allergy. *Cell Immunol* 264(2): 143–149.

O'Shea, J. J. and W. E. Paul (2010). Mechanisms underlying lineage commitment and plasticity of helper CD4+ T cells. *Science* 327(5969): 1098–1102.

Oba, Y. and G. A. Salzman (2004). Cost-effectiveness analysis of omalizumab in adults and adolescents with moderate-to-severe allergic asthma. *J Allergy Clin Immunol* 114(2): 265–269.

Omata, N., Y. Ohshima, et al. (2008). A case of milk-protein-induced enterocolitis associated with enterotoxigenic E. coli and MRSA infections. *Eur J Pediatr* 167(6): 683–684.

Oppenheimer, J. J., H. S. Nelson, et al. (1992). Treatment of peanut allergy with rush immunotherapy. *J Allergy Clin Immunol* 90(2): 256–262.

Orivuori, L., K. Mustonen, et al. (2014). Immunoglobulin A and immunoglobulin G antibodies against beta-lactoglobulin and gliadin at age 1 associate with immunoglobulin E sensitization at age 6. *Pediatr Allergy Immunol* 25(4): 329–337.

Osterlund, P. and H. Suomalainen (2002). Low frequency of CD4+, but not CD8+, T cells expressing interferon-gamma is related to cow's milk allergy in infancy. *Pediatr Allergy Immunol* 13(4): 262–268.

Oyoshi, M. K., R. He, et al. (2009). Cellular and molecular mechanisms in atopic dermatitis. *Adv Immunol* 102: 135–226.

Pajno, G. B., L. Caminiti, et al. (2010). Oral immunotherapy for cow's milk allergy with a weekly up-dosing regimen: a randomized single-blind controlled study. *Ann Allergy Asthma Immunol* 105(5): 376–381.

Palm, N. W., R. K. Rosenstein, et al. (2012). Allergic host defences. *Nature* 484(7395): 465–472.

Patriarca, G., E. Nucera, et al. (2003). Oral desensitizing treatment in food allergy: clinical and immunological results. *Aliment Pharmacol Ther* 17(3): 459–465.

Pecquet, S., L. Bovetto, et al. (2000). Peptides obtained by tryptic hydrolysis of bovine beta-lactoglobulin induce specific oral tolerance in mice. *J Allergy Clin Immunol* 105(3): 514–521.

Perez-Machado, M. A., P. Ashwood, et al. (2003). Reduced transforming growth factor-beta1-producing T cells in the duodenal mucosa of children with food allergy. *Eur J Immunol* 33(8): 2307–2315.

Powe, D. G., T. Groot Kormelink, et al. (2010). Evidence for the involvement of free light chain immunoglobulins in allergic and nonallergic rhinitis. *J Allergy Clin Immunol* 125(1): 139–145 e131–133.

Prescott, S. L. (2013). Early-life environmental determinants of allergic diseases and the wider pandemic of inflammatory noncommunicable diseases. *J Allergy Clin Immunol* 131(1): 23–30.

Prescott, S. L., R. Pawankar, et al. (2013). A global survey of changing patterns of food allergy burden in children. *World Allergy Organ J* 6(1): 21.

Price, A. E., H. E. Liang, et al. (2010). Systemically dispersed innate IL-13-expressing cells in type 2 immunity. *Proc Natl Acad Sci U S A* 107(25): 11489–11494.

Priceman, S. J., M. Kujawski, et al. (2013). Regulation of adipose tissue T cell subsets by Stat3 is crucial for diet-induced obesity and insulin resistance. *Proc Natl Acad Sci U S A* 110(32): 13079–13084.

Redegeld, F. A. and F. P. Nijkamp (2003). Immunoglobulin free light chains and mast cells: pivotal role in T-cell-mediated immune reactions? *Trends Immunol* 24(4): 181–185.

Redegeld, F. A., M. W. van der Heijden, et al. (2002). Immunoglobulin-free light chains elicit immediate hypersensitivity-like responses. *Nat Med* 8(7): 694–701.

Rosser, E. C. and C. Mauri (2015). Regulatory B Cells: Origin, Phenotype, and Function. *Immunity* 42(4): 607–612.

Ruiter, B., E. F. Knol, et al. (2007). Maintenance of tolerance to cow's milk in atopic individuals is characterized by high levels of specific immunoglobulin G4. *Clin Exp Allergy* 37(7): 1103–1110.

Saarinen, K. M., A. S. Pelkonen, et al. (2005). Clinical course and prognosis of cow's milk allergy are dependent on milk-specific IgE status. *J Allergy Clin Immunol* 116(4): 869–875.

Saenz, S. A., M. C. Siracusa, et al. (2010). IL25 elicits a multipotent progenitor cell population that promotes T(H)2 cytokine responses. *Nature* 464(7293): 1362–1366.

Salazar, F. and A. M. Ghaemmaghami (2013). Allergen Recognition by Innate Immune Cells: Critical Role of Dendritic and Epithelial Cells. *Front Immunol* 4: 356.

Salimi, M., J. L. Barlow, et al. (2013). A role for IL-25 and IL-33-driven type-2 innate lymphoid cells in atopic dermatitis. *J Exp Med* 210(13): 2939–2950.

Salmivesi, S., M. Korppi, et al. (2013). Milk oral immunotherapy is effective in school-aged children. Acta Paediatr 102(2): 172–176.

Sampaio, G., S. Marinho, et al. (2005). Transient vs persistent cow's milk allergy and development of other allergic diseases. Allergy 60(3): 411–412.

Savilahti, E. M., M. Kuitunen, et al. (2014). Specific antibodies in oral immunotherapy for cow's milk allergy: kinetics and prediction of clinical outcome. Int Arch Allergy Immunol 164(1): 32–39.

Savilahti, E. M., M. Kuitunen, et al. (2014). Use of IgE and IgG4 epitope binding to predict the outcome of oral immunotherapy in cow's milk allergy. Pediatr Allergy Immunol 25(3): 227–235.

Savilahti, E. M., K. M. Saarinen, et al. (2010). Duration of clinical reactivity in cow's milk allergy is associated with levels of specific immunoglobulin G4 and immunoglobulin A antibodies to beta-lactoglobulin. Clin Exp Allergy 40(2): 251–256.

Savilahti, E. M. and E. Savilahti (2013). Development of natural tolerance and induced desensitization in cow's milk allergy. Pediatr Allergy Immunol 24(2): 114–121.

Schade, R. P., M. M. Tiemessen, et al. (2003). The cow's milk protein-specific T cell response in infancy and childhood. Clin Exp Allergy 33(6): 725–730.

Schade, R. P., A. G. Van Ieperen-Van Dijk, et al. (2000). Differences in antigen-specific T-cell responses between infants with atopic dermatitis with and without cow's milk allergy: relevance of TH2 cytokines. J Allergy Clin Immunol 106(6): 1155–1162.

Schoemaker, A. A., A. B. Sprikkelman, et al. (2015). Incidence and natural history of challenge-proven cow's milk allergy in European children — EuroPrevall birth cohort. Allergy.

Schouten, B., B. C. van Esch, et al. (2012). A potential role for CD25+ regulatory T-cells in the protection against casein allergy by dietary non-digestible carbohydrates. Br J Nutr 107(1): 96–105.

Schouten, B., B. C. van Esch, et al. (2008). Acute allergic skin reactions and intestinal contractility changes in mice orally sensitized against casein or whey. Int Arch Allergy Immunol 147(2): 125–134.

Schouten, B., B. C. van Esch, et al. (2009). Cow milk allergy symptoms are reduced in mice fed dietary synbiotics during oral sensitization with whey. J Nutr 139(7): 1398–1403.

Schouten, B., B. C. Van Esch, et al. (2011). Non-digestible oligosaccharides reduce immunoglobulin free light-chain concentrations in infants at risk for allergy. Pediatr Allergy Immunol 22(5): 537–542.

Schouten, B., B. C. van Esch, et al. (2012). Invariant natural killer T cells contribute to the allergic response in cow's milk protein-sensitized mice. Int Arch Allergy Immunol 159(1): 51–59.

Schouten, B., B. C. van Esch, et al. (2010). Contribution of IgE and immunoglobulin free light chain in the allergic reaction to cow's milk proteins. J Allergy Clin Immunol 125(6): 1308–1314.

Schwartz, R. H. (2003). T cell anergy. Annu Rev Immunol 21: 305–334.

Scott-Taylor, T. H., O. B. H. J, et al. (2010). Correlation of allergen-specific IgG subclass antibodies and T lymphocyte cytokine responses in children with multiple food allergies. Pediatr Allergy Immunol 21(6): 935–944.

Semeniuk, J., M. Kaczmarski, et al. (2009). Histological evaluation of esophageal mucosa in children with acid gastroesophageal reflux. Folia Histochem Cytobiol 47(2): 297–306.

Senti, G., S. von Moos, et al. (2014). Epicutaneous Immunotherapy for Aeroallergen and Food Allergy. Curr Treat Options Allergy 1: 68–78.

Shreffler, W. G., N. Wanich, et al. (2009). Association of allergen-specific regulatory T cells with the onset *of clinical tolerance to milk protein. J Allergy Clin Immunol 123(1): 43–52 e47.*

Silbart, L. K. and D. F. Keren (1989). *Reduction of intestinal carcinogen absorption by carcinogen-specific secretory immunity. Science 243(4897): 1462–1464.*

Skripak, J. M., S. D. Nash, et al. (2008). *A randomized, double-blind, placebo-controlled study of milk oral immunotherapy for cow's milk allergy. J Allergy Clin Immunol 122(6): 1154–1160.*

Smit, J. J., M. Bol-Schoenmakers, et al. (2011). *The role of intestinal dendritic cells subsets in the establishment of food allergy. Clin Exp Allergy 41(6): 890–898.*

Sprikkelman, A. B., H. S. Heymans, et al. (2000). *Development of allergic disorders in children with cow's milk protein allergy or intolerance in infancy. Clin Exp Allergy 30(10): 1358–1363.*

Staden, U., C. Rolinck-Werninghaus, et al. (2007). *Specific oral tolerance induction in food allergy in children: efficacy and clinical patterns of reaction. Allergy 62(11): 1261–1269.*

Steinman, R. M., D. Hawiger, et al. (2003). *Tolerogenic dendritic cells. Annu Rev Immunol 21: 685–711.*

Sun, J. B., C. F. Flach, et al. (2008). *B lymphocytes promote expansion of regulatory T cells in oral tolerance: powerful induction by antigen coupled to cholera toxin B subunit. J Immunol 181(12): 8278–8287.*

Tadmor, T., Y. Zhang, et al. (2011). *The absence of B lymphocytes reduces the number and function of T-regulatory cells and enhances the anti-tumor response in a murine tumor model. Cancer Immunol Immunother 60(5): 609–619.*

Takanaski, S., R. Nonaka, et al. (1994). *Interleukin 10 inhibits lipopolysaccharide-induced survival and cytokine production by human peripheral blood eosinophils. J Exp Med 180(2): 711–715.*

Takatsu, K. and H. Nakajima (2008). *IL-5 and eosinophilia. Curr Opin Immunol 20(3): 288–294.*

Tang, X. Z., J. Jo, et al. (2013). *IL-7 licenses activation of human liver intrasinusoidal mucosal-associated invariant T cells. J Immunol 190(7): 3142–3152.*

Tao, M. H., R. I. Smith, et al. (1993). *Structural features of human immunoglobulin G that determine isotype-specific differences in complement activation. J Exp Med 178(2): 661–667.*

Tedder, T. F. (2015). *B10 cells: a functionally defined regulatory B cell subset. J Immunol 194(4): 1395–1401.*

Tiemessen, M. M., A. G. Van Ieperen-Van Dijk, et al. (2004). *Cow's milk-specific T-cell reactivity of children with and without persistent cow's milk allergy: key role for IL-10. J Allergy Clin Immunol 113(5): 932–939.*

Torgerson, T. R., A. Linane, et al. (2007). *Severe food allergy as a variant of IPEX syndrome caused by a deletion in a noncoding region of the FOXP3 gene. Gastroenterology 132(5): 1705–1717.*

Treiner, E. and O. Lantz (2006). *CD1d- and MR1-restricted invariant T cells: of mice and men. Curr Opin Immunol 18(5): 519–526.*

Turunen, S., T. J. Karttunen, et al. (2004). *Lymphoid nodular hyperplasia and cow's milk hypersensitivity in children with chronic constipation. J Pediatr 145(5): 606–611.*

van den Biggelaar, A. H., R. van Ree, et al. (2000). *Decreased atopy in children infected with Schistosoma haematobium: a role for parasite-induced interleukin-10. Lancet 356(9243): 1723–1727.*

van den Elsen, L. W., L. A. Meulenbroek, et al. (2013). *CD25+ regulatory T cells transfer n-3 long chain polyunsaturated fatty acids-induced tolerance in mice allergic to cow's milk protein. Allergy 68(12): 1562–1570.*

van den Elsen, L. W., B. C. van Esch, et al. (2013). *Dietary long chain n-3 polyunsaturated fatty acids prevent allergic sensitization to cow's milk protein in mice. Clin Exp Allergy 43(7): 798–810.*

van den Hoogen, S. C., A. C. van de Pol, et al. (2014). Suspected cow's milk allergy in everyday general practice: a retrospective cohort study on health care burden and guideline adherence. BMC Res Notes 7: 507.

van der Neut Kolfschoten, M., J. Schuurman, et al. (2007). Anti-inflammatory activity of human IgG4 antibodies by dynamic Fab arm exchange. Science 317(5844): 1554–1557.

van Esch, B. C., B. Schouten, et al. (2010). Depletion of CD4+CD25+ T cells switches the whey-allergic response from immunoglobulin E- to immunoglobulin free light chain-dependent. Clin Exp Allergy 40(9): 1414–1421.

van Houwelingen, A. H., K. Kaczynska, et al. (2007). Topical application of F991, an immunoglobulin free light chain antagonist, prevents development of contact sensitivity in mice. Clin Exp Allergy 37(2): 270–275.

Vanto, T., S. Helppila, et al. (2004). Prediction of the development of tolerance to milk in children with cow's milk hypersensitivity. J Pediatr 144(2): 218–222.

Verhoef, A., C. Alexander, et al. (2005). T cell epitope immunotherapy induces a CD4+ T cell population with regulatory activity. PLoS Med 2(3): e78.

Vignali, D. A., L. W. Collison, et al. (2008). How regulatory T cells work. Nat Rev Immunol 8(7): 523–532.

Visness, C. M., S. J. London, et al. (2009). Association of obesity with IgE levels and allergy symptoms in children and adolescents: results from the National Health and Nutrition Examination Survey 2005–2006. J Allergy Clin Immunol 123(5): 1163–1169, 1169 e1161–1164.

Vocca, I., R. B. Canani, et al. (2011). Peripheral blood immune response elicited by beta-lactoglobulin in childhood cow's milk allergy. Pediatr Res 70(6): 549–554.

Wang, Y. H., K. S. Voo, et al. (2010). A novel subset of CD4(+) T(H)2 memory/effector cells that produce inflammatory IL-17 cytokine and promote the exacerbation of chronic allergic asthma. J Exp Med 207(11): 2479–2491.

Wanich, N., A. Nowak-Wegrzyn, et al. (2009). Allergen-specific basophil suppression associated with clinical tolerance in patients with milk allergy. J Allergy Clin Immunol 123(4): 789–794 e720.

Westerholm-Ormio, M., O. Vaarala, et al. (2010). Infiltration of Foxp3- and Toll-like receptor-4-positive cells in the intestines of children with food allergy. J Pediatr Gastroenterol Nutr 50(4): 367–376.

Williams, J. W., M. Y. Tjota, et al. (2012). The contribution of allergen-specific IgG to the development of th2-mediated airway inflammation. J Allergy (Cairo) 2012: 236075.

Wu, L. C. and A. A. Zarrin (2014). The production and regulation of IgE by the immune system. Nat Rev Immunol 14(4): 247–259.

Xiong, H., J. Dolpady, et al. (2012). Sequential class switching is required for the generation of high affinity IgE antibodies. J Exp Med 209(2): 353–364.

Zaiss, M. M., K. M. Maslowski, et al. (2013). IL-1beta suppresses innate IL-25 and IL-33 production and maintains helminth chronicity. PLoS Pathog 9(8): e1003531.

Zhu, J., H. Yamane, et al. (2010). Differentiation of effector CD4 T cell populations (*). Annu Rev Immunol 28: 445–489.

Chapter 5

Immune Mechanisms in Non-alcoholic Steatohepatitis (NASH)

Akinobu Takaki[1], Nozomu Wada[1], Kazuhide Yamamoto[1]

1 Introduction

Non-alcoholic fatty liver had been believed to be a non-progressive benign disease. However, Ludwig *et al.* described some patients who exhibited progressive steatohepatitis without habitual alcohol drinking (Ludwig *et al.*, 1980) and referred to this disease as non-alcoholic steatohepatitis (NASH). Later, NASH and non-progressive simple steatosis patients were included in the single disease entity of non-alcoholic fatty liver disease (NAFLD). Recently, non-progressive simple fatty liver has been renamed as non-alcoholic fatty liver (NAFL). The differential diagnosis of NAFL and NASH requires liver biopsy interpretation, and it is often difficult to clearly distinguish these two disease. NASH is regarded as a more severe form of NAFLD and is broadly defined by the presence of steatosis with inflammation and progressive fibrosis (Matteoni *et al.*, 1999; Brunt *et al.*, 2009), ultimately leading to cirrhosis and hepatocellular carcinoma (HCC) (Yatsuji *et al.*, 2009; Hatanaka *et al.*, 2007; Fassio *et al.*, 2004; Ono & Saibara, 2006). The mechanisms through which the subset of NAFLD patients develops NASH are poorly understood.

The development of NASH is generally thought of as a "two hit" process (Day & James, 1998). The first hit is the development of hepatic steatosis due to overeating, lack of exercise, or drug use. The second hit includes hepatic damage inducing cellular stresses such as oxidative stress, apoptosis, and gut-derived signals such as lipopolysaccharide (LPS). However, recently uncovered liver fat deposition and pro-inflammatory

---

[1] Department of Gastroenterology and Hepatology, Okayama University Graduate School of Medicine, Dentistry, and Pharmaceutical Sciences, Japan

mechanisms have revealed that inflammation could actually precede steatosis and might contribute to steatosis development. In experimental models, inflammatory macrophages could infiltrate before lipid deposition, and antioxidant treatment reversed inflammatory gene expression before the aberrant lipid metabolism related genes expression reversed (Shiri-Sverdlov *et al.*, 2006). These results have encouraged us to define NASH pathogenesis as a "multiple parallel hits" process (Tilg & Moschen, 2010).

As one of the multiple hits, gut microbiota changes or disease susceptible genetic polymorpohisms genotype could be included. A Western-style diet including high-fat and high-fructose characteristics can induce gut microbiota changes following inflammatory responses in the liver even without fat deposition. Patatin-like phospholipase 3 (PNPLA3) is a NASH susceptibility gene that is involved in hepatic fat metabolism. Although NAFL is usually non-progressive, patients harboring the risk allele (G-allele) of PNPLA3 are at increased risk for NASH progression (Romeo *et al.*, 2008). Such dietary and genetic characteristics can precede the first hit of fat deposition. These components could be involved in the multiple parallel hits process. It is often difficult to distinguish the first and second hits. The multiple parallel hits theory has recently become widely accepted.

Many sources of cellular stress, including oxidative stress, apoptosis, and gut-derived LPS, trigger an inflammatory response and progressive liver damage (Csak *et al.*, 2011). Oxidative stress is increased through the generation of reactive oxygen species (ROS), as well as by defects in redox defense mechanisms involving glutathione, catalase, or superoxide dismutase (Muriel, 2009). Mitochondria are the most important and abundant source of intracellular ROS. Therefore, mitochondrial dysfunction plays a central role in the pathological mechanisms of chronic inflammation and subsequent carcinogenesis in NASH. Although the mechanisms of mitochondrial dysfunction are not clearly understood, emerging data suggest that ROS, lipid peroxidation products, and tumor necrosis factor-α (TNF-α) are involved in the multiple hits, inducing the progression from simple steatosis to NASH (Takaki *et al.*, 2014). ROS can educate adaptive inflammatory cells and induce directional migration of resident hepatic pro-fibrogenic cells, resulting in liver inflammation and fibrosis (Novo *et al.*, 2011; Sutti *et al.*, 2014).

Immune responses and inflammation are involved in metabolic diseases, such as diabetes mellitus, atherosclerosis, and NASH. Adipose tissue–derived cytokines promote metabolic disease progression. In obesity, excessive numbers of proinflammatory, M1-like macrophages accumulate in adipose tissue and the liver (Lanthier *et al.*, 2010). Even in simple fatty liver, macrophage infiltration and the expression of the macrophage attractant chemokine monocyte chemotactic protein 1 (MCP1) are significantly increased (Gadd *et al.*, 2013). Macrophages are an important mediator of inflammation and insulin resistance, which are the common phenomena of NAFLD. In advanced NASH, CD4 (+) and CD8 (+) T-cell infiltration increases, and the levels of inflammatory cytokines, such as IL-6 or IL-8, are also increased (Gadd *et al.*, 2013).

Several studies have suggested that antioxidants such as vitamin E and 1-aminobenzotriazole confer benefits upon NAFLD patients, and the American Association for the Study of Liver Disease recommends the use of high-dose vitamin E for NASH (Chalasani *et al.*, 2012). However, most clinical studies involving the treatment of atherosclerotic diseases with dietary antioxidants have not generated clear results, partly because of the non-selective effects of these anti-oxidative drugs and difficulties associated with cytosolic distribution (Steinhubl, 2008). The clinical findings of antioxidant therapies have not always been favorable and are often associated with worsening pathology (Hackam, 2007). Thus, new treatment strategies are needed.

Here, we review the importance of immune reactions in the current understanding of NAFLD molecular pathogenesis and potential immune-related treatments to be considered in future therapeutic paradigms.

2   NASH Pathogenesis: General Characteristics

The pathogenesis of NASH is unclear. The multiple hits involved in NASH development include hepatic steatosis, gut-derived endotoxins, oxidative stress, or proinflammatory cytokines (Day & James, 1998) (Tilg & Moschen, 2010) (Tiniakos et al., 2010). The following factors are related to NASH progression.

2.1   PNPLA3 Genetic Background

PNPLA3 gene polymorphism is a susceptible genetic factor in NAFLD (Romeo et al., 2008). This genetic polymorphism differentiates between simple steatosis with or without minimal inflammation and fibrosis that progresses to NASH (Valenti et al., 2010; Kawaguchi et al., 2012). Patients with the NASH-sensitive single nucleotide polymorphism rs738409 G/G genotype might progress not only to simple steatosis but also to NASH, probably under the same types of metabolic stimulation. The function of PNPLA3 is not well known, since mice deficient in PNPLA3 develop neither fatty liver nor liver injury. However, the overexpression of sterol-regulated binding protein 1c (SREBP-1c) results in its binding to the transcription start site of the mouse PNPLA3 gene, while PNPLA3 knockdown can decrease the intracellular triglyceride content in primary hepatocytes (Qiao et al., 2011). Thus, PNPLA3 might function as a downstream target gene of SREBP-1c to mediate SREBP-1c stimulation of lipid accumulation. A meta-analysis revealed that this variant is associated with increased liver fat content when compared to weight-matched individuals not harboring the PNPLA2 polymorphism as well as increased risk of severe fibrosis, even in the presence of other etiologies of chronic liver diseases (Singal et al., 2014).

Not all patients with progressive NASH harbor the PNPLA3 risk allele; thus, differences in the characteristics of PNPLA3 risk allele–bearing and –nonbearing NAFLD patients have been demonstrated (Lallukka et al., 2013). PNPLA3-related NAFLD is not characterized by features typical of metabolic syndrome such as hyperinsulinemia, hypertriglyceridemia, and low HDL-cholesterol levels (Sookoian & Pirola, 2011). Obesity-related NAFLD patients exhibit the same distribution of the PNPLA3 genotype as non-obese patients, whereas inflammation-related genes are upregulated in adipose tissue.

2.2   Visceral Obesity and Adipokines

Obesity is a growing global epidemic among adults and children and is associated with many diseases such as hypertension, diabetes mellitus, hyperlipidemia, and NAFLD. Furthermore, obesity, hypertriglyceridemia, and hypertension are predictive risk factors for NAFLD (Tsuneto et al., 2010). Visceral fat accumulation in obesity correlates with various organ pathologies including cerebrovascular diseases, cancer, and NASH. Moreover, visceral fat accumulation is regarded as a significant risk factor for the development of NAFLD and NASH. A study from Japan found that the severity of hepatic steatosis, determined by ultrasound, was positively correlated with visceral fat accumulation and insulin resistance in both obese and non-obese individuals, suggesting that hepatic steatosis is influenced by visceral fat accumulation regardless of obesity (Eguchi et al., 2006).

Adipokines are multifunctional secreted factors that are primarily derived from adipose tissue. Adiponectin is the most abundant adipose tissue–specific adipokine. Mature adipocytes mainly produce adiponectin in white adipose tissue, and expression and secretion levels increase during adipocyte differentiation. Adiponectin levels are inversely correlated with visceral obesity, and insulin resistance and weight loss induce adiponectin synthesis. Proinflammatory adipokines such as TNF-a or IL-6 suppress adiponectin, which has anti-inflammatory, anti-atherogenic, and anti-diabetic properties (Polyzos et al., 2011). Adipose tissue is also the main producer of the adipokine leptin, and its levels directly correlate with body fat mass and adipocyte size (Carbone et al., 2012). Leptin production is mainly regulated by food intake, and hormones related to eating such as insulin increase leptin secretion and vice versa. Proinflammatory endotoxins, IL-1, and TNF-α increase the secretion of leptin, which has central and peripheral effects (Sarraf et al., 1997). Leptin acts on hypothalamic cells, inhibits anabolic pathways, activates catabolic pathways, inhibits appetite, and stimulates energy expenditure. Leptin-deficient (ob/ob) mice and leptin receptor–deficient (db/db) mice are severely obese and have increased pituitary and adrenal hormone production, hyperglycemia, elevated insulin, and decreased immune function (Cohen et al., 2001; Lindstrom, 2007).

Contrary to expectations, several groups have made the controversial observation that serum adiponectin levels are lower in NAFLD than in NASH, or are the same (Shimada et al., 2007; Younossi et al., 2008; Argentou et al., 2009; Lemoine et al., 2009). A meta-analysis of 27 studies of 698 controls and 1545 patients with NAFLD found that serum adiponectin levels were low in NAFLD and much lower in NASH (Polyzos et al., 2011). Since adiponectin and leptin exert antagonistic effects on liver fibrogenesis and inflammation, the ratio of adiponectin to leptin might be a better marker with which to distinguish NASH from NAFLD. Levels of adiponectin receptor II are decreased in human liver biopsy specimens and in mouse models of NASH (Kaser et al., 2005; Matsunami et al., 2011). However, since contradictory results have suggested that lower serum adiponectin levels induce high expression of hepatic adiponectin receptor II as a compensatory response, the function of these novel adipokines and receptors requires further investigation (Nannipieri et al., 2009; Ma et al., 2009).

2.3   Hepatic Steatosis and Oxidative Stress

Fatty liver is the basic feature of NAFLD and NASH. Lipid droplets are now considered as complicated organelles that exhibit many functions such as metabolic, inflammatory, and immunological responses. Lipid toxicity induces multiple effects such as oxidative stress, ER stress, and immune reactions (Takaki et al., 2014). Triglycerides are the main type of lipid stored in the liver of patients with NAFLD. The toxic lipids present in NASH and the non-toxic lipids in simple steatosis could differ (Yamaguchi et al., 2007). Diacylglycerol acyltransferase 2 (DGAT2) catalyzes the final step in hepatocyte triglyceride biosynthesis. Hepatic steatosis and the dietary triglyceride contents induced in a model of obese-simple fatty liver are reduced by DGAT2 antisense oligonucleotides in a manner that does not correlate with changes in body weight, adiposity, or insulin sensitivity (Yu et al., 2005). However, DGAT2 antisense oligonucleotide increased levels of hepatic free fatty acids, lipid oxidant stress, lobular necroinflammation, and fibrosis in mice fed a methionine choline-deficient (MCD) diet that generates inflammation and fibrosis with hepatic steatosis, whereas the hepatic triglyceride content decreased (Yamaguchi et al., 2007).

These results suggest that the pathogenesis and treatment of steatosis in simple fatty liver and in NASH are different. Human genetic variability analysis of lifestyle intervention has shown that the DGAT2 gene polymorphism is related to a decrease in liver fat, while changes in insulin resistance are not correlated (Kantartzis et al., 2009). Since insulin resistance is the key marker for NASH, DGAT2 gene polymorphism might only be associated with non-progressive fatty liver.

Excessive oxidative stress induced by mitochondrial, peroxisomal, and microsomal ROS in NASH results in apoptosis as well as nuclear and mitochondrial DNA damage. Limited antioxidant defenses contribute to the processes of both NASH and hepatocarcinogenesis (Kawai et al., 2012; Bugianesi, 2007). Physiologically low levels of ROS are involved in vital cellular processes, indicating that the balance of oxidative and antioxidative responses is important (Mittler et al., 2011). As mitochondria uptakes long chain fatty acid and provide to β-oxidation pathway and redox pathway finally produces detoxified water and ROS, its dysfunction leads to oxidative stress. Indeed, ultrastructural alterations, impaired ATP synthesis, and increased ROS production have been reported in liver mitochondria from NASH patients as well as in a rodent NASH model (Cortez-Pinto et al., 1999; Serviddio et al., 2008). Excess superoxide is generated within injured mitochondria through electron leakage and the resulting excess of superoxide would be converted to hydrogen peroxide (H_2O_2) by superoxide dismutase. Glutathione peroxidase or catalase can metabolize H_2O_2 to non-toxic H_2O; however, the Fenton and/or Haber-Weiss reactions generate the highly reactive and toxic hydroxyl radical.

Iron is the key mineral that induces oxidative stress produced via the Fenton reaction. Although its role in NASH is not fully understood, iron levels are elevated in NASH, which is an inducer of oxidative stress, and lowering iron levels has resulted in fair outcomes for patients with chronic liver diseases (Nelson et al., 2011). However, one-third of early stage NAFLD patients show iron deficiency correlated with the female sex, obesity, and type 2 diabetes (Siddique et al., 2013). We must wait for long-term, follow-up studies to confirm whether iron-deficient obese patients progress to NASH, as well as the role of iron in NAFLD progression.

Autophagy is a catabolic process that degrades old proteins and cellular organelles such as mitochondria and endoplasmic reticulum (ER). Autophagy deficiency enhances ER stress and ROS production from abnormal mitochondria (Yang *et al.*, 2010). Hepatic steatosis results in markedly decreased hepatic autophagy in chronic obesity mouse models via suppression of autophagy-related Atg7 expression or impairment of autophagosomal acidification and cathepsin expression (Singh *et al.*, 2009; Inami *et al.*, 2011). In human NAFLD liver, hepatic cathepsin expression was decreased and associated with the autophagic dysfunction–related protein P62 (Fukuo *et al.*, 2014).

2.4   Insulin Resistance

Insulin resistance is a state of relative insulin insufficiency due to reduced tissue insulin responsiveness. Under normal physiological conditions, insulin secretion from pancreatic b cells is stimulated by postprandial increases in blood glucose, and insulin circulation generally normalizes blood glucose levels. Insulin stimulates glucose uptake by skeletal muscle and adipose tissue. Insulin also stimulates the liver to convert excess glucose into glycogen and triglyceride for storage. Insulin binds the insulin receptor and stimulates receptor autophosphorylation and internalization, which in turn recruits and activates insulin receptor substrate proteins 1 and 2 (IRS1/2). IRS1/2 can activate phosphatidylinositol 3-kinase, which converts PI bisphosphonate (PIP2) to PIP3. Cell proliferation transcription factor Akt binds PIP3 and is subsequently phosphorylated and activated. In muscle and adipose tissue, Akt stimulates the translocation of glucose transporters to the membrane to allow glucose uptake. In the liver, insulin binding promotes fatty acid synthesis through activation of SREBP 1. Akt kinase pathways have roles in cell growth, cell proliferation, fibrogenesis, and hepatocarcinogenesis (Larter *et al.*, 2010). The gold standard methods to detect insulin resistance are the complexed clamp technique requiring the frequent sampling of intravenous glucose; however, simpler methods, such as the oral glucose tolerance test or homeostatic model assessment, are generally used.

Insulin resistance is concordant with NASH (Larter & Farrell, 2006). In the obese insulin-resistant model *ob/ob* mouse, liver insulin receptor knockout improved hepatic lipogenesis (Haas *et al.*, 2012). This result indicates that insulin receptor signaling is required for hepatic steatosis. Insulin resistance could be induced by Kupffer cells, as depletion of Kupffer cells could attenuate systemic insulin resistance and improve liver autophagy in high-fat diet–fed mice (Zeng *et al.*, 2015).

The NAFIC score is a NASH diagnostic screening tool developed for Japanese NASH patients; its criteria include high levels of ferritin, fasting insulin, and type IV collagen 7S (Sumida *et al.*, 2011). As the fasting serum insulin level was significantly correlated with NASH prevalence, a modified NAFIC score with serum fasting insulin level stepwise refinement was more effective to diagnose NASH (Nakamura *et al.*, 2013).

Insulin resistance is one of the most important factors that characterizes NASH and could be a treatment target.

2.5   Gut Microbiota Change and Toll-Like Receptor (TLR) Signaling in Liver Pathogenesis

Gut microbiota has been accepted as a key factor in several diseases. As healthy stool transplantation was proven to show surprising beneficial effects on *Clostridium difficile* enterocolitis, the clinical impact of gut microbiota on many diseases has been analyzed. NAFLD and hepatocellular carcinoma are obviously included in the relation. Endotoxin or LPS produced by gut microbiota could be delivered to the liver via the portal vein, which raises the question of why such toxic materials are capable of flowing into the portal vein through the intestinal barrier. Patients with biopsy-confirmed NAFLD have increased intestinal permeability with disrupted intercellular tight junctions in the intestine (Miele *et al.*, 2009). These abnormalities are related to increased bacterial overgrowth in the small intestine. Murine NAFLD models of bacterial overgrowth develop compositional changes and increased intestinal permeability with a concurrent reduction in the expression of tight junction proteins (Brun *et al.*, 2007). Plasma endotoxin levels are significantly higher in patients with NAFLD and in murine NASH models (Miele *et al.*, 2009; Cani *et al.*, 2008). A high-fat diet could increase LPS concentrations two- to three-fold (Cani *et al.*, 2007). Proinflammatory inflammasomes induce inflammation in the liver of patients with NAFLD, but an inflammasome-deficient mouse model develops exacerbated hepatic steatosis and inflammation through the influx of TLR4 and TLR9 agonists into the portal vein (Henao-Mejia *et al.*, 2012). The microbiota of these inflammasome-deficient mice differed from the microbiota of wild-type mice with NASH. Furthermore, co-housing inflammasome-deficient and wild-type mice resulted in intestinal inflammation and exacerbated hepatic steatosis in the wild-type mice (Henao-Mejia *et al.*, 2012). This finding suggested that altered microbiota in inflammasome-deficient mice could be transferred to healthy mice, resulting in intestinal inflammation, increased permeability, and NAFLD.

The mechanisms by which commensal gut microbiota trigger hepatic steatohepatitis remain to be investigated. The gut microbiota release pathogen- or damage-associated molecular patterns (PAMPs or DAMPs), which are TLR ligands. TLR2, TLR4, and TLR9 have been intensively investigated and found to be involved in the pathogenesis of NASH (Takaki *et al.*, 2014). TLR2 is a receptor for multiple glycolipids or lipoproteins in bacteria adhering to the cell surface of monocytes, myeloid dendritic cells or mast cells. TLR4 is an LPS receptor located on the surfaces of monocytes, myeloid dendritic cells, mast cells, β cells, and the intestinal epithelium. Toll-like receptor 9 is located on the ER or endosomes of plasmacytoid dendritic cells or β cells, and is regarded as a receptor for unmethylated CpG DNA particles that might be released from bacteria. These molecules have been analyzed in several NAFLD and NASH models. The results of TLR studies in different NASH models notably vary. For example, the choline-deficient amino acid-deficient diet model mouse develops steatosis with relatively mild hepatitis or fibrosis with obesity, whereas the methionine-choline-deficient (MCD) diet model mouse develops steatosis with severe hepatitis and fibrosis without obesity. In the TLR2 knockout mouse model, the choline-deficient amino acid-deficient diet induced mild NASH course improved, while the MCD diet induced severe NASH course worsened (Miura *et al.*, 2013; Rivera *et al.*, 2010). As NAFLD includes heterogenous backgrounds and clinical courses, the pathogenesis should be variable. TLR4 and TLR9 agonists might flow into the portal veins of inflammasome-deficient MCD diet mouse models and thus exacerbate NASH (Henao-Mejia *et al.*, 2012). Inflammasomes are multi-protein complexes composed of nucleotide-binding domain and leucine-rich repeat protein 3, apoptosis-associated speck-like protein containing CARD and procaspase 1, which are DAMP or PAMP sensors. Inflammasome activation leads to the processing and secretion of the proinflammatory cytokines IL1β and IL-18, whereas knockdown results in MCD NASH exacerbation (Henao-Mejia *et al.*, 2012). These perplexing findings indicate that the intestinal DAMP or PAMP barrier function that is disrupted in inflammasome knockout mice overcomes the anti-inflammatory effect in the liver and TLR4 and TLR9 ligand outflow into the portal vein where they stimulate NASH progression.

The gut and oral periodontal status correlates with the progression of liver disease (Tamaki *et al.*, 2011). Levels of the periodontopathic bacteria *Porphyromonas gingivalis* (P. gingivalis) are markedly higher in NASH patients than in NAFL patients and healthy subjects (Yoneda *et al.*, 2012). *In vivo* infection of *P. gingivalis* in the high-fat diet–induced mouse NAFLD model resulted in fibrosis with proliferation of hepatic stellate cells (HSC) and collagen formation (Furusho *et al.*, 2013). Treating periodontitis could improve transaminases in NAFLD and, in fact, several probiotics that control gut microbiota improve NAFLD (Yoneda *et al.*, 2012) (Endo *et al.*, 2013; Xu *et al.*, 2012). Studies using models of hepatocarcinogenesis have found that a high-fat diet increases levels of deoxycholic acid, a gut bacterial metabolite that damages DNA and exacerbates hepatocarcinogenesis (Yoshimoto *et al.*, 2013). Antibiotics could abrogate these effects. Gut microbiota affect not only NAFLD, but also obesity-related hepatocarcinogenesis.

3   NASH Pathogenesis: Multiple Hits and Correlation to Immune Responses

Since the significance of apparently similar fat droplets in simple fatty liver and NASH hepatocytes differs in DGAT2 knockdown experiments, analyzing the molecular pathogenesis of NASH at the cellular level is important. Hepatic inflammation and fibrosis, which are the characteristic features of NASH, involve immune reactions induced by cytokines, chemokines, adipokines, and inflammatory cell infiltrations (Figure 1).

Immune responses and inflammation are involved not only in NASH but also in most metabolic diseases, such as diabetes mellitus and atherosclerosis. Adipose tissue–derived cytokines promote metabolic disease progression. In obesity, excessive numbers of proinflammatory, M1-like macrophages accumulate in adipose tissue and the liver (Lanthier *et al.*, 2010). Even in simple fatty liver, macrophage infiltration and macrophage attractant chemokine MCP-1 expression are significantly increased (Gadd *et al.*, 2013). Macrophages are an important mediator of inflammation and insulin resistance, which are common phenomena in NAFLD. In advanced NASH, CD4 (+) and CD8 (+) T-cell infiltration increases, and the levels of inflammatory cytokines, such as IL-6 or IL-8,

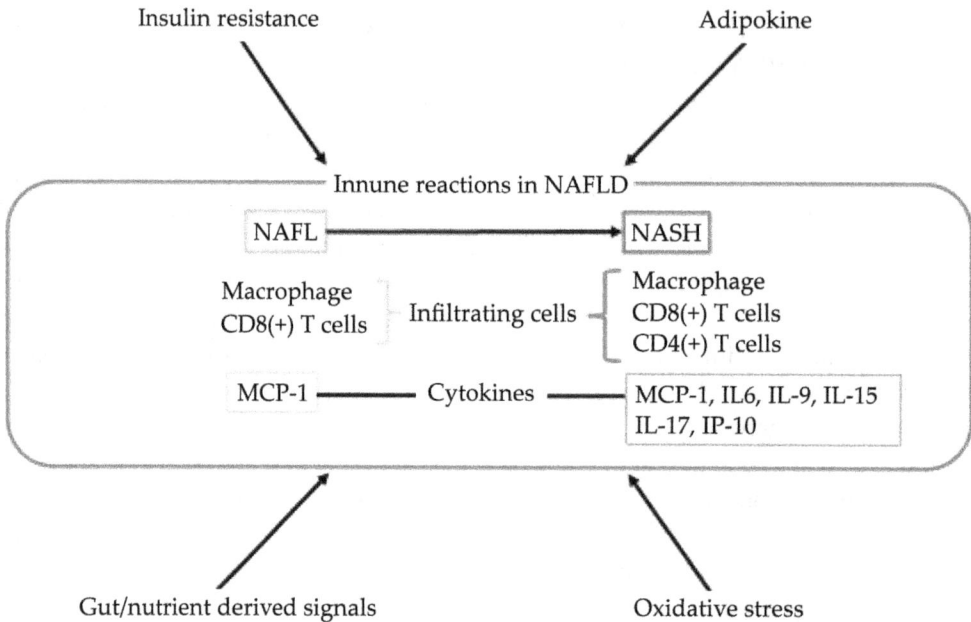

Figure 1: Immune activation in NAFL and NASH

are also increased (Gadd *et al.*, 2013).

3.1   Local Inflammatory Cell Infiltration and Cytokine Milieu

Even in NAFL, several inflammatory cytokines are elevated, evidenced by a report showing that IL-6 or IL-8 mRNA expression in liver biopsy specimens did not significantly differ between NAFL and NASH (Gadd *et al.*, 2013). Inflammation occurs even in NAFL, but some factors exacerbate the inflammation and induce liver fibrosis as well. Fat-induced insulin resistance results in activation of serine kinases such as Jun-N-terminal kinase (JNK), inhibitor of nuclear factor kB (NF-kB) kinase (IKK), and novel isoforms of protein kinase C (Maher *et al.*, 2008). JNK and IKK induce proinflammatory signaling. Excess fat can activate JNK and IKK in hepatocytes resulting in the increased expression of inflammatory cytokines and cell-adhesion molecules (Schattenberg *et al.*, 2006). Hepatic lipid, especially the toxic oxidized lipid-induced oxidative stress product malonyldialdehyde, could be used as immunological antigens to activate proinflammatory cytokine expression in the MCD diet model (Sutti *et al.*, 2014). The NASH characteristic features of insulin resistance and oxidative stress both affect the immune system to activate inflammation in the liver. The infiltrated cells have important correlations with cytokine and chemokine production, resulting in the advancement of steatosis, steatohepatitis, and steato-cirrhosis.

3.1.1   Macrophage and Kupffer Cells

Innate immune responses have great potential for amplification of inflammation in

NAFLD liver. CD68-positive macrophage infiltration and hepatic expression of macro-phage chemotactic factor 1 (MCP1) are increased, even in NAFL, and have important roles in inflammatory cell recruitment and insulin resistance (Lanthier *et al.*, 2010). MCP1 is a major chemokine inducing the recruitment of leukocytes into the liver during inflammation. These changes may be considered to be an early response by fatty liver. In the liver-infiltrated cells, the CD68-positive cells are comprised of inflammatory monocytes and liver resident macrophages, namely Kupffer cells. Kupffer cells are phagocytes of various cellular, viral, or bacterial components and are a source of hepatic pro-inflammatory and pro-fibrogenic cytokines. It is difficult to distinguish these cell types, although a recent report revealed that they could be distinguished by CD11b positivity expression. Kupffer cells might be the initiator of early inflammatory responses in NAFLD through TNF-α production (Tosello-Trampont *et al.*, 2012).

Cholesterol phagocytosis by Kupffer cells can induce their activation along with TLR4 upregulation (Leroux *et al.*, 2012). Aggregation of erythrocytes in inflammatory hepatic sinusoids can be seen in NASH patients. These erythrocytes often express phosphatidylserine on their surface that could be induced by oxidative stress (Otogawa *et al.*, 2007). Such erythrocytes carry hemoglobin and iron that could be easily taken up by Kupffer cells following activation and oxidative stress induction.

Activated Kupffer cells can produce inflammatory monocyte chemoattractant chemokines such as MCP1 or interferon (IFN)-γ inducible protein (IP-10). IP-10 has been reported as a potential NAFLD biomarker that distinguishes NAFL from NASH (Zhang *et al.*, 2014). Additionally, Zhang *et al.* revealed that IP-10 could induce several key in-flammatory cytokines, such as TNF-α, IL-1β, and MCP-1, and the blockade of IP-10 was protective for steatohepatitis development in a mouse model of NASH. IP-10 might be an important biomarker and candidate treatment target. The chemokine- or cytokine-induced recruitment of monocytes accelerates inflammatory responses and activates HSCs to produce pro-fibrotic factors.

3.1.2   Natural Killer (NK) Cells and NKT Cells

NK and NKT cell infiltration is decreased in severe steatosis, and the same phenomenon is observed in a choline-deficient diet–induced mild inflammatory NASH mouse model (Kremer *et al.*, 2010). However, in human advanced fibrotic NASH livers, more NKT cell infiltration occurs than in early fibrotic NASH livers, and NKT cell–deficient mice had less fibrosis than wild-type mice in severe fibrotic NASH model mice fed MCD (Syn *et al.*, 2012). In mild NASH with severe obesity exhibiting KKAy type 2 diabetes mouse model exhibited decreased NKT cell expression and function, especially after high-fat diet supplementation (Yamagata *et al.*, 2013). The function of NK or NKT cells could be different in the degree of obesity, insulin resistance, NAFL, NASH, and advanced NASH. As NAFL and NASH are different diseases, NKT cell function in NAFL and NASH progression is likely to be different.

IL-15 has been identified as a disease preventive cytokine in NAFL but a progression-related cytokine in NASH. IL-15 is an essential survival factor for natural killer (NK) cells, natural killer–like T (NKT) cells, and memory CD8+ T cells (Di Sabatino *et al.*,

2011). The role of NKT cells and related IL-15 in NAFLD is likely that they are preventive in the NAFL stage but disease progressive in fibrotic-stage advanced NASH.

3.1.3   Hepatic Stellate Cells (HSCs)

HSCs play significant roles in the progression of chronic liver inflammation and fibrosis (Rolo *et al.*, 2012). Excess fatty acid accumulation in hepatocytes induces oxidative stress from mitochondria as well as peroxisomes or microsomes. These cytotoxic ROS and lipid peroxidation products are able to diffuse into the extracellular space, affecting Kupffer cells and HSC. Cellular oxidative stresses from hepatocytes and the direct uptake of free fatty acids or free cholesterol in Kupffer cells activates nuclear-factor kB, which induces synthesis of TNF-α and several proinflammatory cytokines such as IL-6 or IL-8 (Hui *et al.*, 2004). Kupffer cells in patients with NASH produce TGF-β, resulting in HSCs acquiring a fibrogenic myofibroblast-like phenotype.

Exposure of primary HSC or HSC cell lines to H_2O_2 leads to increased gene expression of ER chaperone BIP binding transmembrane proteins such as inositol requiring enzyme 1 or activating transcription factor 4. ER stress in HSCs results in increased autophagy and HSC activation to fibrogenic status (Hernandez-Gea *et al.*, 2013).

Levels of free cholesterol (but not of cholesterol ester) are increased in HSC in NAFLD, resulting in increased TLR4 protein levels and fibrogenic HSC (Tomita *et al.*, 2013). Free cholesterol can accumulate in fibrogenic HSC, resulting in an increase in TLR4 by suppressing the endosomal-lysosomal degradation pathway of TLR4. The increased expression of TLR4 sensitizes cells to TGF-β–induced activation (Tomita *et al.*, 2013).

As mentioned in section 2.3 of this article, autophagy is involved in steatosis-related ER stress and oxidative stress. In a mouse model of inflamed NASH liver, activated HSC has been shown to be in autophagy defect condition. However, cytoplasmic lipid droplets are maintained and remain quiescent in autophagy-defective HSCs, indicating that oxidative stress-induced ER stress and autophagy are key events in HSC activation (Hernandez-Gea *et al.*, 2012).

3.1.4   T Cells

In advanced NASH, increases in CD4(+) and CD8(+) T-cell infiltration and inflammatory cytokines, such as IL-6 or IL-8, have been observed (Gadd *et al.*, 2014). Adaptive immune response–linked CD8(+) T cells usually respond after innate immune cell reactions; however, obese adipose tissue could recruit CD8(+) T cells prior to macrophage accumulation (Nishimura *et al.*, 2009). In an obesity-related NASH-hepatocarcinogenesis model, CD4(+) and CD8(+) T cells increased in the NASH condition with strong local activation marker CD44 and CD69 expression (Wolf *et al.*, 2014). Moreover, significant increases in hepatic NKT cells and regulatory T cells were found in this model. Both NKT cells and CD8(+) T cells were necessary for hepatocarcinogenesis, while CD8(+) T cells did not mediate fatty acid uptake or HSC activation as efficiently as NKT cells. Depletion of CD8(+) T cells reversed liver damage but left cholesterol levels unchanged, indicating that CD8(+) T cells are involved in liver inflammation rather than modulating lipid metabolism.

3.1.5   Cytokine Profile in NASH

Visceral obesity induces several cytokines including the inflammatory cytokine inter-leukin-17 (IL-17) (Fabbrini *et al.*, 2013), which induces neutrophil chemokine expression via IL-17 receptor A, which is widely expressed in the liver. Controlling the IL-17–related pathway effectively treats NASH progression in mouse models (Harley *et al.*, 2013). Elevated pre-therapy serum IL-17 levels in patients with HCC correlates with the risk of early recurrence after curative hepatectomy (Wu *et al.*, 2012). Co-cultured HCC cell lines and T cells producing IL-17 *in vitro* augment the proliferation of HCC cells, suggesting the importance of IL-17 for NASH-related HCC pathogenesis.

Interferon (IFN)-γ–inducible protein (IP-10) is a pro-inflammatory cytokine that recruits inflammatory cells to damaged tissue and is associated with lipotoxicity. As mentioned in section 3.1.1. of this articels, IP-10 could be used as NAFL and NASH differential marker. In chronic hepatitis C, intrahepatic IP-10 levels have been correlated with necroinflammatory changes and fibrosis (Zeremski *et al.*, 2008).

4   Treatment for NASH

Since NAFLD and NASH have emerged as lifestyle-associated diseases, lifestyle intervention is an important approach to their treatment. Healthy and Western-style diets differentiate the risk for NAFLD progression (Oddy *et al.*, 2013). A one-year intensive lifestyle intervention, comprised of dietary modifications and physical activity, improved waist circumference, visceral abdominal fat, blood pressure, insulin resistance, and hepatic fat content in obese patients (Goodpaster *et al.*, 2010). Western-style diets, especially those rich in trans-fatty acids, are powerful inducers of obesity and NAFLD and should be avoided (Neuschwander-Tetri *et al.*, 2012). However, maintained compliance with therapeutic measures such as restrained food consumption is mentally challenging, and the opt-out rate is high (Soetens *et al.*, 2008). Such patients require pharmacological therapies.

4.1   Anti-diabetic Therapy

Because the general characteristics of NASH comprise obesity and insulin resistance, anti-insulin resistance therapy has played a significant role. From this viewpoint, the ability of insulin sensitizing anti-diabetic drugs to treat NASH has been analyzed. Among these drugs, the PPAR-γ agonists pioglitazone and metformin have clinically improved NASH, although no histological improvements were shown in one-year studies (Aithal *et al.*, 2008; Bugianesi *et al.*, 2005).

Metformin increases intracellular levels of AMP after the activation of AMPK, which is a highly conserved heterodimeric serine-threonine kinase that serves as an energy sensor in eukaryotic cells and bridges metabolism to carcinogenesis (Hardie *et al.*, 1998). The activation of AMPK suppresses cell proliferation in non-malignant and malignant cells via regulation of the cell cycle, apoptosis, autophagy, and the inhibition of fatty acid synthesis (Motoshima *et al.*, 2006). Phospho (p)-AMPK is downregulated in HCC tissues from patients, and low p-AMPK expression correlates with a poor prognosis, indicating the importance of AMPK signaling in HCC (Zheng *et al.*, 2013). Adding metformin to hepatoma cell lines results in AMPK activation as well as dose- and time-dependent growth inhibition. Metformin might be a good candidate regarding NASH and NASH-related HCC prevention.

Glucagon like peptide-1 (GLP-1) and gastric inhibitory polypeptide (GIP) are both incretins, a group of gastrointestinal hormones that cause increased insulin release from pancreatic β cells, and they represent good potential targets for NASH treatment. A GLP-1 receptor agonist analogue improved metabolic, biochemical, and histopathological indices of NASH in mice by restoring hepatic lipid oxidation (Svegliati-Baroni *et al.*, 2011). Administration of a GLP-1 receptor agonist in type 2 diabetic patients with NAFLD caused a reduction in intrahepatic lipid content that correlated with diabetic control (Cuthbertson *et al.*, 2012). Dipeptidylpeptidase-IV (DPP-IV) degrades GLP-1 and GIP, and thus the inhibition of DPP-IV extends the half-life of endogenous GLP-1 and GIP, resulting in diabetic control. The long-term administration of a DPP-IV inhibitor has reduced liver fat content in animals with diet-induced hepatic steatosis and insulin resistance (Kern *et al.*, 2012).

A recently available anti-diabetic agent, sodium-glucose cotransporter 2 (SGLT2) inhibitor, provides a new treatment approach by lowering blood glucose levels via inhibition of glucose reabsorption from the proximal renal tubule (Kim & Babu, 2012). In type 2 diabetic patients, SGLT2 inhibitor administration induces significant body weight decrease and increased pancreatic β cell function, suggesting that it is a potential treatment for insulin resistance–related NASH (Rosenstock *et al.*, 2012). One of the SGLT2 inhibitors, ipragliflozin, prevented hepatic triglyceride accumulation and large lipid droplet formation (Hayashizaki-Someya *et al.*, 2015). Large clinical trials are needed to evaluate the effect of SGLT2 inhibitors on human NAFLD.

4.2   Anti-oxidant Therapy

The representative antioxidant vitamin E improved the non-alcoholic fatty liver disease activity scores (NAS) for clinical and histological activity within two years but increased insulin resistance and plasma triglyceride levels (Sanyal *et al.*, 2010). However, the recovery of fibrosis progression was not proven (Hoofnagle *et al.*, 2013). Controversy surrounds the value of ROS-scavenging agents because ROS have essential functions for life. Scavengers of ROS consistently exert effective chemical activities *in vitro*, but often not *in vivo* (Bast & Haenen, 2013). Scavenging of ROS is considered effective in preventing cancer development, while recent findings indicate that ROS also contribute to the progression of cancer (Watson, 2013). Stem cell–like cancer cells that express a CD44 variant have a powerful antioxidative phenotype that protects them from oxidative stress and prevents their apoptosis (Yae *et al.*, 2012). The American Association for the

Study of Liver Disease recommends the daily administration of 800 IU of vitamin E, which is higher than that usually administered to treat NASH (Chalasani *et al.*, 2012). This recommendation is based on a two-year randomized study of NASH treatment that resulted in improved ALT and histological activities (Sanyal *et al.*, 2010). Further investigations of longer durations are required to determine the effects of vitamin E on NASH, including hepatocarcinogenesis.

L-carnitine is a precursor of carnitine-palmitoyltransferase 1, the rate-limiting enzyme for mitochondrial β-oxidation that affects mitochondrial function. Any deficiency in the mitochondrial carnitine-dependent transport system results in curtailed fatty acid oxidation. L-carnitine supplementation reduces TNF-α, liver function parameters, plasma glucose levels and histological scores (Malaguarnera *et al.*, 2010).

Dietary intake of tomatoes has been reported to reduce the risk for human cancers (Ip & Wang, 2014). Tomatoes include vitamins A and C and phytochemicals such as carotenoids or flavonoids. Lycopene is the most abundant carotenoid found in tomato, tomato products, and other red fruits. Intake of lycopene inhibits NASH-promoted rat hepatic pre-neoplastic lesions (Ip *et al.*, 2013). Fresh tomato contains 9-oxo-10,12-octadecadienoic acid (9-oxo-ODA), which acts as a PPARα agonist to improve NASH in mice. In addition, processed tomato products such as tomato juice, but not fresh tomato, contains 13-oxo-9,11-octadecadenoic acid (13-oxo-ODA), an isomer of 9-oxo-ODA that improves lipid and carbohydrate metabolism disorders in NAFLD model mice (Kim *et al.*, 2012). Although clinical trials remain necessary, plasma carotenoid levels in NASH patients have been shown to be low, thus suggesting the possibility of a role for tomato intake in NASH prevention.

Molecular hydrogen has been shown to have powerful antioxidant effects with unique features (Ohsawa *et al.*, 2007). In cultured cells, hydrogen scavenges hydroxyl radicals, but not superoxide, hydrogen peroxide (H_2O_2) or nitric oxide (NO), and prevents the decline in mitochondrial membrane potential and the subsequent decrease in cellular ATP synthesis, consistent with antioxidative effects. Kawai *et al.* reported that drinking hydrogen-rich water has favorable effects in NASH models (Kawai *et al.*, 2012). Administration of hydrogen-rich water or the antioxidant pioglitazone reduced plasma transaminase levels, histological NAS, hepatic TNF-α, IL-6, fatty acid synthesis-related gene expression, and the oxidative stress biomarker 8-OHdG in the livers of MCD diet-induced NASH models.

As mentioned above, new antioxidants may be effective in controlling NAFLD progression. However, many investigations into the effects of antioxidants on diseases associated with oxidative stress have been disappointing, and the effects of newer antioxidants could prove similar. More basic and clinical experimentation into this novel potential treatment option is required.

4.3 Other Treatment Possibilities including Immune-targeted Therapy

Pentoxifylline is a methylxanthine derivative that increases red blood cell flexibility, reduces blood viscosity, and decreases platelet aggregation. In addition, pentoxifylline suppresses TNF-α gene transcription and is a hydroxyl and peroxyl radical scavenger with anti-oxidative effects. A randomized controlled trial has proven that pentoxifylline decreases free-radical–mediated lipid oxidation and improves clinical and histological NASH (Zein *et al.*, 2012; Zein *et al.*, 2011).

TNF-α is one of the main cytokines involved in adipocyte-related inflammation including NASH. Powerful anti-TNF-α agents such as infliximab (a chimeric monoclonal antibody), adalimumab (a human monoclonal antibody), and etanercept (a fusion protein) have severe side effects, such as increased risk for tuberculosis, that render them unacceptable as therapies for NAFLD (Ford & Peyrin-Biroulet, 2013). The anti-oxidative agent pentoxifylline also has an anti-TNF-α function that is partially involved in its favorable effects on NASH.

Lipid-lowering drugs such as statins can also improve ALT and radiological steatosis in hyperlipidemic patients with NAFLD; however, histological improvements are not evident (Nelson *et al.*, 2009). Ezetimibe is a Niemann-Pick C1-like protein inhibitor that can reduce the intestinal accumulation of free cholesterol. Ezetimibe showed histological NAS improvement in mice and in 10 patients with NASH, indicating the need for a larger randomized controlled trial (Deushi *et al.*, 2007; Yoneda *et al.*, 2010).

Ursodeoxycholic acid is also reportedly effective in some instances. Several randomized controlled trials have found improvements in ALT but not in liver histology, even at high doses (Leuschner *et al.*, 2010). The combination of ursodeoxycholic acid and vitamin E showed improved ALT and histological NAS scores (Pietu *et al.*, 2012).

A pro-inflammatory intestinal microbiome has been identified in mice and in patients with NASH. Probiotics, such as butyrate-producing agents, reduce hepatic triglyceride content and induce anti-oxidative enzymes that help to prevent the progression of NASH to hepatocellular carcinoma (Endo *et al.*, 2013).

5   Conclusion

Inflammation is a representative finding in NASH pathogenesis. The immune system is an important regulator of the inflammatory process. While NAFL and NASH both present with liver steatosis, these diseases differ in their lipid deposition and infiltrating immune cell function. Thus, differentiating non-progressive NAFL and progressive NASH is a fundamentally important issue that remains to be resolved. Innate immune responses and adaptive immune responses are both involved in NASH-hepatocarcinogenesis mechanisms, while the important cell types differ in different clinical conditions. The treatment approach should be different in different clinical condition. Although vitamin E administration is the only effective treatment currently known, a patient follow-up of longer duration is necessary, as many studies have indicated that caution is required to avoid the potential life-threatening effects of long-term antioxidant therapy. Optimization of treatment protocols warrants further investigation, as does the search for novel therapeutic strategies.

References

Aithal GP, Thomas JA, Kaye PV, Lawson A, Ryder SD, Spendlove I, Austin AS, Freeman JG, Morgan L, Webber J. (2008).Randomized, placebo-controlled trial of pioglitazone in nondiabetic subjects with nonalcoholic steatohepatitis. Gastroenterology 135:1176–84.

Argentou M, Tiniakos DG, Karanikolas M, Melachrinou M, Makri MG, Kittas C, Kalfarentzos F. (2009).Adipokine serum levels are related to liver histology in severely obese patients undergoing bariatric surgery. Obes Surg 19:1313–23.

Bast A, Haenen GR. (2013).Ten misconceptions about antioxidants. Trends Pharmacol Sci 34:430–6.

Brun P, Castagliuolo I, Di Leo V, Buda A, Pinzani M, Palu G, Martines D. (2007).Increased intestinal permeability in obese mice: new evidence in the pathogenesis of nonalcoholic steatohepatitis. Am J Physiol Gastrointest Liver Physiol 292:G518–25.

Brunt EM, Kleiner DE, Wilson LA, Unalp A, Behling CE, Lavine JE, Neuschwander-Tetri BA. (2009).Portal chronic inflammation in nonalcoholic fatty liver disease (NAFLD): a histologic marker of advanced NAFLD-Clinicopathologic correlations from the nonalcoholic steatohepatitis clinical research network. Hepatology 49:809–20.

Bugianesi E, Gentilcore E, Manini R, Natale S, Vanni E, Villanova N, David E, Rizzetto M, Marchesini G. (2005).A randomized controlled trial of metformin versus vitamin E or prescriptive diet in nonalcoholic fatty liver disease. Am J Gastroenterol 100:1082–90.

Bugianesi E. (2007).Non-alcoholic steatohepatitis and cancer. Clin Liver Dis 11:191–207, x–xi.

Cani PD, Amar J, Iglesias MA, Poggi M, Knauf C, Bastelica D, Neyrinck AM, Fava F, Tuohy KM, Chabo C, Waget A, Delmee E, Cousin B, Sulpice T, Chamontin B, Ferrieres J, Tanti JF, Gibson GR, Casteilla L, Delzenne NM, Alessi MC, Burcelin R. (2007).Metabolic endotoxemia initiates obesity and insulin resistance. Diabetes 56:1761–72.

Cani PD, Bibiloni R, Knauf C, Waget A, Neyrinck AM, Delzenne NM, Burcelin R. (2008).Changes in gut microbiota control metabolic endotoxemia-induced inflammation in high-fat diet-induced obesity and diabetes in mice. Diabetes 57:1470–81.

Carbone F, La Rocca C, Matarese G. (2012).Immunological functions of leptin and adiponectin. Biochimie 94:2082–8.

Chalasani N, Younossi Z, Lavine JE, Diehl AM, Brunt EM, Cusi K, Charlton M, Sanyal AJ. (2012).The diagnosis and management of non-alcoholic fatty liver disease: practice Guideline by the American Association for the Study of Liver Diseases, American College of Gastroenterology, and the American Gastroenterological Association. Hepatology 55:2005–23.

Cohen P, Zhao C, Cai X, Montez JM, Rohani SC, Feinstein P, Mombaerts P, Friedman JM. (2001).Selective deletion of leptin receptor in neurons leads to obesity. J Clin Invest 108:1113–21.

Cortez-Pinto H, Chatham J, Chacko VP, Arnold C, Rashid A, Diehl AM. (1999).Alterations in liver ATP homeostasis in human nonalcoholic steatohepatitis: a pilot study. JAMA 282:1659–64.

Csak T, Ganz M, Pespisa J, Kodys K, Dolganiuc A, Szabo G. (2011).Fatty acids and endotoxin activate inflammasome in hepatocytes which release danger signals to activate immune cells in steatohepatitis. Hepatology.

Cuthbertson DJ, Irwin A, Gardner CJ, Daousi C, Purewal T, Furlong N, Goenka N, Thomas EL, Adams VL, Pushpakom SP, Pirmohamed M, Kemp GJ. (2012).Improved glycaemia correlates with liver fat reduction in obese, type 2 diabetes, patients given glucagon-like peptide-1 (GLP-1) receptor agonists.

PLoS One 7:e50117.

Day CP, James OF. (1998).Steatohepatitis: a tale of two "hits"? Gastroenterology 114:842–5.

Deushi M, Nomura M, Kawakami A, Haraguchi M, Ito M, Okazaki M, Ishii H, Yoshida M. (2007).Ezetimibe improves liver steatosis and insulin resistance in obese rat model of metabolic syndrome. FEBS Lett 581:5664–70.

Di Sabatino A, Calarota SA, Vidali F, Macdonald TT, Corazza GR. (2011).Role of IL-15 in immune-mediated and infectious diseases. Cytokine Growth Factor Rev 22:19–33.

Eguchi Y, Eguchi T, Mizuta T, Ide Y, Yasutake T, Iwakiri R, Hisatomi A, Ozaki I, Yamamoto K, Kitajima Y, Kawaguchi Y, Kuroki S, Ono N. (2006).Visceral fat accumulation and insulin resistance are important factors in nonalcoholic fatty liver disease. J Gastroenterol 41:462–9.

Endo H, Niioka M, Kobayashi N, Tanaka M, Watanabe T. (2013).Butyrate-producing probiotics reduce nonalcoholic Fatty liver disease progression in rats: new insight into the probiotics for the gut-liver axis. PLoS One 8:e63388.

Fabbrini E, Cella M, McCartney SA, Fuchs A, Abumrad NA, Pietka TA, Chen Z, Finck BN, Han DH, Magkos F, Conte C, Bradley D, Fraterrigo G, Eagon JC, Patterson BW, Colonna M, Klein S. (2013).Association between specific adipose tissue CD4+ T-cell populations and insulin resistance in obese individuals. Gastroenterology 145:366–74 e1–3.

Fassio E, Alvarez E, Dominguez N, Landeira G, Longo C. (2004).Natural history of nonalcoholic steatohepatitis: a longitudinal study of repeat liver biopsies. Hepatology 40:820–6.

Ford AC, Peyrin-Biroulet L. (2013).Opportunistic Infections With Anti-Tumor Necrosis Factor-alpha Therapy in Inflammatory Bowel Disease: Meta-Analysis of Randomized Controlled Trials. Am J Gastroenterol.

Fukuo Y, Yamashina S, Sonoue H, Arakawa A, Nakadera E, Aoyama T, Uchiyama A, Kon K, Ikejima K, Watanabe S. (2014).Abnormality of autophagic function and cathepsin expression in the liver from patients with non-alcoholic fatty liver disease. Hepatol Res 44:1026–36.

Furusho H, Miyauchi M, Hyogo H, Inubushi T, Ao M, Ouhara K, Hisatune J, Kurihara H, Sugai M, Hayes CN, Nakahara T, Aikata H, Takahashi S, Chayama K, Takata T. (2013).Dental infection of Porphyromonas gingivalis exacerbates high fat diet-induced steatohepatitis in mice. J Gastroenterol 48:1259–70.

Gadd VL, Skoien R, Powell EE, Fagan KJ, Winterford C, Horsfall L, Irvine K, Clouston AD. (2013).The portal inflammatory infiltrate and ductular reaction in human non-alcoholic fatty liver disease. Hepatology.

Gadd VL, Skoien R, Powell EE, Fagan KJ, Winterford C, Horsfall L, Irvine K, Clouston AD. (2014).The portal inflammatory infiltrate and ductular reaction in human nonalcoholic fatty liver disease. Hepatology 59:1393–405.

Goodpaster BH, Delany JP, Otto AD, Kuller L, Vockley J, South-Paul JE, Thomas SB, Brown J, McTigue K, Hames KC, Lang W, Jakicic JM. (2010).Effects of diet and physical activity interventions on weight loss and cardiometabolic risk factors in severely obese adults: a randomized trial. JAMA 304:1795–802.

Haas JT, Miao J, Chanda D, Wang Y, Zhao E, Haas ME, Hirschey M, Vaitheesvaran B, Farese RV, Jr., Kurland IJ, Graham M, Crooke R, Foufelle F, Biddinger SB. (2012).Hepatic insulin signaling is required for obesity-dependent expression of SREBP-1c mRNA but not for feeding-dependent expression. Cell Metab 15:873–84.

Hackam DG. (2007).Review: antioxidant supplements for primary and secondary prevention do not decrease mortality. ACP J Club 147:4.

Hardie DG, Carling D, Carlson M. (1998).The AMP-activated/SNF1 protein kinase subfamily: metabolic sensors of the eukaryotic cell? Annu Rev Biochem 67:821–55.

Harley IT, Stankiewicz TE, Giles DA, Softic S, Flick LM, Cappelletti M, Sheridan R, Xanthakos SA, Steinbrecher KA, Sartor RB, Kohli R, Karp CL, Divanovic S. (2013).IL-17 signaling accelerates the progression of nonalcoholic fatty liver disease in mice. Hepatology.

Hatanaka K, Kudo M, Fukunaga T, Ueshima K, Chung H, Minami Y, Sakaguchi Y, Hagiwara S, Orino A, Osaki Y. (2007).Clinical characteristics of NonBNonC- HCC: Comparison with HBV and HCV related HCC. Intervirology 50:24–31.

Hayashizaki-Someya Y, Kurosaki E, Takasu T, Mitori H, Yamazaki S, Koide K, Takakura S. (2015).Ipragliflozin, an SGLT2 inhibitor, exhibits a prophylactic effect on hepatic steatosis and fibrosis induced by choline-deficient l-amino acid-defined diet in rats. Eur J Pharmacol 754:19–24.

Henao-Mejia J, Elinav E, Jin C, Hao L, Mehal WZ, Strowig T, Thaiss CA, Kau AL, Eisenbarth SC, Jurczak MJ, Camporez JP, Shulman GI, Gordon JI, Hoffman HM, Flavell RA. (2012).Inflammasome-mediated dysbiosis regulates progression of NAFLD and obesity. Nature 482:179–85.

Hernandez-Gea V, Ghiassi-Nejad Z, Rozenfeld R, Gordon R, Fiel MI, Yue Z, Czaja MJ, Friedman SL. (2012).Autophagy releases lipid that promotes fibrogenesis by activated hepatic stellate cells in mice and in human tissues. Gastroenterology 142:938–46.

Hernandez-Gea V, Hilscher M, Rozenfeld R, Lim MP, Nieto N, Werner S, Devi LA, Friedman SL. (2013).Endoplasmic reticulum stress induces fibrogenic activity in hepatic stellate cells through autophagy. J Hepatol 59:98–104.

Hoofnagle JH, Van Natta ML, Kleiner DE, Clark JM, Kowdley KV, Loomba R, Neuschwander-Tetri BA, Sanyal AJ, Tonascia J. (2013).Vitamin E and changes in serum alanine aminotransferase levels in patients with non-alcoholic steatohepatitis. Aliment Pharmacol Ther 38:134–43.

Hui JM, Hodge A, Farrell GC, Kench JG, Kriketos A, George J. (2004).Beyond insulin resistance in NASH: TNF-alpha or adiponectin? Hepatology 40:46–54.

Inami Y, Yamashina S, Izumi K, Ueno T, Tanida I, Ikejima K, Watanabe S. (2011).Hepatic steatosis inhibits autophagic proteolysis via impairment of autophagosomal acidification and cathepsin expression. Biochem Biophys Res Commun 412:618–25.

Ip BC, Hu KQ, Liu C, Smith DE, Obin MS, Ausman LM, Wang XD. (2013).Lycopene metabolite, apo-10'-lycopenoic acid, inhibits diethylnitrosamine-initiated, high fat diet-promoted hepatic inflammation and tumorigenesis in mice. Cancer Prev Res (Phila) 6:1304–16.

Ip BC, Wang XD. (2014).Non-alcoholic steatohepatitis and hepatocellular carcinoma: implications for lycopene intervention. Nutrients 6:124–62.

Kantartzis K, Machicao F, Machann J, Schick F, Fritsche A, Haring HU, Stefan N. (2009).The DGAT2 gene is a candidate for the dissociation between fatty liver and insulin resistance in humans. Clin Sci (Lond) 116:531–7.

Kaser S, Moschen A, Cayon A, Kaser A, Crespo J, Pons-Romero F, Ebenbichler CF, Patsch JR, Tilg H. (2005).Adiponectin and its receptors in non-alcoholic steatohepatitis. Gut 54:117–21.

Kawaguchi T, Sumida Y, Umemura A, Matsuo K, Takahashi M, Takamura T, Yasui K, Saibara T, Hashimoto E, Kawanaka M, Watanabe S, Kawata S, Imai Y, Kokubo M, Shima T, Park H, Tanaka H, Tajima K, Yamada R, Matsuda F, Japan Study Group of Nonalcoholic Fatty Liver D. (2012).Genetic polymorphisms of the human PNPLA3 gene are strongly associated with severity of non-alcoholic fatty liver disease in Japanese. PLoS One 7:e38322.

Kawai D, Takaki A, Nakatsuka A, Wada J, Tamaki N, Yasunaka T, Koike K, Tsuzaki R, Matsumoto K, Miyake Y, Shiraha H, Morita M, Makino H, Yamamoto K. (2012).Hydrogen-rich water prevents progression of nonalcoholic steatohepatitis and accompanying hepatocarcinogenesis in mice. Hepatology 56:912–21.

Kern M, Kloting N, Niessen HG, Thomas L, Stiller D, Mark M, Klein T, Bluher M. (2012).Linagliptin improves insulin sensitivity and hepatic steatosis in diet-induced obesity. PLoS One 7:e38744.

Kim Y, Babu AR. (2012).Clinical potential of sodium-glucose cotransporter 2 inhibitors in the management of type 2 diabetes. Diabetes Metab Syndr Obes 5:313–27.

Kim YI, Hirai S, Goto T, Ohyane C, Takahashi H, Tsugane T, Konishi C, Fujii T, Inai S, Iijima Y, Aoki K, Shibata D, Takahashi N, Kawada T. (2012).Potent PPARalpha activator derived from tomato juice, 13-oxo-9,11-octadecadienoic acid, decreases plasma and hepatic triglyceride in obese diabetic mice. PLoS One 7:e31317.

Kremer M, Thomas E, Milton RJ, Perry AW, van Rooijen N, Wheeler MD, Zacks S, Fried M, Rippe RA, Hines IN. (2010).Kupffer cell and interleukin-12-dependent loss of natural killer T cells in hepatosteatosis. Hepatology 51:130–41.

Lallukka S, Sevastianova K, Perttila J, Hakkarainen A, Orho-Melander M, Lundbom N, Olkkonen VM, Yki-Jarvinen H. (2013).Adipose tissue is inflamed in NAFLD due to obesity but not in NAFLD due to genetic variation in PNPLA3. Diabetologia 56:886–92.

Lanthier N, Molendi-Coste O, Horsmans Y, van Rooijen N, Cani PD, Leclercq IA. (2010).Kupffer cell activation is a causal factor for hepatic insulin resistance. Am J Physiol Gastrointest Liver Physiol 298:G107–16.

Larter CZ, Chitturi S, Heydet D, Farrell GC. (2010).A fresh look at NASH pathogenesis. Part 1: the metabolic movers. J Gastroenterol Hepatol 25:672–90.

Larter CZ, Farrell GC. (2006).Insulin resistance, adiponectin, cytokines in NASH: Which is the best target to treat? J Hepatol 44:253–61.

Lemoine M, Ratziu V, Kim M, Maachi M, Wendum D, Paye F, Bastard JP, Poupon R, Housset C, Capeau J, Serfaty L. (2009).Serum adipokine levels predictive of liver injury in non-alcoholic fatty liver disease. Liver Int 29:1431–8.

Leroux A, Ferrere G, Godie V, Cailleux F, Renoud ML, Gaudin F, Naveau S, Prevot S, Makhzami S, Perlemuter G, Cassard-Doulcier AM. (2012).Toxic lipids stored by Kupffer cells correlates with their pro-inflammatory phenotype at an early stage of steatohepatitis. J Hepatol 57:141–9.

Leuschner UF, Lindenthal B, Herrmann G, Arnold JC, Rossle M, Cordes HJ, Zeuzem S, Hein J, Berg T. (2010).High-dose ursodeoxycholic acid therapy for nonalcoholic steatohepatitis: a double-blind, randomized, placebo-controlled trial. Hepatology 52:472–9.

Lindstrom P. (2007).The physiology of obese-hyperglycemic mice [ob/ob mice]. ScientificWorldJournal 7:666–85.

Ludwig J, Viggiano TR, McGill DB, Oh BJ. (1980).Nonalcoholic steatohepatitis: Mayo Clinic experiences with a hitherto unnamed disease. Mayo Clin Proc 55:434–8.

Ma H, Gomez V, Lu L, Yang X, Wu X, Xiao SY. (2009).Expression of adiponectin and its receptors in livers of morbidly obese patients with non-alcoholic fatty liver disease. J Gastroenterol Hepatol 24:233–7.

Maher JJ, Leon P, Ryan JC. (2008).Beyond insulin resistance: Innate immunity in nonalcoholic *steatohepatitis. Hepatology 48:670–8.*

Malaguarnera M, Gargante MP, Russo C, Antic T, Vacante M, Avitabile T, Li Volti G, Galvano F. (2010).L-carnitine supplementation to diet: a new tool in treatment of nonalcoholic steatohepatitis—a randomized and controlled clinical trial. Am J Gastroenterol 105:1338–45.

Matsunami T, Sato Y, Ariga S, Sato T, Shimomura T, Kashimura H, Hasegawa Y, Yukawa M. (2011).Regulation of synthesis and oxidation of fatty acids by adiponectin receptors (AdipoR1/R2) and insulin receptor substrate isoforms (IRS-1/-2) of the liver in a nonalcoholic steatohepatitis animal model. Metabolism 60:805–14.

Matteoni CA, Younossi ZM, Gramlich T, Boparai N, Liu YC, McCullough AJ. (1999).Nonalcoholic fatty liver disease: a spectrum of clinical and pathological severity. Gastroenterology 116:1413–9.

Miele L, Valenza V, La Torre G, Montalto M, Cammarota G, Ricci R, Masciana R, Forgione A, Gabrieli ML, Perotti G, Vecchio FM, Rapaccini G, Gasbarrini G, Day CP, Grieco A. (2009).Increased intestinal permeability and tight junction alterations in nonalcoholic fatty liver disease. Hepatology 49:1877–87.

Mittler R, Vanderauwera S, Suzuki N, Miller G, Tognetti VB, Vandepoele K, Gollery M, Shulaev V, Van Breusegem F. (2011).ROS signaling: the new wave? Trends Plant Sci 16:300–9.

Miura K, Yang L, van Rooijen N, Brenner DA, Ohnishi H, Seki E. (2013).Toll-like receptor 2 and palmitic acid cooperatively contribute to the development of nonalcoholic steatohepatitis through inflammasome activation in mice. Hepatology 57:577–89.

Motoshima H, Goldstein BJ, Igata M, Araki E. (2006).AMPK and cell proliferation-AMPK as a therapeutic target for atherosclerosis and cancer. J Physiol 574:63–71.

Muriel P. (2009).Role of free radicals in liver diseases. Hepatol Int 3:526–36.

Nakamura A, Yoneda M, Sumida Y, Eguchi Y, Fujii H, Hyogo H, Ono M, Suzuki Y, Kawaguchi T, Aoki N, Okanoue T, Nakajima A, Maeda S, Terauchi Y. (2013).Modification of a simple clinical scoring system as a diagnostic screening tool for non-alcoholic steatohepatitis in Japanese patients with non-alcoholic fatty liver disease. J Diabetes Investig 4:651–8.

Nannipieri M, Cecchetti F, Anselmino M, Mancini E, Marchetti G, Bonotti A, Baldi S, Solito B, Giannetti M, Pinchera A, Santini F, Ferrannini E. (2009).Pattern of expression of adiponectin receptors in human liver and its relation to nonalcoholic steatohepatitis. Obes Surg 19:467–74.

Nelson A, Torres DM, Morgan AE, Fincke C, Harrison SA. (2009).A pilot study using simvastatin in the treatment of nonalcoholic steatohepatitis: A randomized placebo-controlled trial. J Clin Gastroenterol 43:990–4.

Nelson JE, Wilson L, Brunt EM, Yeh MM, Kleiner DE, Unalp-Arida A, Kowdley KV. (2011).Relationship between the pattern of hepatic iron deposition and histological severity in nonalcoholic fatty liver disease. Hepatology 53:448–57.

Neuschwander-Tetri BA, Ford DA, Acharya S, Gilkey G, Basaranoglu M, Tetri LH, Brunt EM. (2012).Dietary trans-fatty acid induced NASH is normalized following loss of trans-fatty acids from hepatic lipid pools. Lipids 47:941–50.

Nishimura S, Manabe I, Nagasaki M, Eto K, Yamashita H, Ohsugi M, Otsu M, Hara K, Ueki K, Sugiura S, Yoshimura K, Kadowaki T, Nagai R. (2009).CD8+ effector T cells contribute to macrophage recruitment and adipose tissue inflammation in obesity. Nat Med 15:914–20.

Novo E, Busletta C, Bonzo LV, Povero D, Paternostro C, Mareschi K, Ferrero I, David E, Bertolani C, Caligiuri A, Cannito S, Tamagno E, Compagnone A, Colombatto S, Marra F, Fagioli F, Pinzani M,

Parola M. (2011).Intracellular reactive oxygen species are required for directional migration of resident and bone marrow-derived hepatic pro-fibrogenic cells. J Hepatol 54:964–74.

Oddy WH, Herbison CE, Jacoby P, Ambrosini GL, O'Sullivan TA, Ayonrinde OT, Olynyk JK, Black LJ, Beilin LJ, Mori TA, Hands BP, Adams LA. (2013).The Western dietary pattern is prospectively associated with nonalcoholic fatty liver disease in adolescence. Am J Gastroenterol 108:778–85.

Ohsawa I, Ishikawa M, Takahashi K, Watanabe M, Nishimaki K, Yamagata K, Katsura K, Katayama Y, Asoh S, Ohta S. (2007).Hydrogen acts as a therapeutic antioxidant by selectively reducing cytotoxic oxygen radicals. Nature Medicine 13:688–694.

Ono M, Saibara T. (2006).Clinical features of nonalcoholic steatohepatitis in Japan: Evidence from the literature. J Gastroenterol 41:725–32.

Otogawa K, Kinoshita K, Fujii H, Sakabe M, Shiga R, Nakatani K, Ikeda K, Nakajima Y, Ikura Y, Ueda M, Arakawa T, Hato F, Kawada N. (2007).Erythrophagocytosis by liver macrophages (Kupffer cells) promotes oxidative stress, inflammation, and fibrosis in a rabbit model of steatohepatitis: implications for the pathogenesis of human nonalcoholic steatohepatitis. Am J Pathol 170:967–80.

Pietu F, Guillaud O, Walter T, Vallin M, Hervieu V, Scoazec JY, Dumortier J. (2012).Ursodeoxycholic acid with vitamin E in patients with nonalcoholic steatohepatitis: long-term results. Clin Res Hepatol Gastroenterol 36:146–55.

Polyzos SA, Toulis KA, Goulis DG, Zavos C, Kountouras J. (2011).Serum total adiponectin in nonalcoholic fatty liver disease: a systematic review and meta-analysis. Metabolism 60:313–26.

Qiao A, Liang J, Ke Y, Li C, Cui Y, Shen L, Zhang H, Cui A, Liu X, Liu C, Chen Y, Zhu Y, Guan Y, Fang F, Chang Y. (2011).Mouse patatin-like phospholipase domain-containing 3 influences systemic lipid and glucose homeostasis. Hepatology 54:509–21.

Rivera CA, Gaskin L, Allman M, Pang J, Brady K, Adegboyega P, Pruitt K. (2010).Toll-like receptor-2 deficiency enhances non-alcoholic steatohepatitis. BMC Gastroenterol 10:52.

Rolo AP, Teodoro JS, Palmeira CM. (2012).Role of oxidative stress in the pathogenesis of nonalcoholic steatohepatitis. Free Radic Biol Med 52:59–69.

Romeo S, Kozlitina J, Xing C, Pertsemlidis A, Cox D, Pennacchio LA, Boerwinkle E, Cohen JC, Hobbs HH. (2008).Genetic variation in PNPLA3 confers susceptibility to nonalcoholic fatty liver disease. Nat Genet 40:1461–5.

Rosenstock J, Aggarwal N, Polidori D, Zhao Y, Arbit D, Usiskin K, Capuano G, Canovatchel W, Canagliflozin DIASG. (2012).Dose-ranging effects of canagliflozin, a sodium-glucose cotransporter 2 inhibitor, as add-on to metformin in subjects with type 2 diabetes. Diabetes Care 35:1232–8.

Sanyal AJ, Chalasani N, Kowdley KV, McCullough A, Diehl AM, Bass NM, Neuschwander-Tetri BA, Lavine JE, Tonascia J, Unalp A, Van Natta M, Clark J, Brunt EM, Kleiner DE, Hoofnagle JH, Robuck PR. (2010).Pioglitazone, vitamin E, or placebo for nonalcoholic steatohepatitis. N Engl J Med 362:1675–85.

Sanyal AJ, Chalasani N, Kowdley KV, McCullough A, Diehl AM, Bass NM, Neuschwander-Tetri BA, Lavine JE, Tonascia J, Unalp A, Van Natta M, Clark J, Brunt EM, Kleiner DE, Hoofnagle JH, Robuck PR, Nash CRN. (2010).Pioglitazone, vitamin E, or placebo for nonalcoholic steatohepatitis. N Engl J Med 362:1675–85.

Sarraf P, Frederich RC, Turner EM, Ma G, Jaskowiak NT, Rivet DJ, 3rd, Flier JS, Lowell BB, Fraker DL, Alexander HR. (1997).Multiple cytokines and acute inflammation raise mouse leptin levels: potential role in inflammatory anorexia. J Exp Med 185:171–5.

Schattenberg JM, Singh R, Wang Y, Lefkowitch JH, Rigoli RM, Scherer PE, Czaja MJ. (2006).JNK1 but not JNK2 promotes the development of steatohepatitis in mice. Hepatology 43:163–72.

Serviddio G, Bellanti F, Tamborra R, Rollo T, Romano AD, Giudetti AM, Capitanio N, Petrella A, Vendemiale G, Altomare E. (2008).Alterations of hepatic ATP homeostasis and respiratory chain during development of non-alcoholic steatohepatitis in a rodent model. Eur J Clin Invest 38:245–52.

Shimada M, Kawahara H, Ozaki K, Fukura M, Yano H, Tsuchishima M, Tsutsumi M, Takase S. (2007).Usefulness of a combined evaluation of the serum adiponectin level, HOMA-IR, and serum type IV collagen 7S level to predict the early stage of nonalcoholic steatohepatitis. Am J Gastroenterol 102:1931–8.

Shiri-Sverdlov R, Wouters K, van Gorp PJ, Gijbels MJ, Noel B, Buffat L, Staels B, Maeda N, van Bilsen M, Hofker MH. (2006).Early diet-induced non-alcoholic steatohepatitis in APOE2 knock-in mice and its prevention by fibrates. J Hepatol 44:732–41.

Siddique A, Nelson JE, Aouizerat B, Yeh MM, Kowdley KV, Network NCR. (2013).Iron Deficiency in Patients With Nonalcoholic Fatty Liver Disease Is Associated With Obesity, Female Gender, and Low Serum Hepcidin. Clin Gastroenterol Hepatol.

Singal AG, Manjunath H, Yopp AC, Beg MS, Marrero JA, Gopal P, Waljee AK. (2014).The Effect of PNPLA3 on Fibrosis Progression and Development of Hepatocellular Carcinoma: A Meta-analysis. Am J Gastroenterol.

Singh R, Kaushik S, Wang Y, Xiang Y, Novak I, Komatsu M, Tanaka K, Cuervo AM, Czaja MJ. (2009).Autophagy regulates lipid metabolism. Nature 458:1131–5.

Soetens B, Braet C, Moens E. (2008).Thought suppression in obese and non-obese restrained eaters: piece of cake or forbidden fruit? Eur Eat Disord Rev 16:67–76.

Sookoian S, Pirola CJ. (2011).Meta-analysis of the influence of I148M variant of patatin-like phospholipase domain containing 3 gene (PNPLA3) on the susceptibility and histological severity of nonalcoholic fatty liver disease. Hepatology 53:1883–94.

Steinhubl SR. (2008).Why have antioxidants failed in clinical trials? Am J Cardiol 101:14D–19D.

Sumida Y, Yoneda M, Hyogo H, Yamaguchi K, Ono M, Fujii H, Eguchi Y, Suzuki Y, Imai S, Kanemasa K, Fujita K, Chayama K, Yasui K, Saibara T, Kawada N, Fujimoto K, Kohgo Y, Okanoue T, Japan Study Group of Nonalcoholic Fatty Liver D. (2011).A simple clinical scoring system using ferritin, fasting insulin, and type IV collagen 7S for predicting steatohepatitis in nonalcoholic fatty liver disease. J Gastroenterol 46:257–68.

Sutti S, Jindal A, Locatelli I, Vacchiano M, Gigliotti L, Bozzola C, Albano E. (2014).Adaptive immune responses triggered by oxidative stress contribute to hepatic inflammation in NASH. Hepatology 59:886–97.

Svegliati-Baroni G, Saccomanno S, Rychlicki C, Agostinelli L, De Minicis S, Candelaresi C, Faraci G, Pacetti D, Vivarelli M, Nicolini D, Garelli P, Casini A, Manco M, Mingrone G, Risaliti A, Frega GN, Benedetti A, Gastaldelli A. (2011).Glucagon-like peptide-1 receptor activation stimulates hepatic lipid oxidation and restores hepatic signalling alteration induced by a high-fat diet in nonalcoholic steatohepatitis. Liver Int 31:1285–97.

Syn WK, Agboola KM, Swiderska M, Michelotti GA, Liaskou E, Pang H, Xie G, Philips G, Chan IS, Karaca GF, Pereira Tde A, Chen Y, Mi Z, Kuo PC, Choi SS, Guy CD, Abdelmalek MF, Diehl AM. (2012).NKT-associated hedgehog and osteopontin drive fibrogenesis in non-alcoholic fatty liver disease. Gut 61:1323–9.

Takaki A, Kawai D, Yamamoto K. (2014).Molecular mechanisms and new treatment strategies for non-alcoholic steatohepatitis (NASH). Int J Mol Sci 15:7352–79.

Tamaki N, Takaki A, Tomofuji T, Endo Y, Kasuyama K, Ekuni D, Yasunaka T, Yamamoto K, Morita M. (2011).Stage of hepatocellular carcinoma is associated with periodontitis. J Clin Periodontol 38:1015–20.

Tilg H, Moschen AR. (2010).Evolution of inflammation in nonalcoholic fatty liver disease: the multiple parallel hits hypothesis. Hepatology 52:1836–46.

Tiniakos DG, Vos MB, Brunt EM. (2010).Nonalcoholic fatty liver disease: pathology and pathogenesis. Annu Rev Pathol 5:145–71.

Tomita K, Teratani T, Suzuki T, Shimizu M, Sato H, Narimatsu K, Okada Y, Kurihara C, Irie R, Yokoyama H, Shimamura K, Usui S, Ebinuma H, Saito H, Watanabe C, Komoto S, Kawaguchi A, Nagao S, Sugiyama K, Hokari R, Kanai T, Miura S, Hibi T. (2013).Free cholesterol accumulation in hepatic stellate cells: Mechanism of liver fibrosis aggravation in nonalcoholic steatohepatitis in mice. Hepatology.

Tosello-Trampont AC, Landes SG, Nguyen V, Novobrantseva TI, Hahn YS. (2012).Kuppfer cells trigger nonalcoholic steatohepatitis development in diet-induced mouse model through tumor necrosis factor-alpha production. J Biol Chem 287:40161–72.

Tsuneto A, Hida A, Sera N, Imaizumi M, Ichimaru S, Nakashima E, Seto S, Maemura K, Akahoshi M. (2010).Fatty liver incidence and predictive variables. Hypertens Res 33:638–43.

Valenti L, Alisi A, Galmozzi E, Bartuli A, Del Menico B, Alterio A, Dongiovanni P, Fargion S, Nobili V. (2010).I148M patatin-like phospholipase domain-containing 3 gene variant and severity of pediatric nonalcoholic fatty liver disease. Hepatology 52:1274–80.

Watson J. (2013).Oxidants, antioxidants and the current incurability of metastatic cancers. Open Biol 3:120144.

Wolf MJ, Adili A, Piotrowitz K, Abdullah Z, Boege Y, Stemmer K, Ringelhan M, Simonavicius N, Egger M, Wohlleber D, Lorentzen A, Einer C, Schulz S, Clavel T, Protzer U, Thiele C, Zischka H, Moch H, Tschop M, Tumanov AV, Haller D, Unger K, Karin M, Kopf M, Knolle P, Weber A, Heikenwalder M. (2014).Metabolic activation of intrahepatic CD8+ T cells and NKT cells causes nonalcoholic steatohepatitis and liver cancer via cross-talk with hepatocytes. Cancer Cell 26:549–64.

Wu J, Du J, Liu L, Li Q, Rong W, Wang L, Wang Y, Zang M, Wu Z, Zhang Y, Qu C. (2012).Elevated pretherapy serum IL17 in primary hepatocellular carcinoma patients correlate to increased risk of early recurrence after curative hepatectomy. PLoS One 7:e50035.

Xu RY, Wan YP, Fang QY, Lu W, Cai W. (2012).Supplementation with probiotics modifies gut flora and attenuates liver fat accumulation in rat nonalcoholic fatty liver disease model. J Clin Biochem Nutr 50:72–7.

Yae T, Tsuchihashi K, Ishimoto T, Motohara T, Yoshikawa M, Yoshida GJ, Wada T, Masuko T, Mogushi K, Tanaka H, Osawa T, Kanki Y, Minami T, Aburatani H, Ohmura M, Kubo A, Suematsu M, Takahashi K, Saya H, Nagano O. (2012).Alternative splicing of CD44 mRNA by ESRP1 enhances lung colonization of metastatic cancer cell. Nat Commun 3:883.

Yamagata H, Ikejima K, Takeda K, Aoyama T, Kon K, Okumura K, Watanabe S. (2013).Altered expression and function of hepatic natural killer T cells in obese and diabetic KK-A(y) mice. Hepatol Res 43:276–88.

Yamaguchi K, Yang L, McCall S, Huang J, Yu XX, Pandey SK, Bhanot S, Monia BP, Li YX, Diehl AM.

(2007).*Inhibiting triglyceride synthesis improves hepatic steatosis but exacerbates liver damage and fibrosis in obese mice with nonalcoholic steatohepatitis. Hepatology 45:1366–74.*

Yang L, Li P, Fu S, Calay ES, Hotamisligil GS. (2010).*Defective hepatic autophagy in obesity promotes ER stress and causes insulin resistance. Cell Metab 11:467–78.*

Yatsuji S, Hashimoto E, Tobari M, Taniai M, Tokushige K, Shiratori K. (2009).*Clinical features and outcomes of cirrhosis due to non-alcoholic steatohepatitis compared with cirrhosis caused by chronic hepatitis C. J Gastroenterol Hepatol 24:248–54.*

Yoneda M, Fujita K, Nozaki Y, Endo H, Takahashi H, Hosono K, Suzuki K, Mawatari H, Kirikoshi H, Inamori M, Saito S, Iwasaki T, Terauchi Y, Kubota K, Maeyama S, Nakajima A. (2010).*Efficacy of ezetimibe for the treatment of non-alcoholic steatohepatitis: An open-label, pilot study. Hepatol Res 40:613–21.*

Yoneda M, Naka S, Nakano K, Wada K, Endo H, Mawatari H, Imajo K, Nomura R, Hokamura K, Ono M, Murata S, Tohnai I, Sumida Y, Shima T, Kuboniwa M, Umemura K, Kamisaki Y, Amano A, Okanoue T, Ooshima T, Nakajima A. (2012).*Involvement of a periodontal pathogen, Porphyromonas gingivalis on the pathogenesis of non-alcoholic fatty liver disease. BMC Gastroenterol 12:16.*

Yoshimoto S, Loo TM, Atarashi K, Kanda H, Sato S, Oyadomari S, Iwakura Y, Oshima K, Morita H, Hattori M, Honda K, Ishikawa Y, Hara E, Ohtani N. (2013).*Obesity-induced gut microbial metabolite promotes liver cancer through senescence secretome. Nature 499:97–101.*

Younossi ZM, Jarrar M, Nugent C, Randhawa M, Afendy M, Stepanova M, Rafiq N, Goodman Z, Chandhoke V, Baranova A. (2008).*A novel diagnostic biomarker panel for obesity-related nonalcoholic steatohepatitis (NASH). Obes Surg 18:1430–7.*

Yu XX, Murray SF, Pandey SK, Booten SL, Bao D, Song XZ, Kelly S, Chen S, McKay R, Monia BP, Bhanot S. (2005).*Antisense oligonucleotide reduction of DGAT2 expression improves hepatic steatosis and hyperlipidemia in obese mice. Hepatology 42:362–71.*

Zein CO, Lopez R, Fu X, Kirwan JP, Yerian LM, McCullough AJ, Hazen SL, Feldstein AE. (2012).*Pentoxifylline decreases oxidized lipid products in nonalcoholic steatohepatitis: new evidence on the potential therapeutic mechanism. Hepatology 56:1291–9.*

Zein CO, Yerian LM, Gogate P, Lopez R, Kirwan JP, Feldstein AE, McCullough AJ. (2011).*Pentoxifylline improves nonalcoholic steatohepatitis: a randomized placebo-controlled trial. Hepatology 54:1610–9.*

Zeng TS, Liu FM, Zhou J, Pan SX, Xia WF, Chen LL. (2015).*Depletion of Kupffer cells attenuates systemic insulin resistance, inflammation and improves liver autophagy in high-fat diet fed mice. Endocr J.*

Zeremski M, Petrovic LM, Chiriboga L, Brown QB, Yee HT, Kinkhabwala M, Jacobson IM, Dimova R, Markatou M, Talal AH. (2008).*Intrahepatic levels of CXCR3-associated chemokines correlate with liver inflammation and fibrosis in chronic hepatitis C. Hepatology 48:1440–50.*

Zhang X, Shen J, Man K, Chu ES, Yau TO, Sung JC, Go MY, Deng J, Lu L, Wong VW, Sung JJ, Farrell G, Yu J. (2014).*CXCL10 plays a key role as an inflammatory mediator and a non-invasive biomarker of non-alcoholic steatohepatitis. J Hepatol.*

Zheng L, Yang W, Wu F, Wang C, Yu L, Tang L, Qiu B, Li Y, Guo L, Wu M, Feng G, Zou D, Wang H. (2013).*Prognostic significance of AMPK activation and therapeutic effects of metformin in hepatocellular carcinoma. Clin Cancer Res 19:5372–80.*

Chapter 6

Cytokine Immunopathogenesis of Enterovirus 71 Infection

Shih-Min Wang[1,2], Ching-Chuan Liu[1,2]

1 Introduction

Humoral mediators including cytokines are the molecular proteins of the innate and specific immune response, play key roles in the pathophysiology of viral infection (Dinarello, 1997). Cytokines, pleiotropic immunological messengers that both boost and sequester inflammation, are produced in response to infections and other stimuli and extend a request to surrounding and/or distant cells for a specific response. Specific cytokines have autocrine, paracrine, and/or endocrine activity and, through receptor binding, can elicit a variety of responses, depending upon the cytokine and the target cell (Tisoncik *et al.*, 2012). Systemic inflammatory response syndrome (SIRS) caused by infection, is a typical condition with in which pro-inflammatory mediators released from infected cells, and persistent hypercytokinemia may result in progression to multiple organ failure (Oda *et al.*, 2005). It is known that activation of cytokine networks increases levels of various cytokines in blood. The burst of cytokine release that follows sepsis, toxin-mediated shock syndrome (eg, *Streptococcus pyogenes* and *Staphylococcus aureus*) (Nakane *et al.*, 1995; Wang *et al.*, 2008), some virus infections such as severe acute respiratory syndrome (SARS) coronavirus (Cameron *et al.*, 2008), influenza virus (Skoner *et al.*, 1999), dengue virus (Lei *et al.*, 2001) and Epstein-Barr virus (Canna *et al.*, 2012) induce an overwhelming stimulation of innate and/or immune responses that storm the physiology of the body. The cytokine response is strong enough to flood beyond the site of infec-

---

[1] Departments of Pediatrics and §Emergency Medicine, National Cheng Kung University and Hospital, College of Medicine, National Cheng Kung University, Tainan, Taiwan

[2] Center of Infectious Disease and Signaling Research, National Cheng Kung University, Tainan, Taiwan

tion, it induces reactions on a systemic level, potentially causing life-threatening tissue damage (Nazinitsky & Rosentha, 2010).

2   Clinical Spectrum of EV71 Brain Stem Encephalitis

Human enterovirus 71 (EV71) is a member of the genus *Enterovirus*, family *Picornaviridae*, which consists of a non-enveloped capsid surrounding a core of single stranded, positive-polarity RNA approximately 7.5 kb in size and 27-30 nm in diameter (Hsiung & Wang, 2000; McMinn, 2002). EV71 produces a broad spectrum of clinical manifestations. The majority of infected individuals have asymptomatic infection. Mild cases characterized as cutaneous diseases such as hand-foot-and-mouth disease (HFMD) and herpangina. However, potentially life-threatening neurological complications such as brain stem encephalitis (BE) are of the greatest clinical and public concern (Wang et al., 1999; Ho et al., 1999; Huang et al., 1999; Lin et al., 2002). EV71 has been recognized as highly neurotropic and associated with a diverse range of neurological diseases, such as aseptic meningitis, BE, encephalomyelitis, acute flaccid paralysis (AFP) and post-infectious neurological syndromes. After the 1998 Taiwan epidemic several clinical stage categories of the disease were developed for the severity of BE to help monitor the clinical course of EV71 infection and to aid management. These systems, however, are not widely accepted, possibly because they are not always simple to follow by primary care physicians. In 2011, World Health Organization Regional Office (WHO) for the Western Pacific and the Regional Emerging Diseases Intervention (REDI) Centre documented guide for clinical management on Hand, Foot, and Mouth Disease, has proposed a simple clinical stages of disease manifestation to describe the disease severity (Wang et al., 2008; Wang et al., 2009). The EV71 BE was stratified into three important critical stages by disease severity, including uncomplicated BE, autonomic nervous system (ANS) dysregulation, and pulmonary edema (PE) (Figure 1), which resulted in high mortality rates (Ho et al., 1999; Huang et al., 1999; Ooi et al., 2010; Solomon et al., 2010; Wang et al., 2014) or long-term neurologic sequelae in survivors (Huang et al., 2006).

The EV71 BE is a continuous and dynamic disease sequence. It may be a reversible disease because each critical stage is a turning point in early period. Through this staging system the pathogenesis of BE was explored and then effective ways to manage the patients was developed. BE is defined as an illness characterized by myoclonus, ataxia, nystagmus, oculomotor palsies, and bulbar palsy in various combinations, with or without neuroimage evidences. ANS dysregulation is defined by the presence of cold sweating, mottled skin, tachycardia, tachypnea, and hypertension. PE is defined as respiratory distress with tachycardia, tachypnea, rales, and frothy sputum that developed after ANS dysregulation, together with a chest radiograph that showed bilateral pulmonary infiltrates without cardiomegaly (Figure 2).

If the diagnosis of EV71 BE once delayed, usually because of the clinical symptoms are not recognized in the early time. Myoclonic jerks are seen more often in EV71 than in other serotypes of the enterovirus in infected patients, and could be an early indicator of brain stem involvement. Diagnostic work-up of EV71 BE should include the

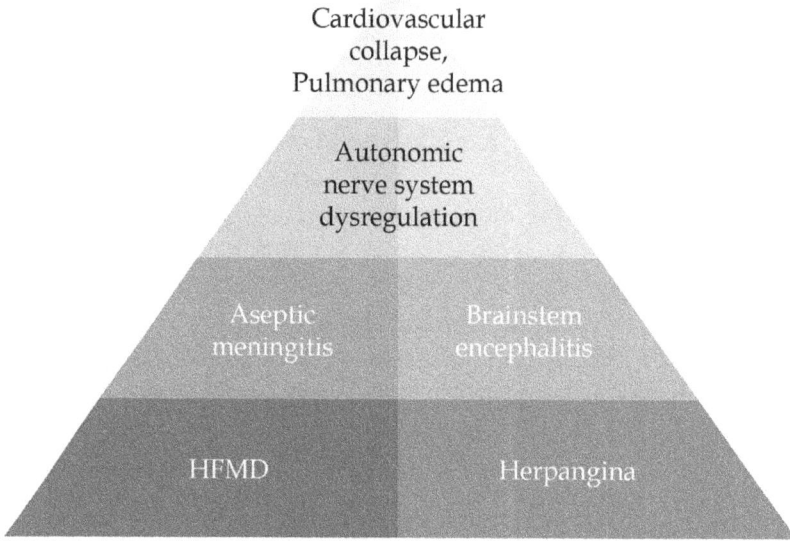

Figure 1: Clinical stages of enterovirus 71 infection by disease severity.

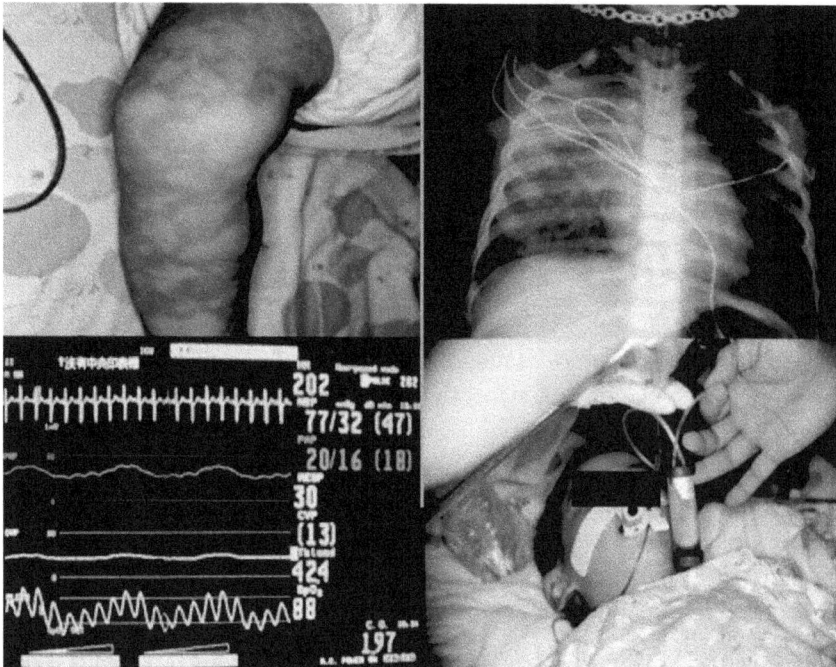

Figure 2: The clinical manifestations of autonomic nervous system (ANS) dys-regulation and pulmonary edema (PE) of enterovirus 71 (EV71) infection. Severe vasoconstriction (left upper), tachycardia and hyperthermia (left lower) in a patient with EV71 associated ANS dysregulation. Radiological evidence (right upper) and frothy tracheal aspirates (right lower) in a patient with EV71 associated PE.

search for one or more neurological symptoms, especially myoclonus jerk and limb paralysis, and the measurement of disease biomarkers, such as peripheral white blood cell count, platelet count, glucose level, inflammatory cytokines and chemokines, immune cell subsets and cerebrospinal fluid analysis (Lin *et al.*, 2002; Chang *et al.*, 1999; Wang *et al.*, 2003; Lin *et al.*, 2003; Wang *et al.*, 2007; Wang *et al.*, 2008).

In the 2008 outbreak of Taiwan, 238 virologically and clinically confirmed severe cases identified, include 41% uncomplicated BE, 44% ANS dysregulation and 15% PE (Wang *et al.*, 2012). The EV of different serotypes has been co circulated in Taiwan yearly. The EV and EV71 isolates distribution by year since 1998 at National Cheng Kung University Hospital was illustrated (Figure 3). EV71 plays a cardinal role among the EV epidemics in 1998, 2000, 2001, 2008 and 2012.

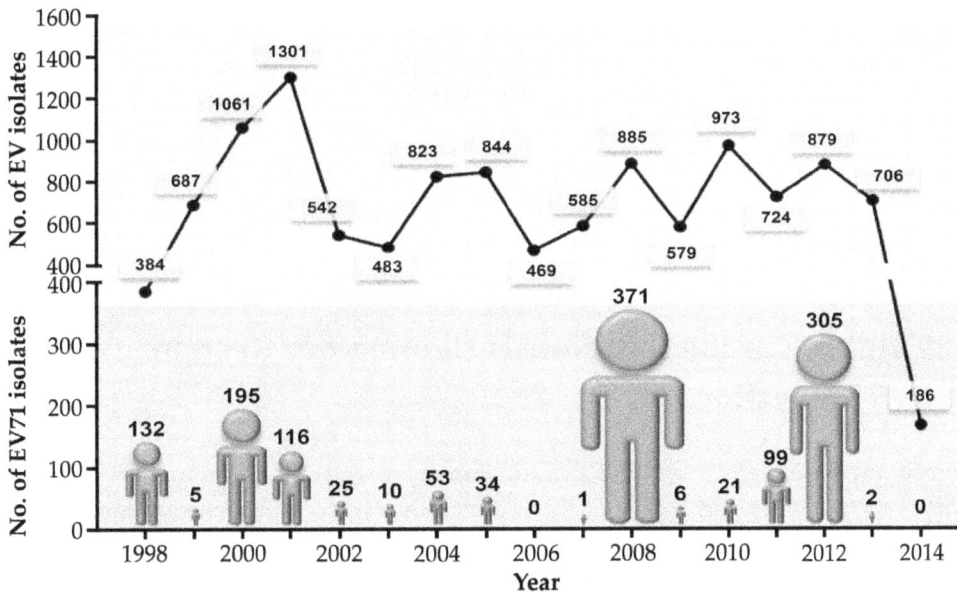

Figure 3: Yearly distribution of enteroviruses and enterovirus 71 isolates of National Cheng Kung University Hospital, Tainan, Taiwan, 1998-2014.

3   Pathogenesis of Complicated EV71 Brain Stem Encephalitis

Both innate and adaptive immune mechanisms are important for host defense against viral infection. The innate immune system provides the first line of defense against virus by activation of adaptive immunity through antigen presentation as well as secretion of pro-inflammatory cytokines. The pathogenesis of PE and hemorrhage in EV71 infections has been studied, with some important findings. Destruction of vasomotor and respiratory centers in the medial, ventral, and caudal medulla by EV71 leads to

ANS dysregulation and PE. It is similar to that observed in bulbar poliomyelitis, produces sympathetic hyperactivity, with surge catecholamine and autonomic dysfunction (Wang *et al.*, 2003; Kao *et al.*, 2004). Abundant catecholamines and strong central nervous system (CNS) inflammatory responses aggravate cytokine storm and pulmonary vascular permeability, causing PE. Catecholamines are among the neurotransmitters that affect immune responses humorally through circulating epinephrine, as well as locally through neuronal release of norepinephrine (NE) (Haskó, 2001). Plasma concentrations of NE and epinephrine (EP) were significantly higher in EV71-infected patients with ANS dysregulation and PE than they were in EV71-infected patients merely with uncomplicated BE. Both α1A- and β2-adrenergic receptors were expressed on A549, RD, SK-N-SH, HL-60, THP-1, Jurkat cells and hPBMCs. NE and EP treatment elevated the percentages of EV71-infected cells in THP-1 and Jurkat cells. α- and β-blockers reduced the percentages of EV71-infected cells with NE or EP treatment. NE and EP may play a role in the pathogenesis of EV71 BE complicated with ANS dysregulation and PE. IL-6 production was enhanced in EV71-infected hPBMCs at a concentration of 10^2 pg/mL NE (Liao *et al.*, 2015). Local release of neuroendocrine mediators coupled with specific receptor expression in immune cells establishes a functional neuroimmune connection capable of modulating various responses, including cytokine production. The excessive sympathetic activation plays a vital role in the pathogenesis and the progression from EV71 BE to PE.

4   Cytokine in the Systemic Inflammatory Response of EV71 Infection

There is increasing evidence that pro-inflammatory and anti-inflammatory cytokines may play a central role in EV71 BE. PE might be the result of increased pulmonary vascular permeability caused by the brain stem lesions and/or a systemic inflammatory response syndrome produced by the release of cytokines and chemokines. The clinical presentation of EV71 PE is caused by a hyperinflammatory syndrome resulting from hypercytokinemia and central nervous system inflammation of various inflammatory mediators. Some studies have shown that pro-inflammatory cytokines (interleukin [IL]-6, tumor necrosis factor [TNF]-α, and IL-1β) are associated with BE that is complicated by PE (Lin *et al.*, 2002; Lin *et al.*, 2003). A significant elevation of plasma IL-10, IL-13, and interferon (IFN)-γ levels are observed in patients with PE (Wang *et al.*, 2003). CD4[+] and CD8[+] T cell, and NK cells were depleted in patients with PE. The depletion of CD4[+] and CD8[+] T cell subsets and NK cells may cause the release of specific cytokines, contributed to the immunopathogenesis of EV71 BE. Human P-selectin glycoprotein ligand-1 (PSGL-1; CD162), a sialomucin membrane protein expressed on leukocytes that has a major role in early stages of inflammation, tethering and rolling of leukocytes on vascular endothelium, was proved as a functional receptor for EV71 infection (Nishimura *et al.*, 2009).The interaction of EV71 with PSGL-1 on lymphocytes may induce production of the inflammatory cytokines involved in BE with PE (Patel & Bergelson, 2009). In an animal study, monkeys were intravenously inoculated with cDNA-derived PSGL-1-

binding (EV71-02363-EG) and PSGL-1-nonbinding (EV71-02363-KE) strains of EV71, respectively. Mild neurological symptoms, transient lymphocytopenia, and inflammatory cytokine responses, were found predominantly in the 02363-KE-inoculated monkeys. In general, cytokine responses were more evident in 02363-KE-inoculated monkeys than those in EG-inoculated monkeys (Kataoka *et al.*, 2015).Mononuclear phagocytic cells are the most important source of IL-6; however, IL-6 is also produced by T and B lymphocytes and numerous other cells (Akira *et al.*, 1993). Elevated plasma level of IL-6 was detected in EV71-infected patient with ANS dysregulation, the priming stage of PE (Wang *et al.*, 2006). The IL-1β, IL-6 and TNF-α levels in fatal patients with encephalitis plus PE were significantly higher than those of uncomplicated patients. Elevated IL-6 may represent the net effect of IL-1β and TNF-α biological actions. IL-6 > 70 pg/ml was suggest as the best predictor of EV71 encephalitis with PE (Lin *et al.*, 2002; Lin *et al.*, 2003).

EV71 infection significantly increased the release of IL-6 from dendritic cells (Lin *et al.*, 2009). IL-6 and T cells are shown to reduce mortality of EV71-infected mice by reducing tissue viral loads in a previous study (Lin *et al.*, 2009). However, Khong and coworkers reported that administration of anti-IL-6 neutralizing antibodies, at day 3 or 6 post-infection, after the onset of the clinical symptoms successfully improved the survival rates and clinical scores of the EV71 infected mice (Khong *et al.*, 2011). Compared to untreated infected controls, anti-IL-6-treated mice displayed reduced tissue damage, absence of splenic atrophy, increased CD4+, CD8+ T cells and B cells activation and markedly elevated systemic levels of IL-10. Further, the anti-IL-6 antibody-mediated protection is independent of the virus load. These findings are justified in treating EV71-infected patients complicated with ANS dysregulation with intravenous immunoglobulin (IVIG) (Lin *et al.*, 2009). However, anti-IL-6 treatment at the time of infection is detrimental to the mice. It means that IL-6 production is beneficial to the host early post-infection to trigger the antiviral host response through attraction of various immune cells; however, sustained high levels of IL-6 may cause tissue damage and immunopathology.

IL-10 initially described as a product of Th2 cells that inhibited cytokine synthesis in Th1 cells. It has emerged as an important immunoregulatory cytokine with multiple biologic effects known to be sourced principally from monocytes/macrophages, dendritic cells, CD4+, CD8+ and Treg lymphocytes during or shortly after antigen presentation (Duell *et al.*, 2012). IL-10 can both impede pathogen clearance and ameliorate immunopathology. Numerous human viral pathogens have been shown to induce IL-10 in various studies. IL-10 was significantly higher in EV71-infected patients with PE than in those with ANS dysregulation or uncomplicated BE (Wang *et al.*, 2003). A close relationship exists between catecholamine and IL-10 release (Grilli *et al.*, 2000). Systemic IL-10 release triggered by sympathetic activation may be an important neuroimmunological mechanism contributing to immunodepression after injury and stress. Woiciechowsky and coworker showed surge of systemic IL-10 and immunodepression closely dependent on brain stem involvement and sympathetic activation (Woiciechowsky *et al.*, 1998). IL-10 can be modulated in several acute and chronic neuropathological conditions. This suggests that IL-10 plays a role in the immune-regulatory functions of the CNS. Thus, the systemic IL-10 increase in patients with PE appears to be triggered by persistent sympathetic activation as a consequence of direct brain stem destruction by the virus. IL-10 inhibits production of several pro-inflammatory mediators, including IL-1, IL-6, IL-8, granulocyte colony stimulating factor and TNF-α, and upregulates the expression of the naturally occurring IL-1 receptor antagonist (Duell et al., 2012). In an animal study of EV71 infection, anti-IL-6 treatment resulted in dramatically increased IL-10/IL-6 ratios, reflecting the upregulation of IL-10 production in the treated animals. Therefore, upregulation of IL-10 likely helped balance between pro-inflammatory and anti-inflammatory cytokines and subsequent tissue damage (Khong et al., 2011). Furthermore, low levels of IL-10 in the bronchoalveolar lavage fluid of patients with acute respiratory distress syndrome were associated with a poor prognosis (Donnelly et al., 1996). Upregulated IL-10 levels may have a protective effect in the development of PE by influencing the pulmonary capillary permeability. IL-10 may play a double-edged role, appears to function as both sword and shield in the response to EV71 infection in the pathogenesis of PE (Wang et al., 2003).

Interferon (IFN)-γ plays a central role in the immune response against infection. IFN-γ, a pleiotropic cytokine, is secreted by both cells of the innate immune system (NK cells, $\gamma\delta$ T-cells) and the adaptive immune system (CD8+ T cells and Th1 CD4+ T cells). NK cells and $\gamma\delta$ T cells provide early sources of IFN-γ during infection (Boehm et al., 1997). Elevated plasma levels of IFN-γ in patients with uncomplicated BE and PE was found. Moreover, the kinetic analysis in patients with PE showed that the production of IFN-γ occurred 24 h after IL-10 production. Increased pulmonary vascular permeability may play a pivotal role in PE. IFN-γ can exhibit enhanced vascular permeability (Martin et al., 1988). IFN-γ-mediated microvascular leakage occurs as a result of the reduced endothelial barrier and tight junction (Corada et al., 1999). IL-10 is a cytokine synthesis inhibitor that will terminate the production of IFN-γ. IFN-γ production appeared later than that of IL-10 in PE patients, which suggests that IFN-γ might play an important role in the development of PE. Recently, IFN-γ was found to be significantly elevated in infected AG129 mice, which lack type I and II interferon receptors, are susceptible to infection with a non-mouse-adapted EV71 strain via both the intraperitoneal and oral routes. The defect in IFN signaling may lead to some compensatory changes in the pattern of immune responses, which implies this model may not accurately reflect the immunopathogenesis seen in immunocompetent patients (Khong et al., 2012). Liao and colleagues demonstrated that the IFN-γ receptor is likely to be critical for protection from EV71 induced paralysis and death by using an IFN-γ receptor knockout (ifngr KO) mouse model. ifngr KO mice, defective only in IFN-γ, not in IFN-α, displayed paralysis and death rates around 80% (Liao et al., 2014). Severe EV71-infected patients with PE have lower numbers of peripheral circulating leukocytes, including natural killer (NK) cells, CD4+ and CD8+ T cells, in comparison with patients of mild disease (Wang et al., 2003). Whereas, invariant natural killer T (iNKT) cells are a distinct subpopulation of T cells that express an invariant $\alpha\beta$ T cell receptor (TCR) and share many cell surface markers in common with NK cells. NK and iNKT cells both produced IFN-γ after mouse-adaptive EV71 infection. Zhu et al. display that EV71 infection primarily activates iNKT cells, and in return, presumably promotes the activation of NK cells. The mouse-adaptive EV71-infected macrophages dramatically induced IFN-γ production by iNKT cells (Zhu *et al.*, 2015).

Polymorphism of some inflammatory mediators associated with the complications and disease severity. Yang et al. reported that IFN-γ + 874 A allele and IL-10-1082 A allele was observed with significantly higher frequency in patients with EV71 encephalitis compared with HFMD patients without complications (Yang *et al.*, 2012). Macrophages, NK cells, dendritic cells and fibroblasts were reported to produce IFN-I (α and β) in response to viral infection or exposure to other microbial pathogens. The early induction and action of IFN-I result in cellular resistance to viral infection, inhibition of viral replication and impediment of viral dissemination (Samuel, 2001). Liu and coworkers showed that polyriboinosinic : polyribocytidylic acid [poly(I : C)], a potent IFN inducer, improved the survival rate and decreased the tissue viral titers after EV71 challenge, which correlated with an increase serum concentration of IFN-α, the percentage of dendritic cells, the expression of major histocompatibility complex class II molecule and IFN-α in spleen of mice (Liu *et al.*, 2005). Type I IFNs represent an essential innate defense mechanism for controlling EV71 infection in mice.

IL-13 is a T-helper type 2 (Th2) cytokine produced predominantly by Th2-polarized CD4+ T cells that has potential anti-inflammatory activity and suppresses the cytotoxic functions of monocytes/macrophages (de Vries *et al.*, 1999). Patients with PE were found to have higher IL-13 levels than those with uncomplicated BE (Wang *et al.*, 2003). High levels of IL-13, which are affected by endogenous IL-4 and required for airway hyper-responsiveness and mucus production, are found in patients with asthma and atopic dermatitis (Brightling *et al.*, 2010). Plasma level of IL-4 was not changed in EV71-infected patients, but IL-13 levels were consistently elevated in all groups, uncomplicated BE, ANS dysregulation and PE. Though IL-13 and IL-4 have partially overlapping effector profiles, that IL-13 may be the more important mediator of the effector at sites of Th2-induced inflammation. IL-13 can act alone in the pulmonary models, overproduction of IL-13 might contribute to the pathogenesis of PE by increasing pulmonary vascular permeability (Wills-Karp, 2004). Further, IL-13 can facilitate the selective recruitment of inflammatory cells from the bloodstream and induces the expression of a myriad of chemokines (Wills-Karp, 2004). Huang and coworkers showed exogenous treatment of IL-6, IL-13, and IFN-γ at day 3 after intracranial infection could induce mild PE and exacerbate pulmonary abnormality of EV71-infected mice. A synergistic pro-inflammatory cytokine responses and damage to specific brain regions may be necessary for the development of EV71-induced PE (Huang *et al.*, 2011). IL-13 upregulation is associated with severe disease of EV71 infection.

Chemokines, a group of small (8-12 kd) proteins, are key regulators of leukocyte migration and involve in numerous aspects of cell growth, differentiation, and activation. Chemokines are distinguished from other cytokines by their ability to act on the superfamily of G-protein-coupled serpentine receptors. Chemokines are classified as homeostatic/constitutive (developmentally regulated) or inducible (inflammatory) by the contexts in which they function. Chemokines are characterized by the presence of 3 to 4 conserved cysteine residues and can be subdivided into 4 families, CC, CXC, CX3C and XC family, based on the positioning of the N-terminal cysteine residues (Rot A &

von Andrian, 2004).

IL-8 was identified as a neutrophil-specific chemotactic factor and later classified as a member of the CXC chemokine family. The major effector functions of IL-8 are activation and recruitment of neutrophils to the site of infection or injury (Kunkel *et al.*, 1991). Patients with ANS dysregulation had higher plasma levels of IL-8 than patients with PE. IL-8 and other cytokines have been proposed to induce alterations in pulmonary permeability. IL-8 is considered the main neutrophil chemoattractant in acute respiratory distress syndrome (ARDS). The levels of IL-8 in ARDS pulmonary edema aspirates and bronchoalveolar lavage fluid (BALF) also correlate with survival and disease severity, as IL-8 levels are lower in survivors compared with nonsurvivors (Baughman *et al.*, 1996). This might account for the elevation of IL-8 in EV71-infected patients with ANS dysregulation and PE. In animal models of acute lung injury, neutralizing IL-8 reduced the severity of lung inflammation and tissue damage (Sekido *et al.*, 1993). Treatment of the rabbits that showed extensive edema in the alveolar lumina with a humanized anti-IL-8 antibody prevented neutrophil infiltration in the lung in association with alleviated acute lung injury syndrome (Bao *et al.*, 2010). These studies provide important information regarding the role that IL-8 play in the pathogenesis of EV71 infection complicated with PE. Because of the known increased expression of IFN-γ in Th1 diseases in children with EV71-associated BE, IFN-γ-induced protein-10 (CXCL10/IP-10), monokine induced by IFN-γ (CXCL9/MIG), and IFN-inducible T cell α chemoattractant were studied. Plasma levels of IP-10, monocyte chemoattractant protein (MCP)-1, and MIG were significantly higher in patients with PE than in those with uncomplicated BE (Wang *et al.*, 2008). IP-10 is recognized as a biomarker that predicts severity of various diseases. IP-10 expression also can be up-regulated by the Th1 cytokine IFN-γ during acute lung inflammation. This is consistent with previous findings that both circulating IFN-γ (Wang *et al.*, 2003) and IP-10 levels were increased in patients with EV71 PE. MCP-1 in the systemic inflammatory response has been suggested. The concentration of MCP-1 has been shown to increase in the plasma of patients with persistent ARDS (Puneet *et al.*, 2005). This may provide an explanation for the increased in MCP levels in plasma when the disease progresses from uncomplicated BE to PE. MIG plays a role in host defense after viral infection (Salazar-Mather *et al.*, 2000). Increased level of MIG in patients with EV71 PE supports the notion that MIG contributes to host defense by promoting a protective Th1 response. Overexpression of the chemokine cascade in the systemic compartment appears to play an important role in the elicitation of the immune response to EV71. Pre-existing antibodies may play a critical role in controlling viral infection or in aggregating the disease severity. Mice that received subneutralizing anti-EV71 IgG before EV71 administration had significantly high serum levels of IFN-γ and monocyte chemoattractant protein-1 (MCP-1) (Chen *et al.*, 2013). These findings support the concept that subneutralizing antibodies directed enhance some cytokines and chemokines production in EV71 infection through antibody-dependent enhancement (ADE) of infectivity pathway in newborn mice model. IL-17A, is a pro-inflammatory cytokine that plays an essential role in host defense against microbial infections and is implicated in various inflammatory conditions. Chen and coworkers reported high expression of acid-related orphan nuclear receptor gamma t (ROR t) in peripheral blood mononuclear cells and elevated serum concentrations of IL-17 and IL-23 of EV71 infections. Further, the frequencies of Th17 cells in blood from EV71-infected children were significantly higher in comparison with controls (Chen *et al.*, 2012).

5   Cytokine in Central Nervous System of EV71 Infection

Cytokines are constitutively expressed in the CNS. Normally, the cellular expression of cytokines in the CNS is highly integrated and under tight regulatory control. However, in certain pathological conditions, cytokine production may become spatially and temporally dysregulated, leading to inappropriate production. Although the blood-brain barrier (BBB) is relatively impermeable to cytokines owing to their size and hydrophilicity, in EV71 BE the integrity of the BBB may be compromised permitting cytokine action within the CNS. The neuroinflammatory cascade activated in response to EV71 BE is mediated by the release of pro- and anti-inflammatory cytokines and chemokines, and the primary source of these inflammatory mediators is in the brain. In the inflammatory process of echovirus 30 meningitis, cytokine network shifts from production of pro-inflammatory cytokines (IL-6, IL-8, and IFN-γ) to that of anti-inflammatory cytokines (IL-10 and TGF-β1) during or after the period when the virus is eliminated from the cerebrospinal cavity (Sato *et al.*, 2003).

Lin and coworkers examined the relationship between level of IL-6 in the cerebrospinal fluid (CSF) and the CNS involvement of EV71 infection (Lin *et al.*, 2003). The median CSF level of IL-6 was significantly higher during the first or second day of CNS involvement. Whereas, CSF levels of IL-6 were not significantly different among EV71-infected patients with different clinical syndromes, PE, encephalitis and/or poliomyelitis-like syndrome and aseptic meningitis during the acute stage of CNS involvement (Lin *et al.*, 2003). However, another study demonstrated the mean CSF concentrations of IL-6 were elevated significantly in children with PE, and ANS dysregulation as compared to children with uncomplicated BE (Wang *et al.*, 2007). The CSF concentrations of IL-6 were elevated by the diseases severity of EV71 infection. The source of IL-6 appears to be the brain, since CSF levels of IL-6 exceed those in plasma. This suggests that IL-6 may contribute to the overwhelming disease process.

Children with EV71 ANS dysregulation or PE had higher IFN-γ levels in CSF than those with isolated BE and echovirus meningitis. This suggests that IFN-γ is responding maximally to severe infection (Wang *et al.*, 2007). IFN-γ is not normally present in the brain parenchyma. IFN-γ appears to promote gliosis and inflammation by its effect on astrocytes. Inflammation protects the brain from infection, but it aggravates injury. This suggests a detrimental effect of IFN-γ on the CNS (Olsson *et al.*, 1994).

IL-1 activates microglia and vascular endothelial cells to recruit peripheral leukocytes and produce neuroinflammation. Elevated IL-1β levels were found only in the CSF and not in the plasma of EV71-infected patients with PE (Wang *et al.*, 2007). Hosoi et al. found increased levels of IL-1β mRNA in the brain in the absence of an increase in circulating IL-1β in rats (Hosoi *et al.*, 2000). These findings support the notion that IL-1β is probably synthesized in the CNS in response to severe EV71 infection. IL-1 can also regulate neurotransmission mediated by amines such as NE and dopamine. The activity of the locus ceruleus, which is the most important source of NE inside the brain, was increased after in vivo IL-1β microinjection in this area; this effect was blocked by IL-1β receptor antagonist (Borsody & Weiss, 2002-2003). This may provide explanation of elevated of IL-1β level in CSF of PE patients, following the stage of ANS dysregulation.

IP-10 and its receptor, CXCR3, are expressed by the CNS and by CNS infiltrating lymphocytes, respectively, only in patients with ongoing CNS inflammation, suggesting an important role for these molecules in the pathogenic process. Increased IP-10 concentration in CSF in patients with enteroviral meningitis was observed (Lahrtz et al., 1998). CSF levels of IP-10 and IL-8 in patients with EV71 BE were significantly higher than the plasma levels in the control subjects (Wang et al., 2008). IP-10 is prominently expressed within the CNS of mice with viral encephalitis (Asensio & Campbell, 1997). Early expression of IP-10 within the CNS after virus infection is important in initiating and maintaining a protective Th1 immune response. This is characterized by high level production of the antiviral cytokine IFN-γ (Asensio & Campbell, 1997; Hoffman et al., 1999). Early expression of IP-10 appears to be beneficial by attracting Th1 T lymphocytes into the CNS, which participate in viral clearance. Shen and colleagues showed that IP-10 deficiency significantly reduced serum levels of MIG, and levels of IFN-γ and the number of CD8 T cells in the mouse brain. Absence of IP-10 significantly increased the mortality of infected mice by 45 %, along with decrease virus clearance in several vital tissues in IP-10 gene knockout mice (Shen et al., 2013).

CSF levels of MIG to be significantly more elevated in patients with EV71 PE than in those with EV71 ANS dysregulation and uncomplicated BE. The CSF to plasma ratio for MIG tended to increase with increasing severity of disease (Wang et al., 2008). In a study of murine brain endothelial cells, MIG was induced following treatment with a cytokine cocktail containing IFN-γ, TNF-α and IL-1β (Ghersa et al., 2002). The coordinate regulation of IP-10 and MIG was mediated by IFN-γ in cultured murine astrocytes and microglia (Carter et al., 2007). This may bolster the previous findings, the increased CSF level of MIG may relate to the increased CSF level of IL-1β and IFN-γ in patients with PE.

6   Modulation of Systemic Inflammatory Response of EV71 Infection

IVIG is a polyclonal immunoglobulin derived from large pools of human serum. IVIG are used not only in replacement therapy in immunodeficient individuals who are unable to mount their own effective immune responses, but also constitute a therapeutic option in patients with autoimmunity. IVIG is being used as a therapeutic modality (in doses higher than for replacement therapy) in certain bacterial or viral infectious diseases. Advantages for IVIG treatment has been demonstrated in patients with sepsis syndrome associated with systemic inflammatory immune responses and organ damage, presumably mediated via an anti-inflammatory effect (Turgeon et al., 2007). The plausible mechanisms of action of IVIG that have been reported to cause an amelioration of inflammatory processes include interaction with Fc receptors, induction of apoptosis, blockade of co-stimulatory molecules, interference with the cytokine network, and neutralization of pathogenic antibodies (Elovaara & Hietaharju, 2010).

IVIG has been used prophylactically and therapeutically against neonatal enterovirus infections and in immunocompromised hosts (Abzug *et al.*, 1995). IVIG injection decreases plasma catecholamines in coxsackievirus B3 myocarditis, suggesting that immunoglobulin exerts its cardioprotective effect through sympathetic modulating actions (Kishimoto *et al.*, 2000). There is considerable evidence linking cytokine-mediated severe systemic inflammatory responses to PE and other the adverse outcomes in patients with EV71-associated BE (Lin *et al.*, 2002; Wang *et al.*, 2003; Wang *et al.*, 2007). Modulating cytokine expression by IVIG may offer a strategy for clinical practice. A previous study demonstrated a decrease in the plasma concentration of IL-6, IL-8, IL-10, IL-13, and IFN-γ following administration of IVIG in patient with ANS dysregulation and PE (Wang *et al.*, 2006). These changes may be responsible for the rapid improvement in symptoms in some treated patients. Patient with ANS dysregulation is the critical timing to receive IVIG infusion. It is possible that a more favorable survival might have been obtained by modulating cytokine storm and reducing sympathetic activity.

Without milrinone treatment, patients with PE have a fatality rate as high as 80-90%. Most patient fatalities occurred within 6-12 hours without prompt care. Milrinone, a bipyridine phosphodiesterase (PDE) III inhibitor, is a member of both inotropic and vasodilatation characters. Milrinone increases cardiac output, and reduces systemic vascular resistance and pulmonary capillary wedge pressure without excessive increases in myocardial oxygen consumption (Shipley *et al.*, 1996). Inhibition of cyclic adenosine 3′, 5′-monophosphate (cAMP) degradation by intracellular PDE3 may attenuate inflammation, reduce edema formation, improve endothelial function and induce pulmonary vasodilation (Hayashida *et al.*, 1999). A pilot study was designed to evaluate the potential therapeutic effect of milrinone in the treatment of patients with EV71-induced PE (Wang *et al.*, 2005). The mortality was lower in the milrinone-treated than non-treated group. Sympathetic tachycardia, white blood cell and platelet counts were decreased. There was a significant decrease in plasma level of IL-13 in milrinone-treated patients compared to controls. The effectiveness and efficacy of milrinone treatment in patients with EV71-related PE has been proven in historically controlled (Wang *et al.*, 2005) and randomized controlled studies (Chi *et al.*, 2013). Milrinone therapy not only increased the expression frequency of CD4$^+$Foxp3$^+$in severe EV71 infection but also reduced the plasma levels of cytokines, IL-6, IL-8 and IL-10. Plasma concentrations of cAMP were significantly decreased in patients with ANS dysregulation or PE compared with patients with HFMD or BE; however, cAMP levels increased after milrinone treatment (Wang *et al.*, 2014). Milrinone therapy provides a useful therapeutic approach for treating life threatening EV71 infections.

7   Conclusions

The production of inflammatory cytokines and chemokines is a unique aspect of the immune responses in the CNS and systemic arms to EV71infection. Cytokines and chemokines released by EV71 infected immune cells contribute directly or indirectly to the disease severity. IVIG and milrinone treatment represents an appropriate approach to the inflammatory responses elicited by severe EV71 infection. Alternative modalities for controlling the cytokine network have been explored experimentally. A better understanding of the fundamental mechanisms and the engaged inflammatory signal-transduction pathways of the cytokines production will be expected to be of value in the treatment of inflammatory responses of EV71 infection.

Acknowledgments

This study was supported by grants from the National Science Council, Taiwan (NSC 101-2314-B-006-014-MY3), Ministry of Science and Technology, Taiwan (MOST 104-2321-B-006-016, MOST 105-2321-B-006-008), and Center of Infectious Disease and Signaling Research, National Cheng Kung University, Taiwan. We thank Ms. Yu-Ting Liao for secretarial assistance.

References

Abzug, M. J., Keyserling, H. L., Lee, M. L., Levin, & M. J., Rotbart, H. A. (1995). Neonatal enterovirus infection: virology, serology, and effects of immune globulin. Clinical Infectious Diseases, 20, 1201–1206.

Akira, S., Taga, T., & Kishimoto, T. (1993). Interleukin-6 in biology and medicine. Advances in Immunology, 54, 1–78.

Asensio, V. C. & Campbell, I. L. (1997). Chemokine gene expression in the brains of mice with lymphocytic choriomeningitis. Journal of Virology, 71, 7832–7840.

Bao, Z., Ye, Q., Gong, W., Xiang, Y., & Wan, H. (2010). Humanized monoclonal antibody against the chemokine CXCL-8 (IL-8) effectively prevents acute lung injury. International Immuno-pharmacology, 10, 259–263.

Baughman, R. P., Gunther, K. L., Rashkin, M. C., Keeton, D. A., & Pattishall, E. N. (1996). Changes in the inflammatory response of the lung during acute respiratory distress syndrome: prognostic indicators. American Journal of Respiratory and Critical Care Medicine, 154, 76–81.

Boehm, U., Klamp, T., Groot, M., & Howard, J. L. (1997). Cellular responses to interferon-gamma. Annual Review of Immunology,15, 749-795.

Borsody, M. K. & Weiss, J. M. (2002–2003). Alteration of locus coeruleus neuronal activity by interleukin-1 and the involvement of endogenous corticotrophin-releasing hormone. Neuroimmuno-modulation, 10, 101–121.

Brightling, C. E., Saha, S., & Hollins, F. (2010). Interleukin-13: prospects for new treatments. Clinical and Experimental Allergy, 40, 42–49.

Cameron, M. J., Bermejo-Martin, J. F., Danesh, A., Muller, M. P., & Kelvin, D. J. (2008). Human immunopathogenesis of severe acute respiratory syndrome (SARS). Virus Research, 133, 13–19.

Canna, S. W. & Behrens, E. M. (2012). Making sense of the cytokine storm: a conceptual framework for understanding, diagnosing, and treating hemophagocytic syndromes. Pediatric Clinics of North America, 59, 329–344.

Carter, S. L., Müller, M., Manders, P. M., & Campbell, I. L. (2007). Induction of the genes for Cxcl9 and Cxcl10 is dependent on IFN-gamma but shows differential cellular expression in experimental autoimmune encephalomyelitis and by astrocytes and microglia in vitro. Glia, 55, 1728–1739.

Chang, L. Y., Lin, T. Y., Hsu, K. H., Huang, Y. C., Lin, K. L., Hsueh, C., Shih, S. R., Ning, H. C., Hwang, M. S., Wang, H. S., & Lee, C. Y. (1999). Clinical features and risk factors of pulmonary edema after enterovirus 71-related hand, foot, and mouth diseases. Lancet, 354, 1682–1686.

Chen, I. C., Wang, S. M., Yu, C. K., & Liu, C. C. (2013). Subneutralizing antibodies to enterovirus 71 induce antibody-dependent enhancement of infection in newborn mice. Medical Microbiology and Immunology, 202, 259–265.

Chen, J., Tong, J., Liu, H., Liu, Y., Su, Z., Wang, S., Shi, Y., Zheng, D., Sandoghchian, S., Geng, J., & Xu, H. (2012). Increased frequency of Th17 cells in the peripheral blood of children infected with enterovirus 71. Journal of Medical Virology, 84, 763–767.

Chi, C. Y., Khanh, T. H., Thoa, le. P. K., Tseng, F. C., Wang, S. M., Thinh, le. Q., Lin, C. C., Wu, H. C., Wang, J. R., Hung, N. T., Thuong, T. C., Chang, C. M., Su, I. J., & Liu, C. C. (2013). Milrinone therapy for enterovirus 71-induced pulmonary edema and/or neurogenic shock in children: a randomized controlled trial. Critical Care Medicine, 41, 1754–1760.

Corada, M., Mariotti, M., Thurston, G., Smith, K., Kunkel, R., Brockhaus, M., Lampugnani, M. G., Martin-Padura, I., Stoppacciaro, A., Ruco, L., McDonald, D. M., Ward, P. A., & Dejana, E. (1999). Vascular endothelial-cadherin is an important determinant of microvascular integrity in vivo. Proceedings of the National Academy of Sciences of the United States of America, 96, 9815–9820.

de Vries, J. E. (1999). The role of IL-13 and its receptor in allergy and inflammatory responses. The Journal of Allergy and Clinical Immunology, 102, 165–169.

Dinarello, C. A. (1997). Proinflammatory and anti-inflammatory cytokines as mediators in the pathogenesis of septic shock. Chest, 112, suppl. 321S–329S.

Donnelly, S. C., Strieter, R. M., Reid, P. T., Kunkel, S. L., Burdick, M. D., Armstrong, I., Mackenzie, A., & Haslett, C. (1996). The association between mortality rates and decreased concentrations of interleukin-10 and interleukin-1 receptor antagonist in the lung fields of patients with the adult respiratory distress syndrome. Annals of International Medicine, 125, 191–196.

Duell, B. L., Tan, C. K., Carey, A. J., Wu, F., Cripps, A. W., & Ulett, G. C. (2012). Recent insights into microbial triggers of interleukin-10 production in the host and the impact on infectious disease pathogenesis. FEMS Immunology and Medical Microbiology, 64, 295–313.

Elovaara, I. & Hietaharju, A. (2010). Can we face the challenge of expanding use of intravenous immunoglobulin in neurology? Acta Neurologica Scandinavica, 122, 309–315.

Ghersa, P., Gelati, M., Colinge, J., Feger, G., Power, C., Papoian, R., & Salmaggi, A. (2012). MIG — differential gene expression in mouse brain endothelial cells. Neuroreport, 13, 9–14.

Grilli, M., Barbieri, I., Basudev, H., Brusa, R., Casati, C., Lozza, G., & Ongini, E. (2000). Interleukin-10 modulates neuronal threshold of vulnerability to ischemic damage. The Europe Journal of Neuroscience, 12, 2265–2272.

Haskó, G. (2001). Receptor-mediated interaction between the sympathetic nervous system and immune system in inflammation. Neurochemical Research, 26, 1039–1044.

Hayashida, N., Tomoeda, H., Oda, T., Tayama, E., Chihara, S., Kawara, T., & Aoyagi, S. (1999). Inhibitory effect of milrinone on cytokine production after cardiopulmonary bypass. The Annals of Thoracic Surgery, 68, 1661–1667.

Ho, M., Chen, E. R., Hsu, K. H., Twu, S. J., Chen, K. T., Tsai, S. F., Wang, J. R., & Shih, S. R. (1999). An epidemic of enterovirus 71 infection in Taiwan. The New England Journal of Medicine, 341, 929–935.

Hoffman, L. M., Fife, B. T., Begolka, W. S., Miller, S. D., & Karpus, W. J. (1999). Central nervous system chemokine expression during Theiler's virus-induced demyelinating disease. Journal of Neurovirology, 5, 635–642.

Hosoi, T., Yasunobu, O., & Nomura, Y. (2000). Electrical stimulation of afferent vagus nerve induce IL-1β expression in the brain and activates HPA axis. American Journal of Physiology Regulatory Integrative and Comparative Physiology, 279, R141–R147.

Hsiung, G. D. & Wang, J. R. (2000). Enterovirus infection with special reference to enterovirus 71. Journal of Microbiology, Immunology and Infection, 33, 1–8.

Huang, C. C., Liu, C. C., Chang, Y. C., Chen, C. Y., Wang, S. T., & Yeh, T. F. (1999). Neurologic complications in children with enterovirus 71 infection. The New England Journal of Medicine, 342, 936–942.

Huang, M. C., Wang, S. M., Hsu, Y. W., Lin, H. C., Chi, C. Y., & Liu, C. C. (2006). Long-term cognitive and motor deficits following enterovirus 71 brainstem encephalitis in children. Pediatrics, 118, e1785–e1788.

Huang, S. W., Lee, Y. P., Hung, Y. T., Lin, C. H., Chuang, J. I., Lei, H. Y., Su, I. J., & Yu, C. K. (2011). Exogenous interleukin-6, interleukin-13, and interferon-gamma provoke pulmonary abnormality with mild edema in enterovirus 71-infected mice. Respiratory Research, 12, 147.

Kao, S. J., Yang, F. L., Hsu, Y. H., & Chen, H. I. (2004). Mechanism of fulminant pulmonary edema caused by enterovirus 71. Clinical Infectious Diseases, 38, 1784–1788.

Kataoka, C., Suzuki, T., Kotani, O., Iwata-Yoshikawa, N., Nagata, N., Ami, Y., Wakita, T., Nishimura, Y., & Shimizu, H. (2015). The role of VP1 amino acid residue 145 of enterovirus 71 in viral fitness and pathogenesis in a cynomolgus monkey model. PLoS Pathogens, 11, e1005033.

Khong, W. X., Foo, D. G., Trasti, S. L., Tan, E. L., & Alonso, S. (2011). Sustained high levels of interleukin-6 contribute to the pathogenesis of enterovirus 71 in a neonate mouse model. Journal of Virology, 85, 3067–3076.

Khong, W. X., Yan, B., Yeo, H., Tan, E. L., Lee, J. J., Ng, J. K., Chow, V. T., & Alonso, S. (2012). A non-mouse-adapted enterovirus 71 (EV71) strain exhibits neurotropism, causing neurological manifestations in a novel mouse model of EV71 infection. Journal of Virology, 86, 2121–2131.

Kishimoto, C., Takamatsu, N., Kawamata, H., Shinohara, H., & Ochiai, H. (2000). Immunoglobulin treatment ameliorates murine myocarditis associated with reduction of neurohumoral activity and improvement of extracellular matrix change. Journal of the American College of Cardiology, 36, 1979–1984.

Kunkel, S. L., Standiford, T., Kasahara, K., & Strieter, R. M. (1991). Interleukin-8 (IL-8): the major neutrophil chemotactic factor in the lung. Experimental Lung Research, 17, 17–23.

Lahrtz, F., Piali, L., Spanaus, K. S., Seebach, J., & Fontana, A. (1998). Chemokines and chemotaxis of leukocytes in infectious meningitis. Journal of Neuroimmunology, 85, 33–43.

Lei, H. Y., Yeh, T. M., Liu, H. S., Lin, Y. S., Chen, S. H., & Liu, C. C. (2001). Immunopathogenesis of dengue virus. Journal of Biomedical Science, 8, 377–388.

Liao, C. C., Liou, A. T., Chang, Y. S., Wu, S. Y., Chang, C. S., Lee, C. K., Kung, J. T., Tu, P. H., Yu, Y. Y., Lin, C. Y., Lin, J. S., & Shih, C. (2014). Immunodeficient mouse models with different disease profiles by in vivo infection with the same clinical isolate of enterovirus 71. Journal of Virology, 88, 12485–12499.

Liao, Y. T., Wang, S. M., Wang, J. R., Yu, C. K., & Liu, C. C. (2015). Norepinephrine and epinephrine enhanced the infectivity of enterovirus 71. PLoS One, 10, e0135154.

Lin, T. Y., Hsia, S. H., Huang, Y. C., Wu, C. T., & Chang, L. Y. (2003). Proinflammatory cytokine reactions in enterovirus 71 infections of the central nervous system. Clinical Infectious Diseases, 36, 269–274.

Lin, T. Y., Chang, L. Y., Hsia, S. H., Huang, Y. C., Chiu, C. H., Hsueh, C., Shih, S. R., Liu, C. C., & Wu, M. H. (2002). The 1998 enterovirus 71 outbreak in Taiwan: Pathogenesis and management. Clinical Infectious Diseases, 34, suppl 2. S52–S57.

Lin, T. Y., Chang, L. Y., Huang, Y. C., Hsu, K. H., Chiu, C. H., & Yang, K. D. (2002). Different proinflammatory reactions in fatal and non-fatal enterovirus 71 infections: implications for early recognition and therapy. Acta Paediatrica, 91, 632–635.

Lin, Y. W., Chang, K. C., Kao, C. M., Chang, S. P., Tung, Y. Y., & Chen, S. H. (2009). Lymphocyte and antibody responses reduce enterovirus 71 lethality in mice by decreasing tissue viral loads. Journal of Virology, 83, 6477–6483.

Lin, Y. W., Wang, S. W., Tung, Y. Y., & Chen, S. H. (2009). Enterovirus 71 infection of human dendritic cells. Experimental Biology and Medicine (Maywood), 234, 1166–1173.

Liu, M. L., Lee, Y. P., Wang, Y. F., Lei, H. Y., Liu, C. C., Wang, S. M., Su, I. J., Wang, J. R., Yeh, T. M., Chen, S. H., & Yu, C. K. (2005). Type I interferons protect mice against enterovirus 71 infection. The Journal of General Virology, 86, 3263–3269.

Martin, S., Maruta, K., Burkart, V., Gillis, S., & Kolb, H. (1988). IL-1 and IFN-gamma increase vascular permeability. Immunology, 64, 301–305.

McMinn, P. C. (2002). An overview of the evolution of enterovirus 71 and its clinical and public health significance. FEMS Microbiology Reviews, 26, 91–107.

Nakane, A., Okamoto, M., Asano, M., Kohanawa, M., & Minagawa, T. (1995). Endogenous gamma interferon, tumor necrosis factor, and interleukin-6 in Staphylococcus aureus infection in mice. Infection and Immunity, 63, 1165–1172.

Nazinitsky, A. & Rosentha, K. S. (2010). Cytokine storms: systemic disasters of infectious diseases. Infectious Diseases in Clinical Practice, 18, 188–192.

Nishimura, Y., Shimojima, M., Tano, Y., Miyamura, T., Wakita, T., & Shimizu, H. (2009). Human P-selectin glycoprotein ligand-1 is a functional receptor for enterovirus 71. Nature Medicine, 15, 794–798.

Oda, S., Hirasawa, H., Shiga, H., Nakanishi, K., Matsuda, K., & Nakamura, M. (2005). Sequential measurement of IL-6 blood levels in patients with systemic inflammatory response syndrome (SIRS)/sepsis. Cytokine, 29, 169–175.

Olsson, T., Kelic, S., Edlund, C., Bakhiet, M., Höjeberg, B., van der Meide, P. H., Ljungdahl, A., & Kristensson, K. (1994). Neuronal interferon-γ immunoreactive molecule bioactivities and purification. European Journal of Immunology, 24, 308–314.

Ooi, M. H., Wong, S. C., Lewthwaite, P., Cardosa, M. J., & Solomon, T. (2010). Clinical features, diagnosis, and management of enterovirus 71. The Lancet neurology, 9, 1097–1105.

Patel, K. P. & Bergelson, J. M. (2009). *Receptors identified for hand, foot and mouth virus. Nature Medicine, 15, 728–729.*

Puneet, P., Moochhala, S., & Bhatiam M. (2005). *Chemokines in acute respiratory distress syndrome. American Journal of Physiology Lung Cellular and Molecular Physiology, 288, L3–L15.*

Rot, A. & von Andrian, U. H. (2004). *Chemokines in innate and adaptive host defense: basic chemokinese grammar for immune cells. Annual Review of Immunology, 22, 891–928.*

Salazar-Mather, T. P., Hamilton, T. A., & Biron, C. A. (2000). *A chemokine to cytokine to chemokine cascade critical in antiviral defense. The Journal of Clinical Investogation, 105, 985–993.*

Samuel, C. E. (2001). *Antiviral actions of interferons. Clinical Microbiology Reviews, 14, 778–809.*

Sato, M., Hosoya, M., Honzumi, K., Watanabe, M., Ninomiya, N., Shigeta, S., & Suzuki, H. (2003). *Cytokine and cellular inflammatory sequence in enteroviral meningitis. Pediatrics, 112, 1103–1107.*

Sekido, N., Mukaida, N., Harada, A., Nakanishi, I., Watanabe, Y., & Matsushima, K. (1993). *Prevention of lung reperfusion injury in rabbits by a monoclonal antibody against interleukin-8. Nature, 365, 654–657.*

Shen, F. H., Tsai, C. C., Wang, L. C., Chang, K. C., Tung, Y. Y., Su, I. J., & Chen, S. H. (2013). *Enterovirus 71 infection increases expression of interferon-gamma-inducible protein 10 which protects mice by reducing viral burden in multiple tissues. The Journal of General Virology, 94, 1019–1027.*

Shipley, J. B., Tolman, D., Hastillo, A., & Hess, M. L. (1996). *Milrinone: basic and clinical pharmacology and acute and chronic management. The American Journal of the Medical Sciences, 311, 286–291.*

Skoner, D. P., Gentile, D. A., Patel, A., & Doyle, W. J. (1999). *Evidence for cytokine mediation of disease expression in adults experimentally infected with influenza A virus. The Journal of Infectious Diseases, 180, 10–14.*

Solomon, T., Lewthwaite, P., Perera, D., Cardosa, M. J., McMinn, P., & Ooi, M. H. (2010). *Virology, epidemiology, pathogenesis, and control of enterovirus 71. The Lancet Infectious Diseases, 10, 778–790.*

Tisoncik, J. R., Korth, M. J., Simmons, C. P., Farrar, J., Martin, T. R., & Katze, M. G. (2012). *Into the eye of the cytokine storm. Microbiology and Molecular Biology Reviews, 76, 16–32.*

Turgeon, A. F., Hutton, B., Fergusson, D. A., McIntyre, L., Tinmouth, A. A., Cameron, D. W., & Hébert, P. C. (2007). *Meta-analysis: intravenous immunoglobulin in critically ill adult patients with sepsis. Annals of Internal Medicine, 146, 193–203.*

Wang, S. M., Chen, I. C., Liao, Y. T., & Liu, C. C. (2014). *The clinical correlation of regulatory T cells and cyclic adenosine monophosphate in enterovirus 71 infection. PLoS One, 9, e102025.*

Wang, S. M., Ho, T. S., Lin, H. C., Lei, H. Y., Wang, J. R., & Liu, C. C. (2012). *Reemerging of enterovirus 71 in Taiwan: the age impact on disease severity. European Journal of Clinical Microbiology & Infectious Diseases, 31, 1219–1224.*

Wang, S. M. & Liu, C. C. (2009). *Enterovirus 71: epidemiology, pathogenesis and management. Expert Review of Anti-Infective Therapy, 7, 735–742.*

Wang, S. M. & Liu, C. C. (2014). *Update of enterovirus 71: epidemiology, pathogenesis and vaccine. Expert Review of Anti-Infective Therapy, 12, 447–456.*

Wang, S. M., Ho, T. S., Shen, C. F, & Liu C. C. (2008). *Enterovirus 71, one virus and many stories. Pediatrics and Neonatology, 49, 113–115.*

Wang, S. M., Lei, H. Y., Huang, K. J., Wu, J. M., Wang, J. R., Yu, C. K., Su, I. J., & Liu, C. C. (2003). *Pathogenesis of enterovirus 71 brainstem encephalitis in pediatric patients: the roles of cytokines and cellular immune activation in patients with pulmonary edema. The Journal of Infectious Diseases, 188,* 564–570.

Wang, S. M., Lei, H. Y., Huang, M. C., Su, L. Y., Lin, H. C., Yu, C. K., Wang, J. L., & Liu, C. C. (2006). *Modulation of cytokine production by intravenous immunoglobulin in patients with enterovirus 71-associated brainstem encephalitis. Journal of Clinical Virology, 37,* 47–52.

Wang, S. M., Lei, H. Y., Huang, M. C., Wu, J. M., Chen, C. T., Wang, J. N., Wang, J. R., & Liu, C. C. (2005). *Therapeutic efficacy of milrinone in the management of enterovirus 71-induced pulmonary edema. Pediatric Pulmonology, 39,* 219–223.

Wang, S. M., Lei, H. Y., Su, L. Y., Wu, J. M., Yu, C. K., Wang, J. R., & Liu, C. C. (2007). *Cerebrospinal fluid cytokines in various severity of enterovirus 71 brainstem encephalitis and echovirus meningitis. Clinical Microbiology and Infection, 13,* 677–682.

Wang, S. M., Lei, H. Y., Yu, C. K., Wang, J. R., Su, I. J., & Liu, C. C. (2008). *Acute chemokine response in the blood and cerebrospinal fluid of children with enterovirus 71-associated brainstem encephalitis. The Journal of Infectious Diseases, 198,* 1002–1006.

Wang, S. M., Liu, C. C., Tseng, H. W., Wang, J. R., Huang, C. C., Chen, Y. J., Yang, Y. J., Lin, S. J., & Yeh, T. F. (1999). *Clinical spectrum of enterovirus 71 infection of children in southern Taiwan, with an emphasis on the neurological complications. Clinical Infectious Diseases, 29,* 184–190.

Wang, S. M., Lu, I. H., Lin, Y. L., Lin, Y. S., Wu, J. J., Chuang, W. J., Lin, M. T., & Liu, C. C. (2008). *The severity of Streptococcus pyogenes infections in children is significantly associated with plasma levels of inflammatory cytokines. Diagnostic Microbiology and Infectious Disease, 61,* 165–169.

Wills-Karp, M. (2004). *Interleukin-13 in asthma pathogenesis. Immunological Reviews, 202,* 175–190.

Woiciechowsky, C., Asadullah, K., Nestler, D., Eberhardt, B., Platzer, C., Schöning, B., Glöckner, F., Lanksch, W. R., Volk, H., & Döcke, W. (1998). *Sympathetic activation triggers systemic interleukin-10 release in immunodepression induced by brain injury. Nature Medicine, 4,* 808–813.

Yang, J., Zhao, N., Su, N. L., Sun, J. L., Lv, T. G., & Chen, Z. B. (2012). *Association of interleukin 10 and interferon gamma gene polymorphisms with enterovirus 71 encephalitis in patients with hand, foot and mouth disease. Scandinavian Journal of Infectious Diseases, 44,* 465–469.

Zhu, K., Yang, J., Luo, K., Yang, C., Zhang, N., Xu, R., Chen, J., Jin, M., Xu, B., Guo, N., Wang, J., Chen, Z., Cui, Y., Zhao, H., Wang, Y., Deng, C., Bai, L., Ge, B., Qin, C. F., Shen, H., Yang, C. F., & Leng, Q. (2015). *TLR3 signaling in macrophages is indispensable for the protective immunity of invariant natural killer T cells against enterovirus 71 infection. PLoS Pathogens, 11,* e1004613.

Chapter 7

Human Papillomavirus (HPV) 16 and 18 Variants in Northern Spain

Laila Sara Arroyo Mühr[1], Nerea Fontecha Urcelay[2],
Miren Basaras Ibarzabal[2], Elixabete Arrese Arratibel[3],
Silvia Hernáez Crespo[4], Daniel Andía Ortiz[5], Ramón Cisterna[6]

1 Introduction

Human papillomaviruses (HPVs) comprise a large and diverse group of small DNA viruses, some of which play a main role in the development of different types of cancer such as oropharyngeal, vulva, penis, anal or cervical cancer (zur Hausen, 2000). For cervical cancer, these viruses are recognized as the cause of nearly all cancer cases, with an estimated 500,000 new cases and 274,000 deaths every year (www.who.int, accessed on 2015–02–23).

Most HPV infections do not cause any lesion or symptoms but if the viral infection persists, cancer may develop. In our region, HPV prevalence is approximately 10.4% among women with normal cytology and up to 69.8% among those with abnor-

[1] Laboratory Medicine, Karolinska Institutet, Sweden

[2] Immunology, Microbiology and Parasitology Department, School of Medicine, University of Basque Country, Spain

[3] Immunology, Microbiology and Parasitology Department, Faculty of Pharmacy, University of Basque Country, Spain

[4] Clinical Microbiology and Infection Control Department, Basurto University Hospital, Spain

[5] Department of Obstetrics and Gynecology, University of Basque Country, Basurto University Hospital, Spain

[6] Clinical Microbiology and Infection Control Department, University of Basque Country, Basurto University Hospital, Spain

mal cervical cytology (de Sanjosé *et al.*, 2007; Delgado *et al.*, 2012), being highest among women aged 18–25 years (Delgado *et al.*, 2012).

Up to date, 205 different HPV genotypes have been completely cloned, sequenced and given an official number at the International HPV Reference Center (http://www.hpvcenter.se, accessed on 2015–07–10), and the number of putative novel HPV types is continuously growing (Bzhalava *et al.*, 2014).

Based on their potential risk to develop cancer, HPVs genotypes can be categorized into 3 groups: "high-risk" types associated with a greater risk of inducing invasive cancer, "low-risk" genotypes associated with benign or low-grade cell abnormalities, but not with cancer, and "probable high-risk" genotypes from which there is not enough evidence in humans about their association with carcinogenicity to classify them (Muñoz *et al.*, 2006).

At least 15 genotypes are considered as high-risk types, and two of them (16 and 18) are responsible for over 70% of all cervical cancer cases (Muñoz *et al.*, 2004; Smith *et al.*, 2007; Muñoz *et al.*, 2003; Crow, 2012). Nucleotide variability of these genotypes has been largely studied, and different molecular variants were described (Ong *et al.*, 1993; Yamada *et al.*, 1997).

The taxonomic status of HPV variants is based on the traditional criteria that the sequence of their *L1* genes should be maximally 2% dissimilar from one another (de Villiers *et al.*, 2004). Some authors may use the name "lineage" or "variant lineage" instead of variant, as all variants within a genotype segregate into phylogenetic trees with major branches or variant lineages. These lineages follow a race related distribution and are named after the geographical origin of the population where they are most prevalent. For example, HPV 18 genotype comprises European, Asian-Amerindian and African variants/lineages.

Epidemiological studies have confirmed that variants within a genotype differ in their biological and chemical properties (Sichero *et al.*, 2007; de Araujo *et al.*, 2009; López-Savedra *et al.*, 2009) and therefore, may become an important risk factor in cervical cancer due to possible differences in pathogenicity. For instance, L1 protein from variant 114K of HPV 16 assembles into virus-like particles (VLP) in a heterologous expression system, whereas the reference (prototype) clone of HPV 16 does not show the same property (Kirnbauer *et al.*, 1992; Kirnbauer *et al.*, 1993). Hecht *et al.*, identified an HPV 18 variant with lower oncogenic potential due to its absence in cervical cancer but presence in 40% of intraepithelial lesions (Hetch *et al.*, 1995) and Rose *et al.*, demonstrated that a single mutation in HPV 18 isolates (A41G) confers increased viral transcription activity (Rose *et al.*, 1998).

In order to identify HPV variants, most authors have relied on the phylogenetic analysis of *L1* gene, which is the most conserved region within the genome and encodes for the major capsid protein (de Villiers *et al.*, 2004). Changes in the L1 region of HPV genomes might be important in defining epitopes relevant to vaccine design as well as for optimizing amplification and genotyping methods for HPV detection. It is of great interest to define nucleotide substitutions, especially those that may lead to an amino acid change that may interfere with the functional or antigenic properties of specific viral proteins.

The main objectives of the present study included: i) to characterize the L1 genetic variability of HPV 16 and HPV 18 genotypes, working with both single infection and multiple HPV infection samples, ii) assess the prevalence of HPV variants in our region and iii) to analyze the relationship between variants and type of cervical lesion.

2   Methods

2.1   Recruitment of Participants

Samples from patients which were remitted from different Hospital Services, especially the Consultation of Sexually Transmitted Diseases and the Department of Obstetrics and Gynecology, from 2007 to 2010, were analyzed at the Clinical Microbiology and Infection Control Department at Basurto University Hospital (Basque Country, North of Spain).

All specimens were collected from women who were subjected to cervical screening and/or showed clinical manifestations of HPV-related infections. No restrictions or requirements were applied for participating in this study.

Collection of samples was performed by physicians, following an endo/ectocervical swabbing with a cytobrush for conventional cytology (Pap smear) and with a Dacron swab for HPV DNA genotyping. Sample handling retaining sterility was ensured for all specimens.

All procedures adhered to the declaration of Helsinki and were approved by the Ethical Review Committees related to our institutions (Basurto University Hospital and University of Basque Country). Written and informed consent was obtained from all participants.

Cervical lesions were classified by pathologists, following the 2014 Bethesda system: negative for intraepithelial lesion or malignancy, epithelial cell abnormalities (both from squamous cells – atypical squamous cells, low-grade squamous intraepithelial lesion (L-SIL), high-grade squamous intraepithelial lesion (H-SIL) and squamous cell carcinoma — and from glandular cells) and other malignant neoplasms.

Molecular genotyping was carried out using "Linear Array HPV Genotyping Test" kit (Roche Molecular Diagnostics). In this study, we analyzed samples that tested positive for HPV genotypes 16 and/or HPV 18 (both single infections and multiple HPV infections).

2.2   Genomic DNA Extraction

DNA was extracted using the QIAamp DNA mini Kit (Qiagen, Hilden, Germany), according to manufacturer's instructions, eluted with 200 µl AE buffer, and stored at −20°C until amplification.

2.3   PCR Amplification and Sequencing

Amplification of HPV 16 and 18 L1 genomic regions was performed using consensus primers MY11/09. Samples that were positive for HPV 18, had already been amplified, sequenced and analyzed in a previous paper (Arroyo et al., 2012) and for HPV 16 specimens, a similar protocol was followed.

PCR was performed using 5 µl of template DNA (or water as a negative control) in a 30 µl reaction mixture containing 10 × PCR buffer, 25 mmol/L MgCl2, 25 mmol/L of each deoxynucleoside, 100 pmol/L of sense and anti-sense primer, and 2,5 U of Taq DNA polymerase (Qiagen). The thermal program started with a denaturing step of 95°C for 15 min, followed by 40 cycles of 95°C for 30s, 55°C for 30s and 72°C for 30s, and a final extension at 72°C for 10 min.

All amplicons (including negative controls) were run on a 2% agarose gel to confirm PCR amplification and discard possible contamination. Afterwards, amplimers were automatically sequenced using the "Big Dye Terminator Cycle Sequencing kit" (Applied Biosystems) according to the manufacturer's instructions.

As MY11/09 primers amplify a broad number of HPVs, specific primers for HPV 16 and HPV 18 were designed according to the genome prototype sequences (GenBank accession numbers K02718 and NC001357 for HPV 16 and 18, respectively), in order to sequence HPV 16 and 18 genomes and not other HPV types present in cases of multiple infections. (5' CACAATAATGGCATTTGTTGGGG for HPV 16 and 5'ACAGTCTCCTG TACCTGG for HPV 18).

2.4   Nucleotide Variations, Variants and Phylogenetic Analysis

HPV sequences were aligned and compared to HPV 16 (GenBank accession number: K02718) and 18 (NC001357) prototype sequences which belong to the European and Asian-Amerindian lineages, respectively, using BioEdit Sequence Alignment Editor v7.0.4.1 and Clustal W (http://www.genome.jp/tools/clustalw/). Any nucleotide substitution detected in less than three isolates, was confirmed by repeating the amplification and sequencing procedures for all samples in which the nucleotide variation was found.

All isolates were then assigned to a lineage based on their similarity to HPV 16 or HPV 18 known variant sequences. For HPV 16 isolates, sequences which belong to Asian-American lineage (GenBank accession numbers: AF402678, AY686579), African (AF472508, AF472509, AF536180) and European lineages (AY686580, AY686581, AY686584, EU118173) were taken into consideration while HPV 18 isolates were assigned to Asian-Amerindian lineage (GenBank accession numbers: EF202143– EF202146), African (EF202152–EF202155) or European lineages (EF202147–EF202151). Phylogenetic trees were built using Maximum likelihood method implemented in MEGA software version 5 (Tamura et al., 2011).

The high sequence similarity within the L1 region between Asian-Amerindian and European HPV 18 variants, made it impossible to properly assign one of the lineages to certain specimens. Therefore, genomic sequences from E6, E7, E4 genes as well as URR were also retrieved from all corresponding specimens from the previous study (Arroyo et al., 2012), and used together with L1 sequencing products for proper classification of variants according to their overall substitutions. Deviation of HPV 18 isolates from all three branches had been studied for possible recombination by using three different methods, RDP, Maxchi, and Chimaera (all implemented in RDP3 software package) (Martin et al., 2010; Smith, 1992). Recombination events for HPV 16 isolates were not studied as they could easily be assigned to a lineage, and all isolates gathered into clusters in the phylogenetic tree.

2.5   Variants, Infection Type and Lesions

Association of type of lesion vs. variants and infection type (single HPV vs. multiple HPV infection) were analyzed. Fisher exact test was used for statistically significant association and a p value < 0.05 was considered as statistically significant.

When studying multiple HPV infections, a possible association of lesion grade with specific genotypes (besides HPV 16 or 18) was also analyzed. "Linear Array HPV Genotyping Test" kit (Roche Molecular Diagnostics) is capable of identifying up to 37 HPV types (6, 11, 16, 18, 26, 31,33, 35, 39, 40, 42, 45, 51, 52, 53, 54, 55,56, 58, 59, 61, 62, 64, 66, 67, 68, 69, 70, 71, 72, 73, 81, 82, 83, 84, IS39, and CP6108). For HPV 52 there is not a specific probe but an "HPVmix" cross-reactive probe that detects HPV genotypes 33, 35, 52 and 58. A specimen was considered to be positive only when the sample was negative for genotypes HPV 33, 35 and 58 individually but positive for the "HPVmix" probe.

3   Results

3.1   Samples Collected

A total of 1085 HPV-positive samples from women were received and analyzed, from 2007 to 2010. HPV 16 was detected in 260 specimens (24%) whereas HPV 18 was confirmed in 65 samples (6%). 13 samples showed the presence of both genotypes.

For HPV 16 analysis, 100 samples that had tested positive for this genotype were collected randomly (45 single infections and 55 multiple infections), and the L1 region was amplified in all specimens. Forty-four patients who tested positive for HPV 18 were included randomly in the study, being 10 single HPV infections (22.7%) and 34 multiple HPV infections (77.3%). We were able to amplify 43/44 specimens for the L1 region.

All PCR products were sequenced, and sequences from each region were submitted to GenBank. Accession numbers are shown in Tables 1 and 2.

3.2   Nucleotide Variations

3.2.1   HPV 16

Genetic variability analysis of MY11/09 region within L1 gene showed a total of 17 nucleotide substitutions and no particular variation was found to be associated with any type of infection (single or multiple HPV infection) (Table 1). 96/100 samples presented a deletion of one amino acid (aspartic acid) at position 465 as well as an insertion of 3 nucleotides (ATC) at nucleotide position 6902 leading to an addition of serine amino acid.

Intratypic variant	Nucleotide position	GenBank accession number	Nº isolates	6992	6968	6953	6952	6951	6948	6926	6901	6863	6860	6852	6801	6740	6730	6719	6693	6690	6642
E	Prototype	K02718		G	C	T	A	G	G	T	C	C	T	C	A	G	G	G	A	G	A
	Known sequences	AY686581				Del	Del	Del			Ins ATC										
		EU118173				Del	Del	Del			Ins ATC										
		AY686580				Del	Del	Del			Ins ATC										
		AY686584				Del	Del	Del			Ins ATC					A					
E	Single infection	KJ152709	22	-	-	Del	Del	Del	-	-	Ins ATC	-	-	-	-	-	-	-	-	-	-
		KJ152710	3	-	-	Del	Del	Del	-	-	Ins ATC	-	-	-	-	-	-	-	-	A	-
		KM030561	3	-	-	Del	Del	Del	-	-	Ins ATC	-	-	-	-	-	-	-	-	-	Del
		KM030568	3	-	-	Del	Del	Del	-	-	Ins ATC	-	-	-	-	-	T	-	-	-	-
		KM030569	3	-	-	Del	Del	Del	-	-	Ins ATC	-	-	-	-	-	T	-	-	A	-
		KM030570	3	-	-	Del	Del	Del	A	-	Ins ATC	-	-	-	-	-	-	-	-	-	-
		KM030562	2	-	-	Del	Del	Del	-	-	Ins ATC	-	-	-	-	-	-	-	-	A	Del
	Multiple infection	KJ152709	30	-	-	Del	Del	Del	-	-	Ins ATC	-	-	-	-	-	-	-	-	-	-
		KJ152711	12	-	-	Del	Del	Del	-	-	Ins AT	-	-	-	-	-	-	-	-	-	-
		KJ152712	4	-	-	-	-	-	-	-		-	-	-	-	-	-	-	-	-	-
		KJ152710	3	-	-	Del	Del	Del	-	-	Ins ATC	-	-	-	-	-	-	-	-	A	-
		KJ152713	3	-	-	Del	Del	Del	-	-	Ins AT	-	-	-	-	-	-	-	-	A	-

Continued on next page…

… Continued from previous page

Lineage	Sample type								Ins ATC		Del	Del	T	A	n	Accession
AA	Known sequences		C	A		T	T	T	Ins ATC		Del	Del	T	A		AF402678
	Known sequences		C	A		T	C	T	Ins ATC		Del	Del	T	A		AY686579
	Single infection	-	-	A	-	T	-	T	Ins ATC	-	Del	Del	T	A	1	KM030571
	Multiple infection	-	C	A	-	T	-	T	Ins ATC	-	Del	Del	T	A	1	KJ152717
	Multiple infection	A	C	A	-	T	-	T	Ins ATC	-	Del	Del	T	A	1	KJ152718
AF	Known sequences		C	A				T	Ins ATC	C	Del	Del	T	A		AF472509
	Known sequences			A		T		T	Ins ATC		Del	Del	T	A		AF472508
	Known sequences			A		T		T	Ins ATC		Del	Del	T	A		AF536180
	Single infection	-	A	A	-	-	-		Ins ATC	-	Del	Del	T	A	3	KM030573
	Multiple infection	-	C	A	-	T	-	T	Ins ATC	-	Del	Del	T	A	2	KM030572
	Multiple infection	-	C	A	-	T	-	T	Ins ATC	-	Del	Del	T	A	1	KJ152720

Table 1: Nucleotide sequence variations within L1 region among HPV 16 isolates. Numbering refers to the first nucleotide of the HPV 16 reference genome (accession number K02718). Isolates were assigned to a lineage based on their similarity to HPV 16 known variant sequences (known sequences). Nucleotide positions where a substitution leads to a change of amino acid are highlighted in gray. AA: Asian- American; AF: African; E: European.

Intratypic variant	Nucleotide position	6749	6842	6917	6986	6987	6993	6998	7000	7001	7007	Nº specimens	GenBank accession number
E	Prototype	G	C	G	A	G	G	A	A	T	T		NC001357
E/AA	European Known sequences												EF202147
													EF202148
													EF202149
													EF202150
							A						EF202151
	Asian-Amerindian Known sequences												EF202144
													EF202145
													EF202143
													EF202146
	Single infection		G									4	JN416262
			G								G	1	JN416267
			G							C		1	JN416298
	Multiple infection		G									8	JN416275
			G							C		6	JN416270
			G					G	T		G	2	JN416290
			G			A	A	G	C			1	JN416265
			G				A	G			G	1	JN416271
			G					T	C	C		2	JN416273
			G					G			G	2	JN416280
			G				A	G	T			1	JN416283
			G			A	A					1	JN416279
			G						C	C		1	JN416291
			G				A					1	JN416292
AF	Known sequences	A		A									EF202153
		A		A									EF202154
		A		A									EF202155
		A		A	G								EF202152
	Single infection	A	G	A	G						G	1	JN416263
		A	G	A							G	1	JN416264
		A	G	A								1	JN416303

Continued on next page…

...Continued from previous page

AF	Multiple	A	G	A									2	JN416282
	infection	A	G	A				G			G		1	JN416269
		A	G	A			A	G	T				1	JN416272
		A	G	A	G					C			1	JN416276
		A	G	A		A	A	G			G		1	JN416278
		A	G	A						C			1	JN416301
		A	G	A	G								1	JN416312

Table 2: Nucleotide sequence variations within L1 region among HPV 18 isolates. Numbering refers to the first nucleotide of the HPV 18 reference genome (accession number NC001357). Isolates were assigned to a lineage based on their similarity to HPV 18 known variant sequences (known sequences). AA: Asian-Amerindian; AF: African; E: European.

Eight nucleotide variations (A6693C, G6719A, A6801T, C6852T, T6860C, C6863T, C6968T and G6992A) were specific to non-European lineages and two of them (A6693C and A6801T) lead to non-synonymous amino acid alterations (Glu/Asp and Thr/Ser, respectively). European isolates presented less number of substitutions compared to the other lineages and G6730T, G6740A and G6948A variations were found to be specific to the European branch. G6730T and G6948A mutations lead to an amino acid change (Arg/Leu and Glu/Lys) and G6730T (detected in 6 isolates) had not been described in literature yet.

3.2.2   HPV 18

Genetic analysis of L1 genomic region revealed a total of 10 non-synonymous nucleotide variations and half of them had not been described in literature yet (G6987A, G6993A, A7000T/C, T7001C, T7007G) (Table 2). Single and multiple infections presented the same pattern of substitutions. Substitution C6842G was detected in all our isolates and varia-tions G6749A and G6917A were found to be specific to African lineage.

It was impossible to assign HPV 18 isolates to either Asian-Amerindian or European lineages as genomic sequence within region MY09/11 did not show any differences among those variants (Table 2).

3.3   HPV Variants

Phylogenetic analysis for HPV 16 isolates showed maximal nucleotide diversity between European variants and non-European lineages and closely related nodes between African and Asian-American lineages (Figure 1). L1 nucleotide variability analysis for HPV 18 showed the impossibility to classify Asian-Amerindian and European variants properly, as L1 sequences from most non-African isolates were 100% identical (Figure 2). Therefore, genomic sequences from E6, E7, E4 genes as well as URR were retrieved from all the corresponding specimens (Arroyo et al., 2012) and used together with L1 sequencing products for a proper classification of HPV 18 variants according to their overall substitutions. Figure 2 shows phylogenetic analysis for L1 HPV 18 isolates where a proper classification of variants (taking in consideration all 5 regions) is written for each isolate.

In contrast to HPV 16, phylogenetic analysis of L1 gene from HPV 18 isolates showed that European and Asian-Amerindian HPV 18 lineages formed closely related nodes and a maximal nucleotide diversity between African and non-African variants (Figure 2).
Phylogenetic analysis of E6, E7, E4, L1 and URR from HPV 18 isolates (Figure 3) showed better differentiation between European and Asian-Amerindian lineages. Furthermore, it detected eight isolates that presented nucleotide diversity from the three branches – S03, S06, M01, M03, M10, M16, M21 and M34 – and, therefore, were analyzed for possible recombination.

HPV 16 and HPV 18 variants showed the same pattern of variant distribution, being European variants the most prevalent variants (91/100 for HPV 16 isolates and 25/43 for HPV 18 specimens), followed by the African (6/100 and 10/43) and the Asian-American/Asian-Amerindian variants (3/100 and 5/43 isolates, respectively).

3.4   HPV Recombination

The presence of recombination was studied in the previous publication (Arroyo et al., 2012) where 8 HPV 18 isolates presented nucleotide diversity from the three branches – S03, S06, M01, M03, M10, M16, M21 and M34 –.

5/8 isolates (M01, M03, M10, M16 and S03) were classified as European. Three of them (M01, M16, and S03 specimens) belonged to the European lineage in all regions. Isolate M03 belonged to the European lineage in all regions but in E6 (Asian-Amerindian) due to the lack of one nucleotide substitution (C549A) and isolate M10 was classified as European in all regions but L1 due to the presence of 2 nucleotide variations specific to African lineage. If only analyzing L1 region, isolate M10 would have been classified as African variant (Figures 2 and 3). The rest of the isolates (3/8, samples M21, M34 and S06) belonged to the African branch in some regions but were classified as European in others (Table 3).

RDP (Martin et al., 2010), Maxchi (Smith, 1992) and Chimaera were used for the detection of recombination in these 8 samples and only 2 of them were found to be recombinant, one single (S06) and one multiple HPV infection (M21) (Table 3). M21 and S06 were classified as recombinant isolates while M34 was classified as X variant (unknown).

3.5   Variants, Type of Lesion and Infection Type

Out of 100 samples positive for HPV 16, 56 were classified by pathologists as negative for intraepithelial lesion or malignancy, 10 were diagnosed as atypical squamous cells of undetermined significance (ASC-US), 16 samples as L-SIL while presence of H-SIL was

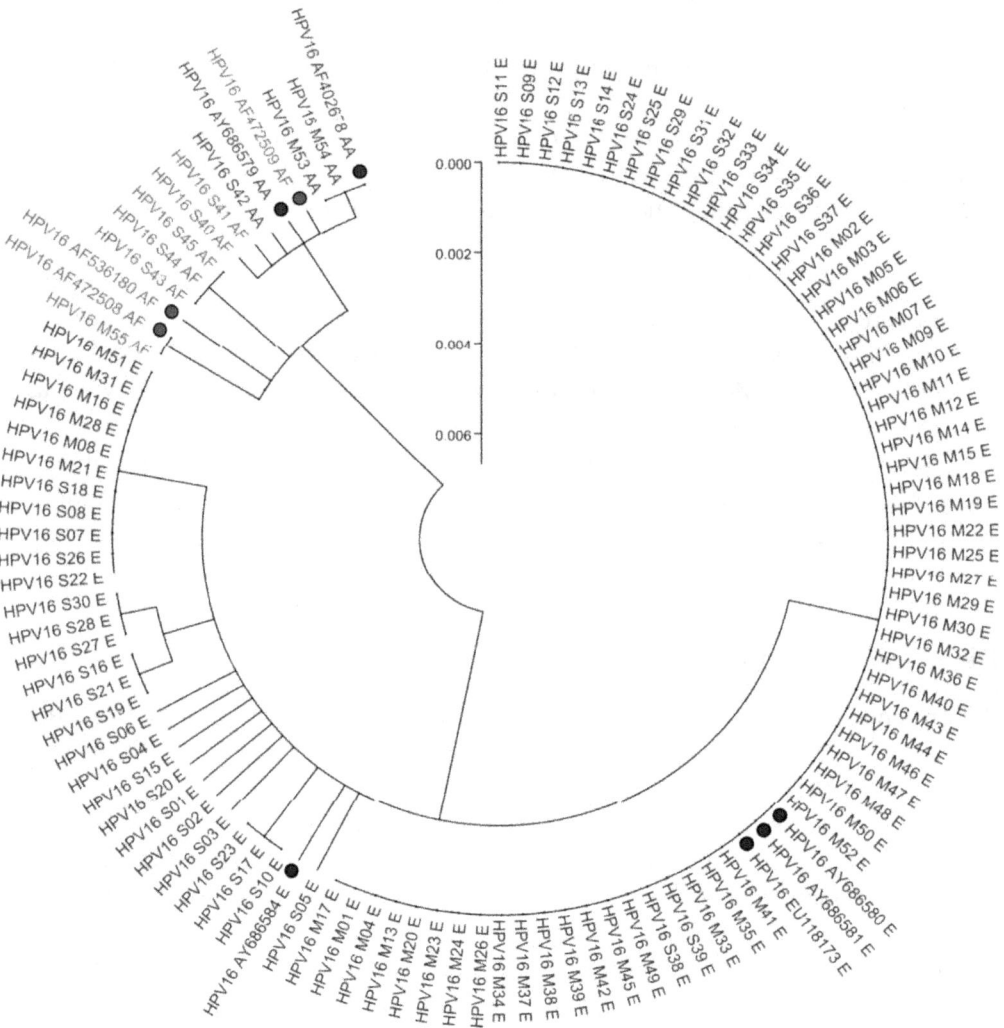

Figure 1: Phylogenetic tree of HPV 16 isolates. Phylogenetic analysis of L1 nucleotide sequences from 100 HPV 16 isolates using the Maximum Likelihood method implemented in MEGA software version 5. European, Asian-American and African isolates are presented in blue, red and green colors, respectively. Isolates are named as follows: "HPV 16" followed by an "M" or "S" (S: Single infection; M: Multiple infection), one number which identifies the sample and letters that specify the lineage (AA: Asian-American; AF: African; E: European). HPV 16 known variant sequences, which belong to Asian-American lineage (GenBank accession numbers: AF402678, AY686579), African (AF472508, AF472509, AF536180) and European lineages (AY686580, AY686581, AY686584, EU118173) are included and marked with a circle.

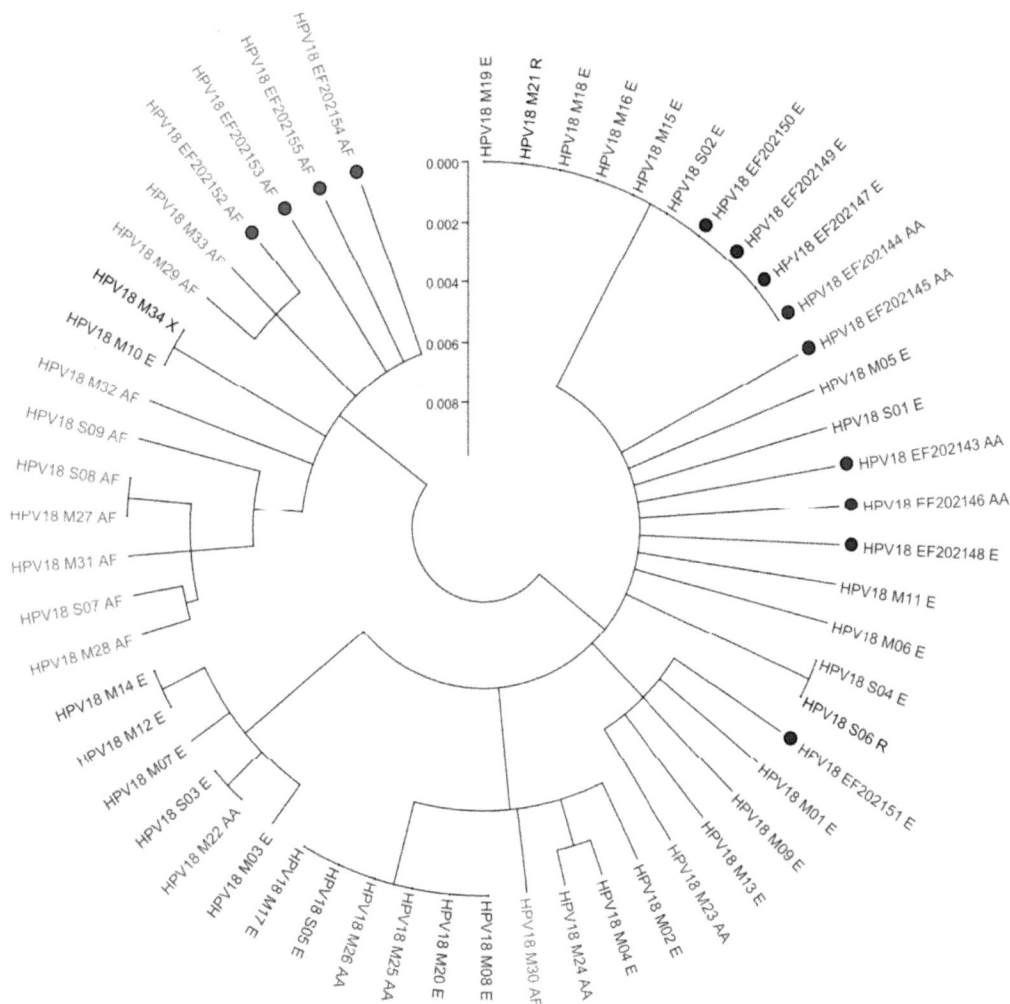

Figure 2: Phylogenetic tree of L1 HPV 18 isolates- Phylogenetic analysis of L1 nucleotide sequences from 43 HPV 18 isolates using the Maximum Likelihood method implemented in MEGA software version 5. European, Asian-American and African isolates are presented in blue, red and green colors, respectively. Isolates are named as follows: "HPV 18" followed by an "M" or "S" (S: Single infection; M: Multiple infection), a number and a letter that identifies the lineage (AA: Asian-Amerindian; AF: African; E: European; R: Recombinant; X: unknown). Isolates EF202143–EF202155 are included as HPV 18 reference variant sequences which belong to Asian-Amerindian, African and European lineages. These known sequences are marked with a circle.

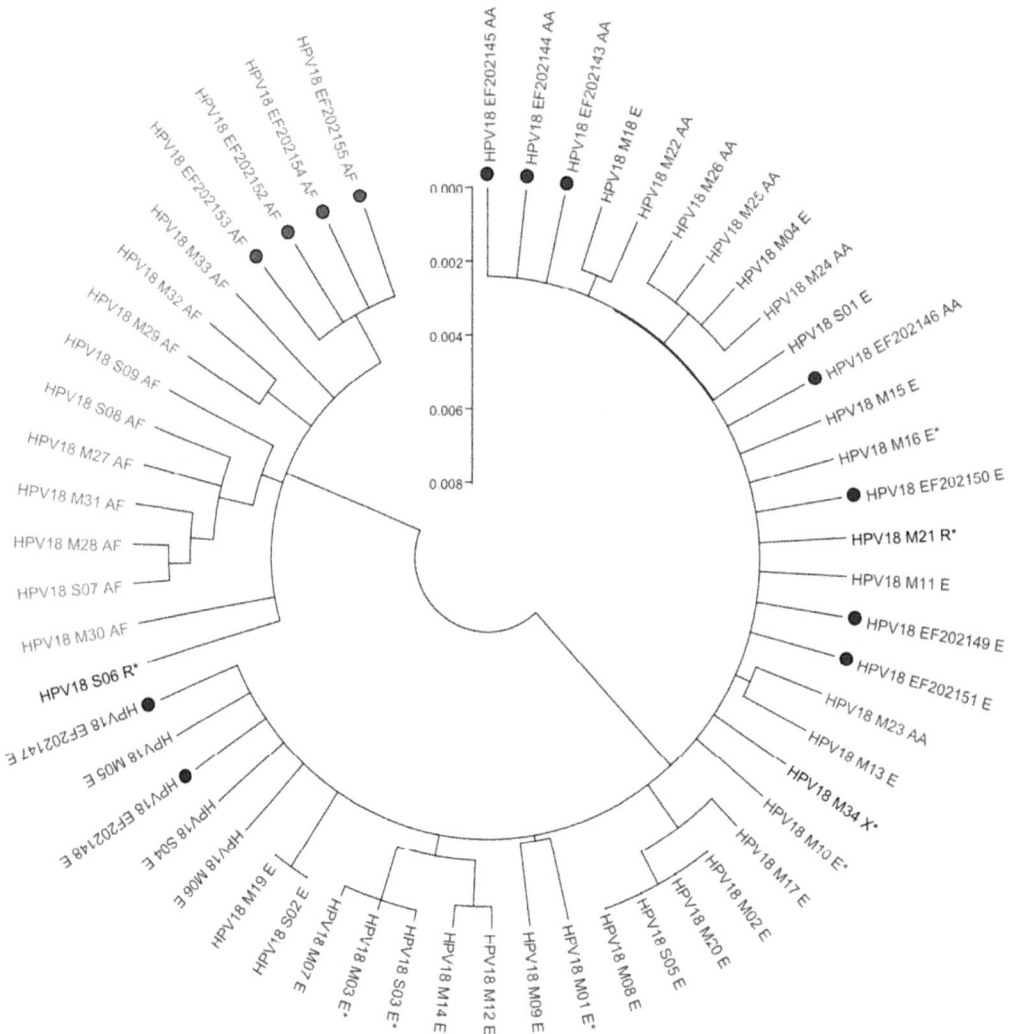

Figure 3: Phylogenetic tree of HPV 18 isolates. Phylogenetic analysis of HPV 18 isolates (E6, E7, E4, L1 and URR nucleotide sequences included) using the Maximum Likelihood method implemented in MEGA software version 5. European, Asian-American and African isolates are presented in blue, red and green colors, respectively. Isolates are named as follows: "HPV 18" followed by an "M" or "S" (S: Single infection; M: Multiple infection), a number and a letter that identi-fies the lineage (AA: Asian-Amerindian; AF: African; E: European; R: Recombi-nant; X: unknown). Asterisk is used for isolates that deviate from all branch-es. Isolates EF202143–EF202155 are included as HPV 18 reference variant se-quences which belong to Asian-Amerindian lineage, African and European line-age. These known sequences are marked with a circle.

Sample/Gene	E6	E7	E4	L1	URR	Program inference	Lineage assigned
S03	E	E	E	E	E	No recombination detected.	E
S06	AA	E	Af	E	Af	Maxchi detected recombination. (M31 and M26 are the donors)	Rec.
M01	E	E	E	E	E	No recombination detected.	E
M03	AA	E	E	E	E	No recombination detected.	E
M10	E	E	E	Af	E	No recombination detected.	E
M16	E	E	E	E	E	No recombination detected.	E
M21	Af	Af	E	E	E	Maxchi detected recombination. (M34 is one of the donors)	Rec.
M34	Af	E	Af	Af	E	No recombination detected.	X

Table 3: Evidence for recombinant samples. Isolates analyzed for possible recombination. Phylogenetic trees were constructed for each sequenced region and isolates were classified as Asian-Amerindian (AsA), European (E) and African (Af) variants for each genomic region. Final assigned lineages included European (E), Recombinant (Rec) and unclassifiable variants (X). RDP, Maxchi and Chimaera were used for the detection of recombination. URR: Upstream regulatory region. Table modified from Arroyo et al., 2012.

Genotype	Variants	Type of lesion				
		Negative	ASC-US	L-SIL	H-SIL	SCC
HPV 16	European	58.2%	8.8%	16.5%	16.5%	0.0%
	Asian-American	66.7%	33.3%	0.0%	0.0%	0.0%
	African	16.7%	16.7%	16.7%	33.3%	16.7%
HPV 18	European	80.0%	12.0%	8.0%	0.0%	0.0%
	Asian-Amerindian	80.0%	0.0%	20.0%	0.0%	0.0%
	African	30.0%	10.0%	40.0%	20.0%	0.0%
	Recombinant	50.0%	0.0%	50.0%	0.0%	0.0%
	X	0.0%	0.0%	0.0%	100.0%	0.0%

Table 4: Human papillomavirus variants vs. type of lesion. All isolates in the study were included in the table (143 samples). Negative: no lesion; ASC-US: atypical squamous cells of undetermined significance; L-SIL: low-grade squamous intraepithelial lesion; H-SIL: high-grade squamous intraepithelial lesion; SCC: squamous cell carcinoma; X: unclassifiable variant.

detected in 17 specimens and only one patient had developed squamous cell carcinoma. For HPV 18, 28 specimens were classified as negative, 4 were diagnosed as ASC-US, 8 samples as L-SIL whereas the presence of H-SIL was detected in 3 specimens.

HPV 16 Asian-American samples were only detected in negative cytology or ASC-US diagnosed specimens, while African variants were mostly present in samples where different lesions were diagnosed. European variants could be found in all types of lesions. However, the majority of them were detected in negative cytology (Table 4). When analyzing HPV 18, high-grade lesions only presented African variants (3 isolates) whereas most European and Asian-Amerindian variants were detected in negative cytology (Table 4).

The presence of lesions associated with African variants was found to be statistically significant for both genotypes HPV 16 and HPV 18 (p=0.045 and p=0.003, respectively). African isolates were more frequently detected in patients that presented epithelial cell abnormalities (ASC-US, L-SIL, H-SIL and SCC) than in those that were classified as negative for intraepithelial lesion or malignancy. Nevertheless, we did not find a statistically significant association between type of infection (single vs. multiple) and presence of lesion (p > 0.1) nor a trend between lesion type and specific genotypes presence in multiple infections.

4 Discussion

Spain has a relatively low incidence rate for cervical cancer incidence (9.1/100,000) (www.eco.iarc.fr, accessed on 2015–07–10) and there are only few national studies that identify natural HPV variants. HPV 16 and 18 genotypes are responsible for approximately 70% of cervical cancer cases, and therefore, variant distribution and nucleotide substitutions in these genotypes are considered extremely helpful for appropriate cervical cancer prevention strategies.

HPV variants segregate based on the geographical origin and therefore, Spain should expect predominance of European variant, followed by African and Asian-American or Asian-Amerindian variants (Xi et al., 2006; de Araujo et al., 2009). Our results are in accordance with this stating: for HPV 16 we detected 91 European variants (91.0%), 6 African (6.0%) and 3 Asian-American variants (3.0%) whereas for HPV 18, 25 European variants (58.1%), 10 African (23.3%) and 5 Asian-Amerindian variants (11.6%) were present. Perez et al., analyzed HPV 18 and 16 variants in Spain and found also a higher prevalence of European variants compared to African isolates for both genotypes (Perez et al., 2014).

Certain genetic nucleotide substitutions have been related with differences in pathogenicity among variants. For HPV 16, many epidemiologic studies have confirmed that non-European variants, specifically the Asian-American variants, tend to be persistent and are associated with cervical lesions and cancer (Kämmer et al., 2000; Illades-Aguiar et al., 2010; Schiffman et al., 2010; Tornesello et al., 2011). This association is also confirmed for HPV 18 where non-European HPV 18 variants persist more frequently and are more associated with pre-invasive lesions (Villa et al., 2000).

Our study results are in accordance with these statements as African variants were most frequently detected in patients that presented epithelial cell abnormalities (p < 0.05 for both genotypes). However, Asian-American (HPV 16) and Asian-Amerindian (HPV 18) variants were mostly detected in cytology where no lesion was diagnosed. These findings do not contradict the fact that non-European variants are persistent as the number of variants classified as Asian-American and Asian-Amerindian in this study was very low (3 and 5 isolates, respectively) and a prospective study has not been performed in order to find persistence. Furthermore, phylogenetic analysis of HPV 16 isolates showed closely related nodes between African and Asian-American lineages as well as maximal nucleotide diversity between European variants and non-European lineages, suggesting that pathogenicity might be similar for those variants included in non-European branches.

Besides the higher oncogenic potential associated with non-European variants, we would like to highlight that European variants were detected among women with and without cervical lesions in the present study, emphasizing the fact that all branches of HPV 16 variants are related to the development of pre-cancer and invasive cancer, although additional factors are likely to have a role in cervical carcinogenesis.

In this study, we observed a high percentage of cases in which the presence of both HPV-16 and/or HPV-18 was positive but a normal cytology was reported (56% and 65%, respectively). Possible explanations for the high rate of negative cytology might include, the limitations of the sampling method, as conventional smears may not always detect cell changes. The Pap test has been reported to produce inherent false-negative results of about 5% (Lieu D, 1996).

The taxonomic status of HPV variants is based on the traditional criteria that the sequence of their L1 genes should differ by no more than 2% from one another (de Villiers et al., 2004). In this study, a 450 bp region (MY09/11) within L1 gene (approx. 1600 bp long) was sequenced, and due to the short amplimer length obtained for sequencing, we found it impossible to differentiate among HPV 18 European and Asian-Amerindian variants. No difference in the nucleotide sequence of MY09/11 PCR products was detected between these two lineages. To overcome this problem, genomic sequences from E6, E7, E4 genes as well as URR were retrieved from the corresponding specimens and used together with L1 sequencing products to classify HPV 18 variants properly according to their overall substitutions (Arroyo et al., 2012).

Authors usually analyze only L1 gene, as it is the region used for classification of HPV genotypes. Taking into consideration only L1 sequences for the phylogenetic analysis, it was obvious that some HPV 18 isolates deviated from the branches, the lineages were not clearly separated from one another and possible recombination was not detected. Burk et al., encouraged authors to classify variant genomes based on a set of complete genomes, as the full extent of the sequence heterogeneity is best summed across the whole genome (Burk et al., 2013). In accordance with his statements, we characterized more than one genomic region in order to classify HPV variants properly and detect recombination (Arroyo et al., 2012).

HPV recombination presence has already been confirmed by other authors (Angulo & Carvajal-Rodríguez, 2007; Jiang et al., 2009). This event may occur due to a homologous recombination or to a repeated infection of the same HPV genotype but different variant and it is more often found since multiple infections with more than one HPV type are becoming a usual finding (Mendez et al., 2005; Nielson et al., 2009; Tinelli et al., 2011).

When analyzing all 5 regions for HPV 18 isolates, we detected 2 HPV 18 recombinant variants (4.7%), one in one single infection and the other one in a multiple HPV infection. These variants might have been missed or wrong classified if only amplifying L1. Moreover, 2 isolates (M10 and M34) presented specific-African variations in L1 whereas their corresponding analysis of URR and/or E7 would have classified these isolates as Europeans. On the contrary, isolate M30 might have been classified as European in L1, but as African in all other genomic regions.

HPV 16 phylogenetic analysis showed all three lineages clearly separated from one another and there was no deviation of any isolate from the clusters. Consequently, variants were assigned to their specific branches without major problems. However, as it happened with HPV 18, possible recombination might have been missed for this genotype. Other authors have found recombination events when studying HPV 16 (Angulo et al., 2007; Jiang et al., 2009) and we would like to highlight that it should be essential to determine HPV variants by analyzing other regions in order to discard recombination completely for this genotype and confirm the variants classification.

To date, only a few studies have reported on the relationship between multiple HPV infections and cervical neoplasia, and their results are not consistent. Some of these studies suggested a possible role for multiple HPV types in the development or progression of cervical neoplasia (Morrison et al., 1991; Ho et al., 1998; Fife et al., 2001; Sasagawa et al., 2001; van der Graaf et al., 2002; Chatuverdi et al., 2005), and a probable protective effect (e.g co-infection of HPV 6 together with genotype 16) (Luostarinen et al., 1999; Arnheim Dahlström et al., 2011;). In our study, no statistical significance was found when analyzing lesion grade vs. type of infection or vs. specific genotypes presence.

Differences in oncogenic potential are due to nucleotide substitutions and, therefore, these variations may play an important role. Some nucleotide changes reported in our study have been previously described, and some of them are of particular importance. In HPV 16 variants for example, mutations A6693C, A6801T, 6901insAC, G6945A and 6950delGT do affect B cell epitopes (Pillai et al., 2009). Furthermore, six "new" nucleotide variations have been detected, and one of them (G6730T in HPV 16) lead to an amino acid change (Arg/Leu). Substitution C6842G was found in all our HPV 18 isolates, and it has been previously reported as an error in the original sequence (Meissner, 1997).

Epidemiologic studies on HPV variants are essential for appropriate cervical cancer prevention strategies. Nucleotide substitutions might increase the viral oncogenic potential as well as they might interfere with the host cellular immune response (HPV infections with a variant may not give immunological protection against other variants of the same genotype), reduce the vaccination success (if substitutions in the amino acids are present on the viral capsid) and escape amplification and genotyping methods for HPV detection (when substitutions in the sequences do not match to designed primers/probes). Nevertheless, studying L1 region solely might not give enough data to classify specimens into a specific lineage. Future studies in the field should take whole genome analysis for proper variant classification and recombination detection (Arroyo et al., 2012, Burk et al., 2013).

Acknowledgements

Authors wish to thank the Department of Health from the Basque Government (project number 2008111058) and Department of Industry from the Basque Government (S-PC11BF002 project) for supporting this project. NFU research staff contract was supported by University of Basque Country, UPV/EHU (PIC 73/14).

References

Angulo, M. & Carvajal-Rodríguez, A. (2007). *Evidence of recombination within human alpha-papillomavirus. Virology Journal, 4, 33.*

Arnheim Dahlström, L., Andersson, K., Luostarinen, T., Thoresen, S., Ögmundsdottir, H., Tryggvadottir, L. Wiklund, F., Skare, G.B., Eklund, C., Sjölin, K., Jellum, E., Koskela, P., Wadell, G., Lehtinen, M. & Dillner, J. (2011). *Prospective seroepidemiologic study of human papillomavirus and other risk factors in cervical cancer. Cancer Epidemiology, Biomarkers & Prevention, 20, 2541–2550*

Arroyo, S.L., Basaras, M., Arrese, E., Hernaez, S., Andia, D., Esteban, V., Garcia-Etxebarria, K., Jugo, B.M. & Cisterna, R. (2012). *Human papillomavirus (HPV) genotype 18 variants in patients with clinical manifestations of HPV related infections in Bilbao, Spain. Virology Journal, 9, 258.*

Burk, R.D., Harari, A. & Chen, Z. (2013). *Human papillomavirus genome variants. Virology, 445, 232–243*

Bzhalava, D., Muhr, L.S.A., Lagheden, C., Ekstrom, J., Forslund, O., Dillner, J. & Hultin, E. (2014). *Deep sequencing extends the diversity of human papillomaviruses in human skin. Scientific Reports, 4, 5807.*

Chaturvedi, A.K., Myers, L., Hammons, A.F., Clark, R.A., Dunlap, K., Kissinger, P.J., & Hagensee, M.E. (2005) *Prevalence and clustering patterns of human papillomavirus genotypes in multiple infections. Cancer Epidemiology, Biomarkers & Prevention, 14, 2439–2445.*

Crow, J.M. (2012). *HPV: The global burden. Nature, 488, 2–3.*

de Araujo Souza, P.S., Sichero, L. & Macia, P.C. (2009). *HPV variants and HLA polymorphisms: the role of variability on the risk of cervical cancer. Future Oncology, 5, 359–370.*

de Sanjosé, S., Diaz, M., Castellsagué, X., Clifford, G., Bruni, L., Muñoz, N. & Bosch, F.X. (2007). *Worldwide prevalence and genotype distribution of cervical human papillomavirus DNA in women with normal cytology: a meta-analysis. The Lancet Infectious Diseases, 7, 453–459.*

de Villiers, E.M., Fauquet, C., Broker, T.R., Bernard, H.U. & Zur, H.H. (2004). *Classification of papillomaviruses. Virology, 324, 17–27.*

Delgado, D., Marín, J.M., de Diego, J., Guerra, S., González, B., Barrios, J.L. & Canut, A. (2012). *Human papillomavirus (HPV) genotype distribution in women with abnormal cervical cytology in the Basque*

Country, Spain. Enfermedades Infecciosas y Microbiología Clínica, 30, 230–235.

Fife, K.H., Cramer, H.M., Schroeder, J.M. & Brown, D.R. (2001). *Detection of multiple human papillomavirus types in the lower genital tract correlates with cervical dysplasia. Journal of Medical Virology, 64, 550–559.*

Hecht, J., Kadish, A., Jiang, G. & Burk, R. (1995). *Genetic characterization of the human papillomavirus (HPV) 18 E2 gene in clinical specimens suggests the presence of a subtype with decreased oncogenic potential. International Journal of Cancer, 60, 369–376.*

Ho, G.Y., Palan, P.R., Basu, J., Romney, S.L., Kadish, A.S., Mikhail, M., Wassertheil-Smoller, S., Runowicz, C. & Burk, R.D. (1998). *Viral characteristics of human papillomavirus infection and antioxidant levels as risk factors for cervical dysplasia. International Journal of Cancer, 78, 594–599*

Illades-Aguiar, B., Alarcón-Romero, L.del C., Antonio-Véjar, V., Zamudio-López, N., Sales-Linares, N., Flores-Alfaro, E., Fernández-Tilapa, G., Vences-Velázquez, A., Muñoz-Valle, J.F. & Leyva-Vázquez, M.A. (2010). *Prevalence and distribution of human papillomavirus types in cervical cancer, squamous intraepithelial lesions, and with no intraepithelial lesions in women from Southern Mexico. Gynecologic Oncology, 117, 291–296.*

Jiang, M., Xi, L.F., Edelstein, Z.R., Galloway, D.A., Olsem, G.J., Lin, W.C-C. & Kiviat N.B. (2009). *Identification of recombinant human papillomavirus type 16 variants. Virology, 394, 8–11.*

Kämmer, C., Warthorst U., Torrez-Martinez N., Wheeler C.M. & Pfister H. (2000). *Sequence analysis of the long control region of human papillomavirus type 16 variants and functional consequences for P97 promoter activity. Journal of General Virology, 81, 1975–1981*

Kirnbauer, R., Booy, F., Cheng, N., Lowy, D. R. & Schiller, J. T. (1992). *Papillomavirus L1 major protein self-assembles into virus-like particles that are highly immunogenic. Proceedings of the National Academy of Sciences, USA 89, 12180–12184.*

Kirnbauer, R., Tabu, J., Greenstone, H., Roden, R., Dürst, M., Gissman, L., Lowy, D. R. & Schiller, J. T. (1993). *Efficient self-assembly of human papillomavirus type 16 L1 and L1–L2 into virus-like particles. Journal of Virology, 67, 6929–6936.*

Lieu, D. (1996) *The papanicolau smear: its value and limitations. The Journal of Family Practice, 42, 391– 399.*

López-Savedra, A., González-Maya, L., de Ponce León, S., García-Carranca, A., Mohar, A. & Lizano, M. (2009). *Functional implication of sequence variation in the long control region and E2 gene among human papillomavirus type 18 variants. Archives of Virology, 154, 747–754.*

Luostarinen, T., af Geijersstam, V., Bjorge, T., Eklund, C., Hakama, M., Hakulinen, T., Jellum, E., Koskela, P., Paayonen, J., Pukkala, E., Schiller, J.T., Thoresen, S., Youngman, L.D., Dillner, J. & Lehtinen, M. (1999). *No excess risk of cervical carcinoma among women seropositive for both HPV 16 and HPV 6/11. International Journal of Cancer, 80, 818–822.*

Martin, D.P., Lemey, P., Lott, M., Moulton, V., Posada, D. & Lefeuvre, P. (2010). *RDP3: a flexible and fast computer program for analyzing recombination. Bioinformatics, 26, 2462–2463.*

Meissner, J. (1997) *Sequencing errors in reference HPV clones. In Human papillomaviruses. A compilation and analysis of nucleic acid and amino acid sequences. 3rd edition. Edited by Myers G, Baker C, Munger K. Los Alamos (NM): Theoretical Biology and Biophysics, Los Alamos National Laboratory, 110–123.*

Méndez, F., Muñoz, N., Posso, H., Molano, M., Moreno, V., van den Brule, A.J., Ronderos, M., Meijer, C. & Munoz, A. (2005). *Cervical coinfection with human papillomavirus (HPV) types and possible implications for the prevention of cervical cancer by HPV vaccines. The Journal of Infectious Diseases, 192, 1158–1165.*

Morrison, E.A., Ho, G.Y., Vermund, S.H., Goldberg, G.L., Kadish, A.S., Kelley, K.F. & Burk, R.D. (1991). Human papillomavirus infection and other risk factors for cervical neoplasia: a case-control study. International Journal of Cancer,49, 6–13

Muñoz, N., Bosch, F.X., Castellsagué, X., Díaz, M., de Sanjose, S., Hammouda, D., Shah, K.V. & Meijer C.J. (2004). Against which human papillomavirus types shall we vaccinate and screen? The international perspective. International Journal of Cancer, 111, 278–285.

Muñoz, N., Castellsague, X., de Gonzalez, A.B. & Gissmann, L. (2006). HPV in the etiology of human cancer. Vaccine, 24, 1–10.

Muñoz, N., Bosch, F.X., de Sanjosé, S., Herrero, R., Castellsagué, X., Shah, K.V., Snijders, P.J. & Meijer, C.J. (2003).Epidemiologic classification of human papillomavirus types associated with cervical cancer. The New England Journal of Medicine, 348, 518–27.

Nielson, C.M., Harris, R.B., Flores, R., Abrahamsen, M., Papenfuss, M.R., Dunne, E.F., Markowitz, L.E. & Giuliano, A.R. (2009). Multiple-type human papillomavirus infection in male anogenital sites: prevalence and associated factors. Cancer Epidemiology, Biomarkers & Prevention, 18, 1077–1083.

Ong, C.K., Chan, S.Y., Campo, M.S., Campo, M.S., Fujinaga, K., Mavromara-Nazos, P., Labropoulou, V., Pfister, H., Tay, S.K., ter Meulen, J. & Villa, L.L. (1993). Evolution of human papillomavirus type 18: an ancient phylogenetic root in Africa and intratype diversity reflect coevolution with human ethnic groups. Journal of Virology, 67, 6424–6431.

Pillai, M.R., Hariharan, R., Babu, J. M., Lakshmi, S., Chiplunkar, S.V., Patkar, M., Tongaonkar, H., Dinshaw, K., Jayshree, R.S., Reddy, B.K.M., Siddiqui, M., Roychoudury, S., Saha, B., Abraham, P., Gnanamony, M., Peedicayil, A., Subhashini, J., Ram, T.S., Dey, B., Sharma, C., Jain, S.K. & Singh, N. (2009). Molecular variants of HPV-16 associated with cervical cancer in Indian population. International Journal of Cancer, 125, 91–103.

Rose, B., Steger, G., Dong, X.P., Thompso, C., Cossart, Y., Tattersall, M. & Pfister, H. (1998). Point mutations in SP1 motifs in the upstream regulatory region of human papillomavirus type 18 isolates from cervical cancers increase promoter activity. Journal of General Virology, 79, 1659–1663.

Sasagawa, T., Basha, W., Yamazaki, H. & Inoue, M. (2001). High-risk and multiple human papillomavirus infections associated with cervical abnormalities in Japanese women. Cancer Epidemiology, Biomarkers & Prevention, 10, 45–52.

Schiffman, M., Rodriguez, A.C., Chen, Z., Wacholder, S., Herrero, R., Hildesheim, A., Desalle, R., Befano, B., Yu, K., Safaeian, M., Sherman, M.E., Morales, J., Guillen, D., Alfaro, M., Hutchinson, M., Solomon, D., Castle, P.E. & Burk, R.D. (2010). A population-based prospective study of carcinogenic human papillomavirus variant lineages, viral persistence, and cervical neoplasia. Cancer Research, 70, 3159–3169.

Sichero, L., Ferreira, S., Trottier, H., Duarte-Franco, E., Ferenczy, A., Franco, E.L. & Villa, L.L. (2007). High grade cervical lesions are caused preferentially by non-European variants of HPVs 16 and 18. International Journal of Cancer, 120, 1763–1768.

Smith, J.S., Lindsay, L., Hoots, B., Keys, J., Franceschi S., Winer, R. & Clifford, G.M. (2007). Human papillomavirus type distribution in invasive cervical cancer and high-grade cervical lesions: a meta-analysis update. International Journal of Cancer, 121, 621–632.

Smith, J. (1992). Analyzing the mosaic structure of genes. Journal of Molecular Evolution, 34, 126–129.

Tamura, K., Peterson, D., Peterson, N., Stecher, G., Nei, M. & Kumar, S. (2011). MEGA5: Molecular Evolutionary Genetics Analysis using Maximum Likelihood, Evolutionary Distance, and Maximum Parsimony Methods. Molecular Biology and Evolution, 28, 2731–3739.

Tinelli, A., Leo, G., Dell'Edera, D., Storelli, F., Galante, M.M., Guido, M., Hudelist, G. & Malvasi, A. (2011) Molecular methods for a correct diagnosis of multiple HPV infections and clinical implications for vaccine. International Journal of Gynecological Cancer, 21, 545–550.

Tornesello, M.L., Losito, S., Benincasa, G., Fulciniti, F., Botti, G., Greggi, S., Buonaguro, L. & Buonaguro, F.M. (2011). Human papillomavirus (HPV) genotypes and HPV 16 variants and risk of adenocarcinoma and squamous cell carcinoma of the cervix. Gynecologic Oncology, 121, 32–42.

van der Graaf, Y., Molijn, A., Doornewaard, H., Quint, W., van Doorn, L.J. & van den Tweel, J. (2002). Human papillomavirus and the long-term risk of cervical neoplasia. American Journal of Epidemiology ,156,158–64.

Villa, L.L., Sichero, L., Rahal, P., Caballero, O., Ferenczy, A., Rohan, T. & Franco, E.L. (2000). Molecular variants of human papillomavirus types 16 and 18 preferentially associated with cervical neoplasma. Journal of General Virology, 81, 2959–2968.

Xi, L.F., Kiviat, N.B., Hildesheim, A., Galloway, D.A., Wheeler, C.M., Ho, J. & Koutsky, L.A. (2006). Human papillomavirus type 16 and 18 variants: race-related distribution and persistence. Journal of the National Cancer Institute, 98, 1045–1052.

Yamada, T., Manos, M.M., Peto, J., Greer, C.E., Munoz, N., Bosch, F.X. & Wheeler, C.M. (1997). Human papillomavirus type 16 sequence variation in cervical cancers: a worldwide perspective. Journal of Virology, 71, 2463–2472.

zur Hausen, H. (2000). Papillomaviruses causing cancer: Evasion from host-cell control in early events in carcinogenesis. Journal of the National Cancer Institute, 92, 690–698.

Chapter 8

Nanomedicine: Basics and Applications in Antimicrobial Resistance and Aids

Feroz Alam[1], Mehar Aziz[1], Mohammed Naim[1], Murad Ahmed[1]

1   Nanotechnology and Medicine

Nanotechnology is the study and use of structures between 1 nanometer (nm) to 100 nanometers in size. This is probably the simplest and generally agreed upon definition of nanotechnology. According to National Nanotechnology Initiative (NNI, a multia-gency US government program initiated in 2001), nanotechnology is broadly defined as the science and engineering involved in the design, synthesis, characterization, and ap-plication of materials and devices with at least one of the dimensions in the nanoscale (typically 1–100 nanometers) (NNI, 2005). Presently nanotechnology is being increasing-ly used in nearly every aspect of life, medicine, clothing, cosmetics, sports, energy, elec-tronics, aero-space, military & security, food, water, air to name a few. In the United States, 2013 Federal Budget provides $1.8 billion for the National Nanotechnology Initi-ative (NNI), reflecting steady growth in the NNI investment. Although difficult to measure accurately, estimates from 2008 show the governments of the European Union (EU) and Japan invested approximately $1.7 billion and $950 million, respectively, in nanotechnology research and development. The governments of China, Korea, and Taiwan invested approximately $430 million, $310 million, and $110 million, respective-ly (NNI-FAQ, 2013). While the evolvement of nanotechnology has the potential to take several decades, and the early developers are likely to be sizeable institutions with great wealth that can produce considerable advancement efforts, in the long term nanotech-nology is going to affect a large variety of people. There will definitely be many other future implications and practical applications of nanotechnology as more and more pos-

[1] Department of Pathology, J.N Medical College, Aligarh Muslim University, India

sibilities and opportunities will keep on continuously coming to light as the branch develops further.

1.1   Role of Nanotechnology in Medicine

Nanomedicine deals with the concept of manipulation and assembly of the matter at the nanoscale for applications at the clinical level of medical sciences. In a broad sense, nanomedicine is the application of nanoscale technologies to the practice of medicine. This enables the miniaturization of many current devices, resulting in faster operation or integration of several operations. Furthermore, at this scale, man-made structures match typical sizes of natural functional units in living organisms. This allows them to interact with the biology of living organisms at the smallest structural level. Nanomedicine has been an important part of nanotechnology from the very beginning, and since nanotechnology began as a visionary enterprise, nanomedicine started by applying mainly nano-mechanical concepts to the body. The 2004 presentation of the cancer nanotechnology initiative in the United States revolves around the goal of "eliminating death and suffering from cancer by 2015" (NCI, 2004). The 2006 European Technology Platform on Nanomedicine is more subtle than this. It speaks of a "revolution in molecular imaging in the foreseeable future, leading to the detection of a single molecule or a single cell in a complex biological environment" (ECR, 2006). Nanomedicine, in other words, is disease centered, trying to do better and on a molecular level what physiology, pathology, and the various other specialized medical sciences have been doing so far. Table 1 summarizes some to the main advantages of nanomedicine over conventional medicine

Improved pharmaco-kinetic & pharmaco-dynamic profile of drugs
Low toxicity & fewer adverse effects of drugs
Targeted delivery of therapeutic agents
Combining of multiple therapeutic agents in a single nano-scale entity
Combining of diagnostic & therapeutic agents in a single nano-scale entity (theranostics)
More precise, less time and labour consuming

Table 1: Advantages of Nanomedicine over conventional medicine.

1.2   Preventive Medicine

New diagnostic tests making use of nanotechnology to quantify disease-related biomarkers could offer an earlier and more personalized risk assessment before symptoms show up. In general, these analyses must be cost-effective, sensitive, and reliable. The test itself should inflict only minimal discomfort to the patient. Supported by such an analysis and bioinformatics, health professionals could advise patients with an increased risk to take up a personalized prevention program. People with an increased risk for a certain disease could benefit from regular personalized check-ups to monitor changes in the pattern of their biomarkers. Nanotechnology could improve in vitro diagnostic tests by providing more sensitive detection technologies or by providing better nano-labels that can be detected with high sensitivity once they bind to disease-specific molecules present in the sample. Nanotechnology could also improve the ease-of-use of in vitro diagnostic tests done by untrained users or even by patients at home. For example a relatively painless minimally invasive sampling technique would greatly improve patient comfort. Diseases with no secretion of biomarkers into blood or urine will require imaging procedures of high specificity for their early detection. One well-known example used already is x-ray mammography for the early detection of breast cancer. Novel targeted imaging agents, precisely homing in on diseased cells, promise a much higher sensitivity than today's imaging procedures making possible the detection of cancer at an even earlier stage.

1.3   Diagnosis

If a medical check-up had found an indication or a hint of symptoms for a disease, it is important that "false positives" are excluded by applying more specific diagnostic procedures. These can be more laborious and expensive as they are applied to a smaller number of patients. In this case, molecular imaging, which makes use of specific targeted agents, plays a crucial role for localization and staging of a disease, or – equally important – for ascertaining the health of a patient. Here, nanotechnology could help to design a plethora of very specific imaging agents over the next few years. Miniaturized imaging systems will make it possible to perform image-based diagnostics everywhere and not only in research centers. Automatic methods will give diagnostic results without an onsite expert. Conceptually a novel method, combining biochemical techniques with advanced imaging and spectroscopy provide insight to the behavior of single diseased cell and its microenvironment for the individual patient. This could lead to personalized treatment and medication tailored to the specific needs of a patient. Often, the differences between healthy and diseased or pre-disease states are very small, and the ability to detect single molecules or small changes in the behavior of a cell is required for diagnosis. Nanotechnology capable of measuring single binding events or interactions is a great asset for diagnostics. Nanotechnology hence may enhance disease diagnosis by improving sensitivity, selectivity, decreasing time to diagnosis, and the availability of highly accurate testing equipment.

1.4   Therapy

In many cases, therapy is not restricted to medication only but requires more severe therapeutic action such as surgery or radiation treatment. Planning of therapeutic interventions is based on imaging, or may be performed under image guidance. Here, nanotechnology can lead to a miniaturization of devices that enable minimally invasive procedures and new ways of treatment. The possibilities range from minimally invasive catheter based interventions to implantable devices. Targeted delivery systems and nanotechnology-assisted regenerative medicine will play a central role in future therapy. Targeted delivery agents allows localized therapy which targets only the diseased cells, thereby increasing efficacy while reducing unwanted side effects. Pleuripotent stem cells and bioactive signaling factors will be essential components of smart, multifunctional implants which can react according to the changes in surrounding micro-environment. Imaging and biochemical assay techniques will be used to monitor drug release or to follow the therapy progress. This therapeutic logic will lead to the development of novel, disease modifying treatments that will not only significantly increase quality of life but also dramatically reduce societal and economic costs related to the management of permanent disabilities.

1.5   Follow-up and Monitoring

Medical reasons may call for monitoring of the patient after completing the acute therapy. This might be a regular check for recurrence, or, in the case of chronic diseases, a frequent assessment of the actual disease status and medication planning. Continuous medication could be made more convenient by implants, which release drugs in a controlled way over an extended period of time. In vitro diagnostic techniques and molecular imaging play an important role in this part of the care-process, as well. Biomarkers could be systematically monitored to pick up early signs of recurrence, complemented by molecular imaging where necessary. Oncology is one of the areas where these techniques are already being evaluated today. Also, in the case of drug resistance, signs of disease progression can be immediately picked up and alternative treatments can be prescribed.

Although, still in its infancy, but nanomedicine has all the potential and is going to grow exponentially in the coming future. The global nanomedicine market reached $43.2 billion in 2010 and $50.1 billion in 2011. The market is expected to grow to $96.9 billion by 2016 at a compound annual growth rate (CAGR) of 14.1% between years 2011 and 2016. The anticancer products market reached $4.7 billion in 2010 and $5.5 billion in 2011. It is expected to reach $12.7 billion by 2016, a CAGR of 18.2% between years 2011 and 2016 (BCC report, 2013).

2   Basics of Nanomedicine

Particles in the size of nanoscale known as nanoparticles (NPs) have unique operating ability in the complex bio-environment of the body to interact at the level of biomolecules (McNeil, 2005). This interaction of the NPs is facilitated by nm size of the organic and inorganic molecules and atoms in the body (for e.g. DNA 2.5 nm, Na atom 0.2nm). For unique size, optical, electrical, magnetic, chemical, and ligands carrying properties nanoparticles can be targeted to the cells with specificity and monitored efficiently with extreme precision in real-time (Yang *et al.*, 2012). The blood vessel endothelial gaps facilitate extravasations and circulation of NPs of <5nm size. Glomerular membrane allows clearance of NPs <6 nm size. Liver cells do uptake the NPs >8 nm size. The NPs with specific surface properties such as charge and hydrophobicity are phagocytosed by the Kupffer cells and cleared into the biliary system (Longmire *et al.*, 2008). Surface modifications of NPs may prevent opsonization by the reticulo-endothelial system (RES), and facilitates their retention in blood circulation. For these reasons the nanoparticles have enhanced permeability and retention (EPR) and longer circulation time in the body (Chatterjee *et al.*, 2008). The nanoparticle-EPR in a tumor is increased due to relative lack of lymphatic drainage, and over expression of vascular endothelial growth factor (VEGF) by tumor-cells promoting disorganized angiogenesis producing more permeable/leaky blood vessels. It leads to retention and accumulation of the nanoparticles in the tumor, and gives advantages of using nano-particulate contrast agents for tumor diagnostic magnetic resonance imaging (MRI), optical imaging, photo acoustic imaging, as well as NP delivered therapy (Jain, 2008).

Nanoparticles can be used to carry multiple chemotherapeutic, anti-angiogenic, and gene therapy agents simultaneously to the tumor site for synergistic therapeutic effect. Also the imaging as well as therapy agents can be co-delivered for integrated molecular/cellular diagnosis, therapy, and follow-up, referred as *theranostics*. The multimodal utility of nanoparticle for therapy and diagnosis may be further enhanced by constructs capable of combining multiple functionalities into a single nano-scale entity. A nanoparticle-tagged reporter, such as an apoptotic marker, may help signals about the payload delivery of the drug and reaching of the desired therapeutic effect in a patient. Nano-biotechnology, thus, may facilitate the means for *"personalized medicine"* as per the diagnostic and cure requirements of the individual patient (Fernandez *et al.*, 2011).

2.1   Targeting Strategies for Nanoparticles

Nanotechnology may use neutrally charged particles of average diameter of 10–100 nm and molecular weight around 30 kDa, it is referred as 'Passive targeting', which may be limited in utility for its low specificity, thereby, lower than required concentration at the target (Fernandez *et al.*, 2011). Desired specificity and concentration hence, may require 'Active targeting' of the nano- vehicle with moieties such as small ligands, antibodies, and biomarkers capable of specific binding to the cell expressed molecular receptors, facilitating efficient cellular uptake, internalization and receptor-mediated endocytosis resulting in elevated concentrations inside the cells (Figure-1) (Fernandez *et al.*, 2011). Monoclonal antibodies (mAbs) in their engineered chimeric humanized and clinically non antigenic forms are being presently widely applied for the active targeting. Several mAbs based nano-therapies like trastuzumab, cetuximab, rituximab, and bevacizumab had been already under trials. Aptamers can also be used for nanotechnology based active targeting, they derive their name from a Latin word "aptus" meaning "to fit". Aptamers are single-stranded DNA/RNA oligonucleotides (with a molecular weight of 5–40 kDa) which can fold into well defined 3-dimensional structure and binds to their target molecules with high affinity and specificity. For active targeting, the aptamers can be selected against a wide range of targets such as proteins, phospholipids, sugars, nucleic acids or even whole cells. The most important advantage of aptamers over antibodies is that they does not require a biological system for their production and can be synthesized chemically. Furthermore, due to their small size and similarity to endogenous molecules, aptamers exhibit superior tissue penetration and are believed to be less immunogenic than antibodies (Drolet *et al.*, 2000). The aptamers may be modified to prevent nuclease degradation by replacing naturally occurring nucleotides with modified nucleotides (i.e. 2'-F pyrimidines, 2'- OCH3 nucleotides) that are poor substrates for endo- and exonuclease degradation. RNA aptamers to the vascular endothelial growth factor (VEGF) isoform with 2'-O-methylpurine and 2'-F pyrimidines are known to show anti-angiogenic properties, and the aptamer Pegaptanib had been FDA approved for the treatment of neovascular macular degeneration. Besides, many tissue biomarkers also have been identified as possible targets of NPs, including the transferrin receptor, epidermal growth factor receptor, folate receptor, and human epidermal receptor 2 (HER-2) (Fernandez *et al.*, 2011).

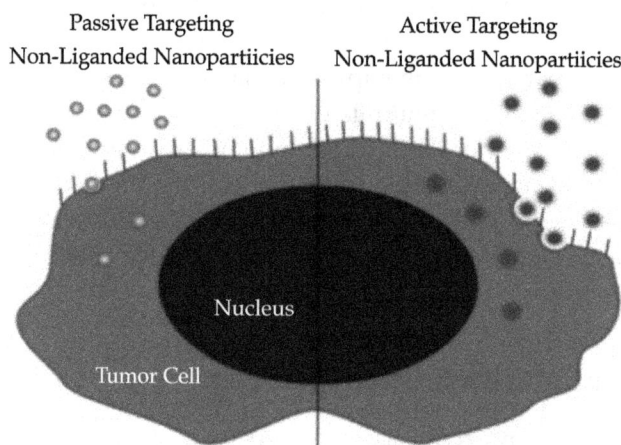

Figure 1: Active and passive targeting of nanoparticles.

Nanotechnology manifests itself in a wide range of materials that can be useful in the field of medicine (Zhang, 2002). The nanoparticles are designed with a chemically modifiable surface to attach a variety of ligands that can turn them into biosensors, molecular-scale fluorescent tags, imaging agents, targeted molecular delivery vehicles, and other useful biological tools. Diagnosis and treatment of cancer are the two most important fields that can be revolutionized with the help of nanotechnology. Nanotechnology's applications in cancer diagnosis include tumor localization, tumor margin detection, identification of important adjacent structures, mapping of sentinel lymph nodes, and detection of residual tumor cells or micro metastases (Singhal *et al.*, 2010). From the point of view of treatment the nanoparticles target the delivery of drugs, radiotherapy, phototherapy, immunotherapy more precisely to the tumor cells (Davis *et al.*, 2008; Zhang *et al.*, 2008; Park *et al.*, 2009; Wang *et al.*, 2011).

2.2   Application in Diagnostics

Studies in gene and related protein expressions (*genomics and proteomics*) have made it possible to trace such changes in tissue for the purpose of early cell molecular diagnosis of the disease for preventive and therapeutic purposes (Ray *et al.*, 2012).Both the *in vitro* and *in vivo* molecular tests are being worked out. *In vitro* patients' genetic material (DNA) samples are examined for gene expression in terms of RNA production, single nucleotide polymorphisms (SNPs), and corresponding protein expressions with single amino acid variations for genetic molecular diagnosis of the disorders and sensitivity to chemical substances for the purpose of theranostics (Kimchi *et al.*, 2007; Huang & Dolan, 2010). DNA analysis chips devised for DNA analysis are currently available for the scientific biomedical research, awaiting clinical applications. DNA chip comprises of an inert support carrying microarrays of thousands of single strand DNA molecules with different base sequences. DNA from tissue sample is labeled with suitable radioactive or fluorescent material and can be identified on the basis of its binding spot on the DNA chip, (Shrivastava & Dash, 2009). The Dutch Cancer Institute has been using such a DNA chip since 2003 to predict the spread of breast tumors on the basis of gene expression profiles. This information makes it much easier than it was in the past to determine which patients would benefit from supplementary chemotherapy after the tumor has been surgically removed. Similar chips are also being developed for the diagnosis of leukemias and mouth and throat tumors (Shrivastava & Dash 2009). The bio-chip is a micro-fluidic device, in fact a lab on chip and promising hope for future pocket size bio-chip laboratory, or at-clinic or at-home non-laboratory settings for diagnosis of diseases particularly cancer based on nano analytic procedures with advantages of minimized analytical procedures, applications, transport, micro measurements and instrumentations (Gambari *et al.*, 2003).

The application of nanotechnology to cancer imaging is subdivided into two main areas: (i) nanodetection for sensing protein and cancer cells and (ii) nanoparticle or nanovector formulation for high-contrast imaging. (McCarthy & Weissleder, 2008; Ferrari, 2005; Yang *et al.*, 2007; Medarova *et al.*, 2007; Hirsch *et al.*, 2006; Hirsch *et al.*, 2003; McCarthy *et al.*, 2007). Nanoparticles have been successfully used to selectively tag a wide range of medically important targets, including bacteria, biomarkers and individual molecules such as proteins and DNA (Sanvicens & Marco 2008). Nanoparticle devices are currently being developed for the early detection of cancer cells in body fluids such as blood and serum. Capturing circulating tumor cells is of great interest and current systems are limited in their ability to accurately select and collect sufficient numbers of these cancer cells for analysis. On average there are only 1–2 cancer cells per milliliter of blood. The nanoparticle devices being evaluated are conjugated with cancer-specific antibodies or ligands that may improve the yield of cancer cells captured (Dinh *et al.*, 2007; Nie *et al.*, 2007). Nanoparticles also offer fluorescent nano platforms and it is possible to image a single cell or an entire organism *in vivo* (Kumar *et al.*, 2008). Dual-mode nanoparticles can be imaged with MR and optical imaging to increase accuracy by cross evaluation and detection of breast, lung, colon, prostate, and ovarian cancers hidden or overt metastatic colonies at the time of presentation (Menon & Jacobs, 2000). Advances in nanotechnology may lead to a nanoparticle-based MRI, positron emission tomography (PET), single photon emission tomography, and computed tomography (CT) enhancing sensitivity and specificity for tumor imaging (Wang *et al.*, 2008).

3   Weapons of Nano-Arsenal

Applications of nanotechnology in various disciplines of medicine are becoming increasingly popular so much so that the process of replacing traditional health-care by nanomedicine had already begun. Nanomedicine focuses on the formulations of imaging, diagnostic and therapeutic agents, which can be carried by biocompatible nanoparticles, for the purpose of disease management. One of the major advantages, which nanomedicine offers is the specific site targeted delivery of the theranostic agents, lowering the risk of toxicity to the normal tissues around the lesion and other organs of the patient. Nanomaterials and devices, which have been worked out and presently applicable in disease imaging, diagnosis and therapy (theranostics) are classifiable on the basis of the carrying nanoparticles as liposomes, polymeric-micelles, dendrimers, nanocantilevers, carbon nanotubes, quantum dots, magnetic-nanoparticles, gold nanoparticles (AuNPs), silver nanoparticles and miscellaneous nanoparticles based nanotheranostic products. Here, we present a brief introduction of the structure, function and utilities of the various nanodevices applicable in the disease care and medicine.

3.1   Liposomes

The liposomes are 50–100 nm size, single or multi lamellar phospholipid-vesicles having anionic, cationic or neutral charges and composed of lipid layers surrounding a central aqueous space or core (Jesorka & Orwar, 2008; Irache *et al.*, 2011).The nanoliposomes are used for encapsulating the lipophilic and hydrophilic drugs within their lipid layers or in the aqueous core, for delivery to the specific target site, thus, minimizing biodistribution toxicity (Allen & Moase, 1996). Liposome based theranostic systems can have advantages of, cell specific targeting, pH and reductive environmental sensitivity, temperature sensitivity and long circulation half-life due to the surface modifiable lipid composition. However, there are issues of stability, batch to batch reproducibility and sterilization limiting their wider utilities (Mansoori *et al.*, 2012). Liposome based theranostic products had been in a good number approved for the clinical practice and now widely used for cancer/diseases managements, besides many new ones, which are under trail (Chang *et al.*, 2012).

3.2   Polymeric Micelles

These are nanoparticles of 10–100 nm size made up of polymer chains having a hydrophobic or ionic core and shell structure, capable of carrying drug, diagnostic, or imaging molecules, and the shell is capable of interacting with the fluid vehicle for stability. The lipophilic anticancer drugs, as paclitaxel (a potent microtubule growth inhibitor) has low water solubility (0.0015 mg/ml), therefore, on intravenous (i.v.) administration may undergo rapid drug aggregation and cause capillary embolisms. By encapsulation of such drugs in micelles, the solubility may be increased to the magnitude of 0.0015–2 mg/ml to prevent drug aggregation and embolism (Torchilin *et al.*, 2003; Soga *et al.*, 2005). Flourophores for detection of various microbes can be attached to the polymeric nanoparticles core, the shell can be functionalized with various molecules such as amines, carboxylic acids and esters which helps in attachment of these nanoparticles to the microbial target molecule. These fluorescent polymers can be detected with the help of a fluorescence spectrometer, flow cytometer, and fluorescence-recording microtiter plate reader (Zhao *et al.*, 2004; Qin *et al.*, 2008).

3.3   Dendrimers

The dendrimers are polymers of regularly branched macromolecules measuring 2–10 nm in size and spherical in shape. Dendrimer structures can be divided into three main components: the core, the interior, and the shell. The core affects the 3D shape of the dendrimer, the interior affects the host–guest properties of the dendrimer. The surface of the dendrimer can be further polymerized or modified with functional peripheral groups. Both the core and the number/type of interior branching units affect the overall dendrimer morphology. Dendrimers having an isohydrophillic end-group like a car-boxyl group are water soluble. Dendrimers are easily modifiable and can be loaded with drugs in their core cavities through hydrophobic interactions, hydrogen bonds, or chemical linkages. It is also possible to design a water-soluble dendrimer with internal hydrophobicity allowing it to carry a hydrophobic drug in its interior (Cheng *et al.*, 2011). The most commonly studied system has been the family of polyamidoamine (PAMAMs) dendrimers, but the list of the variety of building blocks is fast growing (Sakthivel & Florence, 2003). Dendrimers have also found use in clinical settings as anti-viral agents. VivaGel® (SPL7013, Starpharma), a topical vaginal microbicide is currently undergoing phase II clinical trials. The compound inhibits HIV-1 and HSV-2 infections by binding to gp120 glycoprotein receptors on the surface of these viruses, thus prevent-ing the viruses from binding to CD4+ receptors on human T-cells (O'Loughlin *et al.*, 2010). The ability to conjugate gadolinium chelating agents onto the surface of den-drimers has allowed for their use as MRI contrast agents. The success of such research studies is reflected by the clinical use of Gadomer-17, which is currently in phase II clin-ical trials (Herborn *et al.*, 2003).

3.4   Nanocantilevers

The nanocantilevers are lithographic semi-conductors producing flexible microscopic beams resembling a row in the diving boards. Cantilevers may be coated with the mole-cules for detection by the microarray methods, providing indispensable tool for detec-tion of cancer expressions, molecular diagnosis and genome research and drug discov-ery. The tiny bars anchored at one end of cantilever can be engineered to bind diagnos-tic molecules, which in turn may bind to the specific deoxyribonucleic acid (DNA) pro-teins. When this bio-specific interaction occurs between a receptor immobilized on the cantilever and a ligand in solution, the cantilever bends, which is detectable optically to tell that a molecule is present, thereby, helping in molecular diagnosis. The deflection of cantilever beam depends on the amount of DNA protein bound to the cantilever surface. The deflection can be observed directly using laser light or by measurement of perturbations in their resonant vibration frequency. Wu *et al.* used micro-cantilevers to detect single-nucleotide polymorphisms in a 10-mer DNA target oligonucleotide without the use of extrinsic fluorescent or radioactive labeling. They coated the surface of the micro-cantilever with antibodies specific to prostate specific antigen (PSA). When the micro-cantilever was made to interact with the blood sample of the prostate cancer patient the antigen antibody complex formed and the cantilever bent due to the adsorbed mass of the complex. The nanometer bending of cantilever was detected optically by a low power laser beam with sub-nanometer precision using a photo detector. This nanocantilever based assay was more sensitive than the conventional biochemical techniques for detection of PSA. The technique is good and potentially better than enzyme-linked immunosorbent assay. Moreover, the cost per assay is less as there are no requirements for any fluorescent tags or radiolabel molecules (Wu *et al.*, 2001).

3.5   Quantum Dots (QDs)

QD is spherical crystalline semiconductor nanoparticle of <10 nm size made of 200–1000 atoms. Structurally QD consists of a semiconductor core coated by shell having optical properties, covered by a cap enabling solubility in the aqueous buffers. The proto-type QD has been cadmium selenide. Recently, QDs have attracted research attention in view of their scientific and technological applications in microelectronics, optoelectronics and cell imaging (Ferrari, 2005; Nie *et al.*, 2007; Grodzinski *et al.*, 2006; Rhyner *et al.*, 2006). These semiconductors are characterized by composition-dependent band-gap energy. The band-gap energy is the minimal-energy required to excite an electron from its orbit to a higher level. As the election relaxes and returns back to the ground orbit, a photon gets emitted, leading to a visible fluorescence. The band gap energy is dependent on the size of the semiconductor nanoparticle; hence the optical characteristics of QD can be tuned by adjusting its size (Smith *et al.*, 2008). Increase in the QD size improves optical penetration of the tissue and reduces the background fluorescence at near infrared (NIR) wave lengths. The QDs demonstrate 10–100 times improved signal brightness, compared with the other fluorescent proteins and organic dyes. They also display greater resistance against photo-bleaching (Nagasaki *et al.*, 2004); thus, affording longer stability to the probes. In addition, single QD light source is capable of exciting multiple expressions simultaneously producing different identifiable fluorescence colors (Fountaine *et al.*, 2006). This broad absorption and narrow emission characteristics of the QDs, make it possible, to perform multicolor imaging with a single excitation source. This makes them suitable for various biomedical applications such as sensing and detection of biomarkers including antigens and pathogens, immunolabelling of cells and tissues. QD imaging have been used for detection of breast cancer metastasis/micro-metastasis (Alam & Yadav, 2013), pancreatic cancer, ovarian cancer and prostate cancer (Gao *et al.*, 2005; Michalet *et al.*, 2005; Peng & Li, 2010). The QDs can directly transfer energy to oxygen by photodynamic reactions, but act better synergistically in conjugation with routine photosensitizers used for photodynamic therapy of cancer cells. QDs may also be used as versatile nano-scale scaffolds for designing multifunctional imaging cum therapeutic nanoparticles. The QDs because of their intense fluorescent signals and multiplexing capabilities also hold great promise for intra-operative tumor imaging (Bera *et al.*, 2010).

3.6   Magnetic Nanoparticles

These are magnetic nanomaterials. The iron oxides either magnetite (Fe_3O_4) or maghemite (γ-Fe_2O_3) are the most often used magnetic nanoparticles (10–100 nm size) used in the biomedical operations. One of their main envisaged applications has been the targeted chemotherapeutic-drug delivery to the tumors. Magnetic nanoparticles coated with the drug are injected intravenously and can be retained at the tumor site by application of an external magnetic field gradient, to ensure requisite prolonged release of drug at the tumor site (Vatta *et al.*, 2006; Häfeli, 2004). An important extension of this technique is the use of implanted magnetized cardiac stents (Rosengart *et al.*, 2005; Yellen *et al.*, 2005). Another interesting therapeutic application is in the field of cancer hyperthermic (Jordan *et al.*, 1999) and photodynamic therapy (Qiao, 2012). Magnetic nanoparticles conjugated to antibodies have been used for the immunomagnetic separation of nucleic acids, proteins, viruses, bacteria and cells (Jain, 2005; Rosi & Mirkin, 2005). Surface modification of magnetic nanoparticles can facilitate the addition of functional groups (such as amino and carboxylic acids), making subsequent conjugations with peptides, small molecules, proteins, antibodies and nucleic acids easy. Therefore, iron oxide nanoparticles have been used for the identification and quantification of several targets, including mRNA, DNA, viruses, bacteria and cells (Nath *et al.*, 2009; Kaittanis *et al.*, 2007; Lee *et al.*, 2008; Perez *et al.*, 2002; Perez *et al.*, 2003). The superparamagnetic nanoparticles are also useful contrast agents for magnetic resonance imaging (MRI) to better enhance the image-contrast between normal and diseased tissue and indicate the status of organ function and blood flow. Small super-paramagnetic iron oxides have been developed for use in imaging of the liver metastases and to distinguish loops of bowel from the other abdominal structures.

3.7   Gold Nanoparticles

Gold nanoparticles (AuNPs) are versatile particles of <50 nm size and can be prepared in different geometries such as nanospheres, nanoshells, nanorods and nanocages. These are widely used as conjugates for attaching oligonucleotides, antibodies and proteins etc., for biotechnological applications (Moyano & Rotello, 2011). On binding with the analytes the physicochemical properties of AuNPs such as surface plasmon resonance (SPR), conductivity and the redox behavior are altered leading to detectable signals (Uehara, 2010). They are also useful as platforms for therapeutic agents due to their high surface area allowing binding of drugs and targeting agents. The spherical AuNPs have better useful attributes of size-shape related opto electronic properties, surface-to volume ratio, SPR, efficiency to quench fluorescence, excellent biocompatibility, low toxicity, range of colors (brown, orange, red and purple) in aqueous solution with the increase of core-size 1–100 nm and size relative absorption peak at 500–550 nm. The AuNPs play a critical role in the "bio-barcode assay" (Nam *et al.*, 2007), which is an ultra-sensitive method for detecting the target proteins and nucleic acids. The optical and electronic properties of AuNPs have been employed for cell imaging using the computed tomography (CT), dark-field light scattering, optical coherence tomography (OCT), photothermal heterodyne imaging and Raman spectroscopy techniques. Effective targeting and delivery strategies using AuNPs have been developed for therapeutic applications in photothermal therapy, genetic regulation and drug treatment (Brown *et al.*, 2010). AuNPs have also been exploited as attractive large surface area scaffolds for making transfection agents for gene therapy of cancer and genetic disorders.

3.8   Silver Nanoparticles

Silver nanoparticles are 1–100 nm size particles of silver having unique properties which are utilized for molecular diagnostics, therapeutics, as well as in several medical devices. Anti-microbial property is the most commonly utilized therapeutic application of nanosilver, though its anti-inflammatory property has also gained reputation. Silver nanoparticles are bactericidal in many ways, they accumulate and anchors to the bacterial cell wall and subsequently penetrate it, forming pores which increases the membrane permeability ultimately leading to cell death (Sondi & Salopek, 2004). Free radical generation is another mechanism by which the bacterial cell membrane is damaged, forming pores and finally leading to the death of bacteria (Danilcauk *et al.*, 2006; Kim *et al.*, 2007). It has also been proposed that there can be release of silver ions by the nanoparticles (Feng *et al.*, 2008), and these ions can interact with the thiol groups of many vital enzymes and inactivate them (Matsumura *et al.*, 2003). The bacterial cells which are in contact with silver nanoparticles, imbibes silver ions which inhibit several functions in the cell and damages the cell. Inside the bacteria, the silver ions inhibit respiratory enzyme causing generation of reactive oxygen, which damage bacterial cell. The anti-inflammatory effects of nanosilver may be attributed to the reduction of local matrix metalloproteinase (MMP) activity and increase in neutrophil apoptosis. It has been suggested that the MMP can induce inflammation and hence cause non-healing wounds (Kirsner *et al.*, 2001). In a mouse model with burn injury, a reduction in the levels of pro-inflammatory cytokines was noticed when silver nanoparticles were applied (Tian *et al.*, 2007). Silver nanoparticles are also known to inhibit the activities of interferon gamma and tumor necrosis factor alpha which have a proven role in inflammation (Shin *et al.*, 2007). Though these studies prove the anti-inflammatory effects of silver nanoparticles, the precise mechanism of action remains to be elucidated.

3.9   Toxicity of Nanoparticles

Nanoparticles can translocate from entry portals (e.g. skin, lungs, and the gastro-intestinal tract) into the circulatory and lymphatic systems, and ultimately to body tissues and organs where they can produce irreversible damage to cells. Although, not all nanoparticles produce adverse cellular effects — the toxicity of nanoparticles depends on various factors, including: size, aggregation, composition, crystallinity, surface functionalization, etc. In addition, the toxicity of any nanoparticle to an organism is also determined by the individual's genetic complement. Free radical/oxidative activity of nanoparticles has been reported to cause oxidative stress and lung inflammation, and may likely cause genotoxicity. The Kupffer cells in liver are portal of nanoparticle clearance and are affected by NPs oxidative stress to produce inflammatory mediators such as TNFα. In rat liver, the nano drugs were reported to cause oxidative stress and cell injury, leading to inflammation, alterations in hepatic production of clotting factors, and systemic thrombosis (Alam *et al.,* 2014). Several nanoparticles are able to cross blood brain barrier through intravenous route and may cause neurotoxicity. There were already some reports of nanoparticle neurotoxicity both in the vitro and *in vivo*, and are under further investigations.

With the help of above mentioned nanoparticles and several other nanoparticles also, the field of pathogen detection is being revolutionized. Several specific signature markers of bacteria/viruses can be utilized for the purpose of organism identification. The numerous receptors, glycoproteins, glycopeptides, lipoproteins, carbohydrates, and lipids etc present on the microbial surface can be the targets for organism identification. In nature these epitopes are recognized by a specific antigen-antibody reaction. Nanotechnological modalities also use this antigen-antibody reaction for rapid and precise microbial identification (Zhao *et al.,* 2004; Valanne *et al.,* 2005). As the genome of every organism is unique in itself, an organism's genome sequence is also a very attractive construct used for organism identification with the help of nucleic acid tagged nanoparticle (Bailey *et al.,* 2003; Storhoff *et al.,* 2004; Darbha *et al.,* 2008). Toxins and other biomarkers secreted by pathogenic organisms are also being identified with the help of nanotechnology (Nagy *et al.,* 2008; Shim *et al.,* 2007; Tang *et al.,* 2007).

4   Antimicrobial Resistance and Nanotechnology

Antimicrobial resistance (AMR) is resistance of a microorganism to an antimicrobial medicine to which it was originally sensitive. Resistant organisms (they include bacteria, fungi, viruses and some parasites) are able to withstand attack by antimicrobial medicines, such as antibiotics, antifungals, antivirals, and antimalarials, so that standard treatments become ineffective and infections persists increasing risk of spread to others. The evolution of resistant strains is a natural phenomenon that happens when microorganisms are exposed to antimicrobial drugs, and resistant traits can be exchanged between certain types of bacteria. The misuse of antimicrobial medicines accelerates this natural phenomenon. Poor infection control practices encourage the spread of AMR. The death rate for patients with serious infections treated in hospitals is about twice that in patients with infections caused by non-resistant bacteria. New resistance mechanisms, such as enzymes produced by the bacteria that destroy last generation antibiotics, have emerged among several Gram-negative bacilli and have rapidly spread to many countries. This can render ineffective, the powerful antibiotics, which are often the last defense against multi-resistant strains of bacteria. This new resistant mechanism is encountered in ordinary human pathogens (e.g. *Escherichia coli*) that cause common infections such as urinary tract infection.

In 2011 there were an estimated 6,30,000 cases of Multi-drug resistant tuberculosis (MDR-TB) among the world's 12 million cases of TB. Globally, 3.7% of new cases and 20% of previously treated cases are estimated to have MDR-TB. The average cost of treating a patient with MDR-TB is estimated to be about US $9000 as compared to $19 for drug-sensitive TB. Extensively drug-resistant TB (XDR-TB, defined as MDR-TB plus resistance to any fluoroquinolone and any second-line injectable drug) has been identified in 84 countries globally. A high percentage of hospital-acquired infections are caused by highly resistant bacteria such as methicillin-resistant *Staphylococcus aureus* (MRSA) and vancomycin or multidrug-resistant enterococci (Antimicrobial resistance 2013). MRSA infections lead to an estimated $3 billion to $4 billion of additional health care costs per year. The use/misuse of antibiotics is the single most important factor leading to antibiotic resistance around the world. Antibiotics are among the most commonly prescribed drugs used in human medicine. However, up to 50% of all the antibiotics prescribed for people are not needed or are not optimally effective as prescribed. Antibiotics are also commonly used in food animals to prevent, control, and treat disease, and to promote the growth of food-producing animals. The use of antibiotics for promoting growth is not necessary, and the practice should be phased out. Recent guidance from the U.S.Food and Drug Administration (FDA) describes a pathway toward this goal (Guidance for industry 2013). It is difficult to directly compare the amount of drugs used in food animals with the amount used in humans, but there is evidence that more antibiotics are used in food production. The other major factor in the growth of antibiotic resistance is spread of the resistant strains of bacteria from person to person, or from the non-human sources in the environment, including food. Bacteria will inevitably find ways of resisting the antibiotics we develop, which is why aggressive action is needed now to keep new resistance from developing and to prevent the resistance that already exists from spreading.

4.1   Nano-based Identification of MDR Bacteria

The present, routinely employed methods of microbial detection are time-consuming and laborious to perform; nanotechnology offers several rapid, economical and very accurate methods for microbial detection. A solution-based circuit chip has been developed that can rapidly detect and identify types of infectious bacteria. This nanotechnology based electronic chip can analyze samples for groups of infectious bacteria in a very fast time and confirm the identity of the pathogen within a few minutes with the use of biomolecule-specific microsensors. These microsensors are functionalized with nucleic acid probes to target specific region of pathogens. This multiplexed technique is also capable of distinguishing different bacterial strains like *S. aureus* and *E. coli*, as well as markers of bacterial resistance (Lam *et al.*, 2001). Another modality is the popcorn-shaped iron-magnetic core gold plasmonic shell nanoparticles, used for surface-enhanced Raman spectroscopy (SERS) detection and photothermal destruction of MDR Salmonella bacteria. The central sphere of the nanoparticle acts as an electron reservoir, whereas the tips are capable of focusing the field at their apexes, resulting in a huge field enhancement of the SERS-scattering signal. The same nanoparticle can be used as "light-directed nanoheaters" for the hyperthermic destruction of MDR bacteria by using NIR light on the gold coating. The plasmonic gold coating is very useful for stabilizing the high-magnetic-moment nanoparticles in corrosive biological conditions. The gold coating also eliminates the possible toxicity of iron nanoparticle and also aids in easy bio-conjugation (Fan *et al.*, 2013).

NanoELIwell device for MDR-TB diagnosis based on a combination of mycobacteria antigen immunoassay (ELISA) and microwell technologies has been developed. The major advantage of combining these technologies is significant increase in the sensitivity and shortening of the analytical time by confining the cytokines released from cultured cells within a nano-liter chamber for ELISA assay. NanoELIwell device can successfully culture mycobacteria in a nano-liter chamber and analyze the antigen secretion within 48 hours, the device also successfully differentiates between drug-susceptible and resistant mycobacteria (Nguyen *et al.*, 2012). A molecular method detects rifampicin-resistant M.tuberculosis based on padlock probes (a type of linear oligonucleotides) and magnetic nanobeads. The padlock probes were designed to target the most common mutations associated with rifampicin resistance in M. tuberculosis, i.e. at codons 516, 526 and 531 in the gene rpoB. For detection of the wild type sequence at all three codons simultaneously, a padlock probe and two gap-fill oligonucleotides were used in a novel assay configuration. The assay also includes a probe for identification of the M. tuberculosis complex. Circularized probes were amplified by rolling circle amplification. Amplification products were coupled to oligonucleotide-conjugated magnetic nanobeads and detected by measuring the frequency-dependent magnetic response of the beads using a portable AC susceptometer (Engstorm *et al.*, 2013). A graphene based nanosensor has been developed to detect pathogenic bacteria at the surface of biomaterials like tooth enamel. The specificity for bio-recognition was achieved by attaching odoranin-HP (OHP–an antimicrobial peptide) peptide on graphene monolayers, which has a broad-spectrum activity towards pathogenic bacteria like MRSA (Mannoor *et al.*, 2012). Nanomaterial based on zeolite L was shown to target, label, and photo-inactivate pathogenic and antibiotic-resistant bacteria. A highly green-luminescent dye was inserted into the channels of zeolite L nanocrystals for imaging and to label the cells. The outer surface was functionalized with a photosensitizer that forms toxic singlet oxygen upon red-light irradiation and with amino groups for targeting the living microorganisms. The resulting trifunctional nanomaterial therefore shows intense green fluorescence and efficient $^1O_2$ photo-production. These zeolite L nanocrystals has been shown to target, label, and photo-inactivate antibiotic resistant *E.coli* and *N.gonorrhoeae* (Strassert *et al.*, 2009).

4.2   Nano-based Delivery of Antibiotics against MDR Bacteria

Many new nano-vehicles have been developed for the targeted delivery of antibiotics to

MDR bacteria increasing the therapeutic efficacy and reducing side effects. Nano-hydroxyapatite (nHA) pellets were used as carriers for vancomycin in the treatment of chronic osteomyelitis and bone defects caused by MRSA strains. Vancomycin loaded nHA pellets released high levels of antibiotics locally over a prolonged period, stimulated the reconstruction of new bone and provided effective antimicrobial activity. These nHA pellets were shown to successfully repair bone defects and control infection and also proved to be an effective and safe controlled-release vancomycin carrier for chronic osteomyelitis with bone defects induced by MRSA (Jiang *et al.*, 2012). Another study reported the synergistic effect of chitosan NPs with sulfamethoxazole against resistant *P. aeruginosa*. The exact mechanism of this synergism was not known, yet the potential for use of such combinations clinically is huge since it may be able to make some un-treatable resistant infections treatable at currently recommended dosages that are often marginally effective against resistant strains when used alone (Tin *et al.*, 2009). In another method of drug delivery, an antibiotic was put inside nanofibers made of polyvinyl alcohol and polyethylene oxide. The antibiotics wrapped inside these nanofibers were highly effective in killing a variety of disease causing bacteria and fungi, including *E. coli* and *P. aeruginosa*. The fibers by themselves, doesn't have any anti-bacterial properties but they aid in killing the bacteria by enhancing the local delivery and prolonging the duration of drug action (ACS-2011). In a research at Madras University India, the fungus Trichoderma viride was used for the extracellular biosynthesis of silver nano-particles (AgNPs) from silver nitrate solution. The nanoparticles were evaluated for their increased antimicrobial activities with various antibiotics against gram-positive and gram-negative bacteria. The antibacterial activities of ampicillin, kanamycin, erythromycin, and chloramphenicol were increased in the presence of AgNPs against test strains. The highest enhancing effect was observed for ampicillin against test strains. The ampicillin molecules acted on the cell wall, which leads to cell wall lysis and thus increased the penetration of AgNPs into the bacterium. The AgNP-ampicillin complex also reacted with bacterial DNA and prevented DNA unwinding, resulting in more serious damage to bacterial cells (Fayaz *et al.*, 2010). Recently, spherical silver and gold nanoparticles (AuNPs) were synthesized and then functionalized with ampicillin, and the capacity of gold nanoparticles (AuNPs) to serve as an alternative to silver nanoparticles (AgNPs) as a drug delivery system was compared. It was found that ampicillin-functionalized AuNP and ampicillin-functionalized AgNP were comparable as bactericides and killed pathogenic *Escherichia coli, Vibrio cholerae,*and multiple-drug-resistant bacteria such as *Pseudomonas aeruginosa, Enterobacter aerogenes*, and a methicillin-resistant isolate of *Staphylococcus aureus* (Brown *et al.*, 2012). Vancomycin capped gold nanoparticles have also shown enhanced in vitro antibacterial activities against vancomycin-resistant enterococci (Gu *et al.*, 2003).

Nanotechnology based approaches have also been utilized for targeted delivery (monocytes & macrophages) and sustained release of anti-tubercular drugs in both blood plasma & organ tissue. (Fawaz, 1998; Anisimova, 2000; Pandey *et al.*, 2003). These chemotherapy regimens with superior sustained release pharmokenetic profiles, targeted delivery, and improved bioavailability can significantly reduce regimen duration, dose frequency, and dose load. This can greatly increase compliance in drug-susceptible

TB patients, in turn improving cure rates and eliminating the possibility of a drug re-sistant re-infection. Though there are no first-line MDR- or XDR-TB drugs, nanotech-nology can be applied to several second line drugs (Pandey & Ahmad, 2011). Although, resistance profiles in drug resistant TB vary greatly, there is a growing body of evidence demonstrating that increased levels of drug-susceptible TB chemotherapy, namely high-level INH, can be used to overcome MDR-TB (Katiyar, 2008; Leimane *et al.*, 2005). How-ever, this has only been investigated in conventional methods of drug delivery and pos-es little actual potential. Various nanocarriers have also been evaluated to deliver anti-malarial drugs targeting the Plasmodium infected cells. Considering the peculiarities of malarial parasites, the focus is placed mainly on lipid-based and polymer-based nanocarriers. These nanocarriers are known to improve the efficacy of currently availa-ble antimalarial drugs and also contribute to the formulation and delivery of new chem-ical entities (Santos & Mosqueira, 2010).

4.3   Miscellaneous Nano-biotics against MDR bacteria

As mentioned earlier, nanomaterials have unique physical and chemical properties with respect to larger-sized counterparts, such as increased surface-to-volume ratio, greater chemical reactivity and useful optical features (e.g. strong visible fluorescence). Such properties are being exploited for a wide array of new bio-medical products including anti-microbial agents. Recently a new class of nanomaterials has been introduced that has generated keen interest in the fight against MDR bacteria. These nanotechnology based macromolecular antimicrobial polymers (MAPs) are synthesized by metal-free organocatalytic ring opening polymerization of functional cyclic carbonate. These na-noparticles selectively disrupt microbial walls/membranes, thus inhibiting the growth of gram-positive bacteria, MRSA and fungi. These bio-degradable MAPs can be synthe-sized in large quantities at low cost, raising hope for treating life-threatening MDR bac-terial infections (Nederberg, 2011). Since these nano-MAPs directly destroy microbial walls/ membranes without targeting any specific step of the microbial metabolic path-way (as is the mechanism of action of several antibiotics), there may be less opportunity for mutations or other alterations in the microbe to impart drug resistance. This may be responsible for the decreased resistance of the pathogens to these nano-MAPs (Brogden, 2005).

Nitric oxide (NO), a diatomic free radical that plays a key role in the natural im-mune system response to infection, is also an attractive molecule for designing antibac-terial nanoparticles. NO-releasing silica nanoparticles were synthesized as novel anti-bacterial agents against *Pseudomonas aeruginosa*. Comparison of the bactericidal efficacy of the NO-releasing nanoparticles to a small molecule NO donor, demonstrated en-hanced bactericidal efficacy of nanoparticle-derived NO and reduced cytotoxicity to healthy cells (mammalian fibroblasts). Confocal microscopy also revealed that fluores-cently labeled NO-releasing nanoparticles were associated more with the bacterial cell, providing rationale for the enhanced bactericidal efficacy of these nanoparticles (Hetrick *et al.*, 2008). In another study, NO releasing nanoparticles had shown broad spectrum antibacterial effect on antibiotic resistant *K. pneumonia*, *E. faecalis*, *Str. pyogenes*, *E. coli* and *P. aeruginosa*. NO altered peripheral and integral structures on the bacterial plasma membrane, particularly membrane-bound proteins and lipids. Formation of peroxynitrite from interaction with superoxides further disrupted the microbial membrane through lipid peroxidation, accelerating degradation of cellular integrity. Furthermore, as a lipophilic, uncharged molecule, NO transverse the lipid bilayer to reach important metabolic enzymes and DNA, crippling essential biological processes (Friedman *et al.*, 2011).

Recently, it has been shown that the magnetic properties of superparamagnetic iron oxide nanoparticles (SPION) and antibacterial properties of silver can be combined to design unique silver-conjugated SPION. For the first time, it is demonstrated that MRSA biofilms can be eradicated by these silver-conjugated SPION without resorting to the use of antibiotics. The SPION anti-biofilm efficacy can be further improved by application of an external magnetic field. Under the influence of an external magnetic field the magnetic core of the silver-conjugated SPION allowed for deeper penetration into the bio-film. The anti-biofilm property of silver-conjugated SPION treatment is due to the significant increases in intracellular or membrane-bound iron, sulfur and silver concentrations (Durmus & Webster, 2013). Photodynamic therapy (PDT) has been investigated as an alternative antimicrobial therapy for treating microbial infections. Cellulose nanocrystals modified with porphyrin-derived photosensitizer were used to mediate bacterial photodynamic inactivation. These crystals were capable of inducing photodynamic inactivation of multidrug resistant *Acinetobacter baumannii* (MDRAB) and MRSA upon illumination with visible light (Carpenter *et al.*, 2012). The anti-microbial silver carbene complexes (SCCs) encapsulated in poly(ethylene glycol)-poly(lactic acid) (PEG-PLA) nanoparticle complexes act as controlled release systems and were found to be active against various antibiotic resistant forms of bacteria like MRSA, *P. aeruginosa*, *B. cepacia*, *K. pneumonia* (Leid *et al.*, 2012).

Nanotechnology is emerging as a powerful weapon in the fight against MDR organisms. The most important advantage is their unique and different approach to damage multiple necessary microbial cell functions, rather than focusing upon a particular biochemical process. These multiple lethal blows may make it more difficult for microbes to withstand or develop resistance. Secondly, as drug carriers NPs offer the possibility of more efficient and targeted delivery of antibiotic agents over prolonged periods lowering the likelihood of sublethal dosing of antibiotics as well as broad spectrum microbial exposures, which in turn could reduce the development of resistance to NPs attached antibiotics.

5   Nanotechnology and HIV/AIDS therapy

Presently used drugs for anti-retroviral (ARV) therapy of HIV/AIDS are broadly classified as nucleoside reverse transcriptase inhibitors (NRTIs), nucleotide reverse transcriptase inhibitors (NtRTIs), non-nucleoside reverse transcriptase inhibitors (NNRTIs), protease inhibitors (PIs), and more recently fusion and integrase inhibitors (Rathbun *et al.*, 2006). These ARV drugs have several limitations like extensive first pass metabolism, low bioavailability, short half-life and side-effects related to toxicity leading to patient non-compliance and rebound viral replication (Richman *et al.*, 2009). High genetic diversity of HIV-1 and the continuous mutation it undergoes may lead to development drug resistance even with good regimen adherence (Sax *et al.*, 2007). Moreover, complete eradication is prevented since the 'latent reservoirs' of the virus are present within memory CD4+ T cells and cells of the macrophage–monocyte lineage (Richman *et al.*, 2009). The cells that harbor these latent HIV are typically concentrated in specific anatomic sites, such as secondary lymphoid tissue, testes, liver, kidney, lungs, gut and the CNS (Richman *et al.*, 2009). The eradication of this latent viral pool is necessary for effective long term treatment of HIV/AIDS patients. Nanotechnology can be utilized to improve the pharmacokinetic profile and targeted delivery of ARV drugs, holding promise for complete viral destruction from host body.

Active targeting strategies have been utilized for ARV drug delivery. Macrophages (one of the HIV reservoir cells), have various receptors on their surface such as formyl peptide, mannose, galactose and Fc receptors, which could be utilized for receptor-mediated internalization. The drug stavudine was encapsulated using various liposomes conjugated with mannose and galactose, resulting in increased cellular uptake compared with free drug or plain liposomes, and generating significant level of the drug in liver, spleen and lungs (Garg *et al.*, 2006; Garg *et al.*, 2007; Garg *et al.*, 2008). Zidovudine, has also been encapsulated in a mannose targeted liposome made from stearylamine, showing increased localization in lymph node and spleen (Kaur *et al.*, 2008). Immunoliposomes have the targeting specificity of antibodies on their surface e.g., anti-HLA-DR monoclonal antibodies which target follicular dendritic cells, B cells and macrophages which express the HLA-DR determinant of MHC-II molecule. Such immunoliposomes have been shown to enhance accumulation of indinivar in mice lymph nodes (Gagne *et al.*, 2002). Other lipid based nano-systems carrying indinavir achieve about 22 times higher concentration of the drug in lymph nodes compared to plasma, and 10-fold reduction in peak plasma concentrations (Kinman *et al.*, 2003; Choi *et al.*, 2008). Furthermore, highest drug levels in lymph nodes were seen on surface modification with polyethylene glycol (Kinman *et al.*, 2006). In latently infected cells (resting CD4+ T cells) lipid based nanoparticles loaded with bryostatin-2 (a protein kinase C activator), were able to activate primary CD4+ T cells and stimulate HIV replication. Moreover, upon addition of an antiretroviral agent such as nelfinavir, the multifunctional nanoparticles simultaneously activated latent virus and also inhibited viral spread (Kovochich *et al.*, 2011). Similar to liposomes, poly-(lactic-co-glycolic acid) polymeric nanoparticles containing ritonavir, lopinavir, and efavirenz resulted in longer intracellular peak levels in peripheral blood mononuclear cells compared to free drug (Destache *et al.*, 2009). Mannosylated fifth-generation poly(propyleneimine) dendrimers targeting lectin receptors of macrophage surface have also been shown to increase the uptake of lamivudine (Dutta & Jain, 2007) and efavirenz (Dutta *et al.*, 2007). Tuftsin (a natural macrophage activator tetrapeptide), when conjugated to poly(propyleneimine) dendrimers (TuPPI), increased the cellular uptake of efavirenz (Dutta *et al.*, 2008). In addition to active targeting of ARV drugs, various fullerene (C-60) based structures, dendrimers and inorganic nanoparticles, such as gold and silver, have been shown to have anti-HIV activity *in vitro* (Mamo *et al.*, 2010).

Gene therapy is another promising technology for HIV/AIDS treatment, in which a gene is inserted into a cell to interfere with viral infection or replication. Other nucleic acid-based compounds, such as DNA, siRNA, RNA decoys, ribozymes and aptamers or protein-based agents such as fusion inhibitors and zinc-finger nucleases can also be used to interfere with viral replication (Rossi *et al.*, 2007, Haasnoot *et al.*, 2007). In addition to poor pharmacokinetic profile, nucleic acid delivery by vector methods has also posed potential safety concerns due to their oncogenic, inflammatory and immunogenic effects (Gao & Huang, 2009). Numerous methods for non-viral delivery of therapeutic DNA and RNA have been explored. Several of these approaches have been adopted for the delivery of anti-HIV RNA and DNA therapeutics. In general, the nucleic acid is condensed with a cationic reagent via electrostatic interactions. The cationic reagent (which may be a peptide, liposome or dendrimer) protects the nucleic acid against degradation and facilitates cellular uptake by endocytosis (Parboosing *et al.*, 2012).

Immunotherapy for AIDS aims at modulating the host immune response against HIV. The various immunotherapy approaches for HIV/AIDS could be based on delivering cytokines (such as IL-2, IL-7 and IL-15) or antigens. The development of cellular immunity, and to a large degree humoral immunity, requires antigen-presenting cells (APCs) to process and present antigens to CD4+ and CD8+ T cells. Dendritic cells (DCs) are the quintessential professional APCs responsible for initiating and orchestrating the development of cellular and humoral (antibody) immunity. Protein/peptide antigens or DNA immunogens (which lead to endogenous protein expression) could then be delivered to endogenous or *ex vivo*-generated DCs. Nanotechnology platforms for delivery of immune-modulatory factors and targeting antigens to DC surface receptors *in vivo* provide immense opportunities in the fight against HIV/AIDS. The most clinically advanced application of nanotechnology for immunotherapy of HIV/AIDS is the DermaVir patch. DermaVir is a targeted nanoparticle system based on polyethyleimine mannose (PEIm), glucose and HIV antigen coding DNA plasmid formulated into nanoparticles (~100 nm) and administered under a patch after a skin preparation. The nanoparticles are delivered to epidermal Langerhans cells that trap the nanoparticles and mature to become highly immunogenic on their way to the lymph nodes. Mature DCs containing the nanoparticles present antigens to T cells inducing cellular immunity (Mamo *et al.*, 2010).

Vaccines based on nanotechnological modalities for HIV/AIDS are also showing potential in early studies. Their ability to target specific cells and release antigens in a controlled and sustained manner makes nanoparticles a great alternative to viral vectors. Lipid- and polymer-based nanoparticles have been shown to induce HIV-specific antibody and cellular immune responses in animal studies. Despite the progress so far, preclinical studies remain important to ensure a clear understanding and optimization of mechanisms involved in the nanoparticle induction of strong humoral and cellular immunity. In addition to continued efforts in vaccine development, research into microbicide development remains important. Nanotechnology can play a major role in microbicide development by providing innovative strategies for nanoparticle-based delivery of therapeutic molecules or RNAi (Mamo *et al.*, 2010).

Nanotechnology can hugely impact the treatment and prevention of HIV/AIDS with various innovative approaches. Various nanosystems have shown the ability to simplify drug regimens, enhancing antiretroviral activity, while reducing their toxicity and increasing patient's compliance, preventing development of drug resistance. Targeted nanoparticles have been used to target macrophages, and latent viral reservoirs resulting in better viral suppression. Newer treatment approaches, such as gene therapy, immunotherapy, vaccine development and local microbicides can be enhanced with nanotechnology. Overall the multi-faceted anti-retroviral effects shown by different nano-agents hold great promise for treatment of AIDS pandemic.

Funding source

No funding was received from anywhere and this is a purely institutional work.

Conflict of interest

The authors declare that they have no conflict of interest.

References

ACS press release (2011): Antibiotics wrapped in nanofibers turn resistant disease-producing bacteria into ghosts. Available at: http://www.acs.org/content/acs/en/pressroom/newsreleases/2011/march/antibiotics-wrapped-in-nanofibers-turn-resistant-disease-producing-bacteria-into-ghosts.html

Alam F, Yadav N (2013). Potential applications of quantum dots in mapping sentinel lymph node and detection of micrometastases in breast carcinoma. J Breast Cancer 16 :1–11.

Alam F, Naim M, Aziz M, Yadav N (2014). Unique roles of nanotechnology in medicine and cancer. Indian J Cancer (article in press).

Allen TM, Moase EH (1996). Therapeutic opportunities for targeted liposomal drug delivery. Adv Drug Deliv Rev21:117–133.

Anisimova YV (2000). Nanoparticles as antituberculosis drugs carriers: effect on activity against Mycobacterium tuberculosis in human monocyte-derived macrophages. J Nanopart Res 2:165.

Anti microbial resistance (2013). Media centre W.H.O. Available at: http://www.who.int/mediacentre/factsheets/fs194/en/

Bailey RC, Nam JM, Mirkin CA, Hupp JT (2003). Real-time multicolor DNA detection with hemoresponsive diffraction gratings and nanoparticle probes. J Am Chem Soc 125:13541–13551.

BCC report (2013). Nanotechnology in Medical Applications: The Global Market. Available at http://www.bccresearch.com/report/nanotechnology-medical-applications-global-market-hlc069b.html

Bera D, Qian L, Tseng TK, Holloway PH (2010). Quantum dots and their multimodal applications: A review. Materials3:2260–2345.

Brogden KA (2005).Antimicrobial peptides: pore formers or metabolic inhibitors in bacteria?Nat Rev

Microbiol 3: 238–250.

Brown AN, Smith K, Samuels TA, Lu J, Obare SO, Scott ME (2012). Nanoparticles Functionalized with Ampicillin Destroy Multiple- Antibiotic-Resistant Isolates of Pseudomonas aeruginosa and Enterobacter aerogenes and Methicillin-Resistant Staphylococcus aureus. Appl Environ Microbiol 782768–2774.

Brown SD, Nativo P, Smith JA, Stirling D, Edwards PR, Venugopal B, et al (2010). Gold nanoparticles for the improved anticancer drug delivery of the active component of oxaliplatin. J Am Chem Soc 132:4678–4684.

Carpenter BL, Feese E,Sadeghifar H, Argyropoulos DS, Ghiladi RA (2012). Porphyrin-cellulose nanocrystals: a photobactericidal material that exhibits broad spectrum antimicrobial activity. Photochem. Photobiol 88: 527–536.

Chang HI, Cheng MY, Yeh MK (2012). Clinically-proven liposome-based drug delivery: Formulation, characterization and therapeutic efficacy. Open Access Sci Rep 1:195. Available at: http://www. omicsonline.org/scientific-reports/2155-983X-SR195.pdf. Last accessed 29 November 2013.

Chatterjee DK, Fong LS, Zhang Y (2008). Nanoparticles in photodynamic therapy: An emerging paradigm. Adv Drug Deliv Rev60:1627–1637.

Cheng Y, Zhao L, Li Y, Xu T (2011). Design of biocompatible dendrimers for cancer diagnosis and therapy: Current status and future perspectives. Chem Soc Rev40:2673–2703.

Choi SU, Bui T, Ho RJ (2008). pH-dependent interactions of indinavir and lipids in nanoparticles and their ability to entrap a solute. J Pharm Sci97: 931–943.

Danilcauk M, Lund A, Saldo J, Yamada H, Michalik J (2006). Conduction electron spin resonance of small silver particles. Spectrochimaca Acta Part A 63:189–191.

Darbha GK, Rai US, Singh AK, Ray PC (2008). Gold-nanorod-based sensing of sequence specific HIV-1 virus DNA by using hyper-Rayleigh scattering spectroscopy. Chemistry 14:3896–3903.

Davis ME, Chen Z, Shin DM (2008). Nanoparticle therapeutics: An emerging treatment modality for cancer. Nat Rev Drug Discov 7:771-782.

Destache CJ, Belgum T, Christensen K, Shibata A, Sharma A, Dash A (2009). Combination antiretroviral drugs in PLGA nanoparticle for HIV-1. BMC Infect Dis 9: 198.

Dinh P, Sotiriou C, Piccart MJ (2007). The evolution of treatment strategies: Aiming at the target. Breast 16:S10–16.

Drolet DW, Nelson J, Tucker CE, Zack PM, Nixon K, Bolin R, et al (2000). Pharmacokinetics and safety of an anti-vascular endothelial growth factor aptamer (NX1838) following injection into the vitreous humor of rhesus monkeys. Pharm Res 17:1503–1510.

Durmus NG and Webster TJ (2013). Eradicating antibiotic-resistant biofilms with silver-conjugated superparamagnetic iron oxide nanoparticles.Adv Healthc Mater 2:165–171.

Dutta T, Agashe HB, Garg M, Balasubramanium P, Kabra M, Jain NK (2007). Poly (propyleneimine) dendrimer based nanocontainers for targeting of efavirenz to human monocytes/macrophages in vitro. J Drug Target 15: 89–98.

Dutta T, Garg M, Jain NK (2008). Targeting of efavirenz loaded tuftsin conjugated poly (propyleneimine) dendrimers to HIV infected macrophages in vitro. Eur J Pharm Sci34:181–189.

Dutta T, Jain NK (2007). Targeting potential and anti-HIV activity of lamivudine loaded mannosylated poly (propyleneimine) dendrimer. BBA Gen Subjects1770: 681–686.

ECR (2006), Nanomedicine: Nanotechnology for Health – European Technology Platform. Brussels: European Commission, Research DG, p. 12.

Engstrom A, de la Torre TZG, Stromme M, Nilsson M, Herthnek D (2013). Detection of Rifampicin Resistance in Mycobacterium tuberculosis by Padlock Probes and Magnetic Nanobead-Based ReadoutPlos One 8:4. doi:10.1371/journal.pone.0062015.

Fan Z, Senapati D, Khan SA, Singh AK, Hamme A, Yust B et al (2013). Popcorn-Shaped Magnetic Core– Plasmonic Shell Multifunctional Nanoparticles for the Targeted Magnetic Separation and Enrichment, Label-Free SERS Imaging, and Photothermal Destruction of Multidrug-Resistant Bacteria.Chem Eur J 19: 2839–2847.

Fawaz F, Bonini F, Maugein J, Lagueny AM (1998).Ciprofloxacin-loaded polyiso-butylcyanoacrylate nanoparticles: pharmacokinetics and in vitro antimicrobial activity. Int J Pharm168:255–259.

Fayaz AM, Balaji K, Girilal M, Yadav R, Kalaichelvan PT, Venketesan R (2010). Biogenic synthesis of silver nanoparticles and their synergistic effect with antibiotics: a study against gram-positive and gram-negative bacteriaNanomedicine 6 :103–109.

Feng QL, Wu J, Chen GQ, Cui FZ, Kim TN, Kim JO (2008). A mechanistic study of the antibacterial effect of silver ions on Escherichia coli and Staphylococcus aureus. J Biomed Mater Res 52: 662–668.

Fernandez-Fernandez A, Manchanda R, McGoron AJ (2011). Theranostic applications of nanomaterials in cancer: Drug delivery, image-guided therapy, and multifunctional platforms. Appl Biochem Biotechnol 165:1628–1651.

Ferrari M (2005). Cancer nanotechnology: Opportunities and challenges. Nat Rev Cancer 5:161—171.

Fountaine TJ, Wincovitch SM, Geho DH, Garfield SH, Pittaluga S (2006). Multispectral imaging of clinically relevant cellular targets in tonsil and lymphoid tissue using semiconductor quantum dots. Mod Pathol 19:1181–1191.

Friedman A, Blecher K, Sanchez D, Vernon CT, Gialanella P, Friedman JM et al (2011). Susceptibility of Gram-positive and –negative bacteria to novel nitric oxide-releasing nanoparticle technology. Virulence 2: 217–221.

Gagné JF, Désormeaux A, Perron S, Tremblay MJ, Bergeron MG (2002). Targeted delivery of indinavir to HIV-1 primary reservoirs with immunoliposomes. Biochim Biophys Acta 1558: 198–210.

Gambari R, Borgatti M, Altomare L, Manaresi N, Medoro G, Romani A, et al (2003). Applications to cancer research of "lab-on-a-chip" devices based on dielectrophoresis (DEP). Technol Cancer Res Treat 2:31–40.

Gao K, Huang L (2009). Nonviral methods for siRNA delivery. Mol Pharm 6: 651–658.

Gao X, Yang L, Petros JA, Marshall FF, Simons JW, Nie S (2005). In vivo molecular and cellular imaging with quantum dots. Curr Opin Biotechnol 16:63–72.

Garg M, Asthana A, Agashe HB, Agrawal GP, Jain NK (2006). Stavudine-loaded mannosylated liposomes: In-vitro anti-HIV-1 activity, tissue distribution and pharmacokinetics. J Pharm Pharmacol 58:605– 616.

Garg M, Dutta T, Jain NK (2007). Reduced hepatic toxicity, enhanced cellular uptake and altered pharmacokinetics of stavudine loaded galactosylated liposomes. Eur J Pharm Biopharm 67:76–85.

Garg M, Garg BR, Jain S, et al (2008). Radiolabeling, pharmacoscintigraphic evaluation and antiretroviral efficacy of stavudine loaded 99mtc labeled galactosylated liposomes. Eur J Pharm Sci 33: 271–281.

Grodzinski P, Silver M, Molnar LK (2006). Nanotechnology for cancer diagnostics: Promises and *challenges. Expert Rev Mol Diagn 6:307–318.*

Gu H, Ho PL,Tong E, Wang L, Xu B (2003). *Presenting Vancomycin on Nanoparticles to Enhance AntimicrobialActivities.Nano Lett 3:1261–1263.*

Guidance for industry (2013). *Available at: http://www.fda.gov/downloads/AnimalVeterinary/Guidance ComplianceEnforcement/GuidanceforIndustry/UCM299624.pdf*

Haasnoot J, Westerhout EM, Berkhout B (2007). *RNA interference against viruses: strike and counterstrike. Nat Biotechnol 25:1435–1443.*

Häfeli UO (2004). *Magnetically modulated therapeutic systems. Int J Pharm 277:19–24.*

Herborn CU, Barkhausen J, Paetsch I, Hunold P, Mahler M, Shamsi K,et al (2003). *Coronary arteries: contrast-enhanced MR imaging with SH L 643A — experience in 12 volunteers. Radiology 229: 217–223.*

Hetrick EM, Shin JH, Stasko NA, Johnson CB, Wespe DA, Holmuhamedov E et al (2008). *Bactericidal Efficacy of Nitric Oxide-Releasing Silica Nanoparticles. ACS Nano 2:235–246.*

Hirsch LR, Gobin AM, Lowery AR, Tam F, Drezek RA, Halas NJ, et al(2006). *Metal nanoshells. Ann Biomed Eng 34:15–22.*

Hirsch LR, Stafford RJ, Bankson JA, Sershen SR, Rivera B, Price RE, et al(2003). *Nanoshell-mediated near-infrared thermal therapy of tumors under magnetic resonance guidance. ProcNatlAcadSci USA 100:13549–13554.*

Huang RS, Dolan ME (2010). *Approaches to the discovery of pharmacogenomic markers in oncology: 2000-2010-2020. Pharmacogenomics 11:471–474.*

Irache JM, Esparza I, Gamazo C, Agüeros M, Espuelas S (2011). *Nanomedicine: Novel approaches in human and veterinary therapeutics. Vet Parasitol 180:47–71.*

Jain KK (2005). *Nanotechnology in clinical laboratory diagnostics. Clin Chim Acta358:37–54.*

Jain RK (2008). *Lessons from multidisciplinary translational trials on anti-angiogenic therapy of cancer. Nat Rev Cancer 8:309–316.*

Jesorka A, Orwar O (2008). *Liposomes: Technologies and analytical applications. Annu Rev Anal Chem (Palo Alto Calif)1:801–832.*

Jiang JL, Li YF, Fang TL, Zhou J, Li XL,Wang YC and Dong J (2012). *Vancomycin-loaded nano-hydroxyapatite pellets to treat MRSA-induced chronic osteomyelitis with bone defect in rabbits.Inflamm Res 61: 207–215.*

Jordan A, Scholtz R, Wust P, Fähling H, Felix R (1999). *Magnetic fluid hyperthermia (MFH): Cancer treatment with AC magnetic field induced excitation of biocompatible superparamagnetic nanoparticles. J Magn Magn Mater 201:413–419.*

Kaittanis C, Naser SA, Perez JM (2007). *One-step, nanoparticle-mediated bacterial detection with magnetic relaxation. Nano Lett 7:380–383.*

Katiyar SK (2008). *A randomised controlled trial of high-dose isoniazid adjuvant therapy for multidrug-resistant tuberculosis. Int J Tuberc Lung Dis12:139.*

Kaur CD, Nahar M, Jain NK (2008). *Lymphatic targeting of zidovudine using surface-engineered liposomes. J Drug Target 16:798–805.*

Kim JS, Kuk E, Yu K, Kim JH, Park SJ, Lee HJ, et al (2007). *Antimicrobial effects of silver nanoparticles. Nanomedicine 2007; 3: 95–101.*

Kimchi-Sarfaty C, Oh JM, Kim IW, Sauna ZE, Calcagno AM, Ambudkar SV, et al (2007). A silent polymorphism in the MDR1 gene changes substrate specificity. Science 315:525–528.

Kinman L, Brodie SJ, Tsai CC, Bui T, Larsen K, Schmidt A, et al (2003). Lipid-drug association enhanced HIV-1 protease inhibitor indinavir localization in lymphoid tissues and viral load reduction: A proof of concept study in HIV-2287-infected macaques. J Acquir Immune Defic Syndr34: 387–397.

Kinman L, Bui T, Larsen K, Tsai CC, Anderson D, Morton WR et al (2006). Optimization of lipid-indinavir complexes for localization in lymphoid tissues of HIV-infected macaques. J Acquir Immune Defic Syndr 42: 155–161.

Kirsner R, Orsted H, Wright B (2001). Matrix metalloproteinases in normal and impaired wound healing: a potential role of nanocrystalline silver. Wounds 13: 5–10.

Kovochich M, Marsden MD, Zack JA (2011). Activation of latent HIV using drug-loaded nanoparticles. PLoS One6: e18270.

Kumar R, Roy I, Ohulchanskyy TY, Goswami LN, Bonoiu AC, Bergey EJ, et al (2008). Covalently dye-linked, surface-controlled, and bioconjugated organically modified silica nanoparticles as targeted probes for optical imaging. ACS Nano 2:449–456.

Lam B, Das J, Holmes RD (2001). Solution-based circuits enable rapid and multiplexed pathogen detection. Nat Commun.4. Available at: http://www.nature.com/ncomms/2013/130612/ncomms3001/full/ncomms 3001.html

Lee H, Sun E, Ham D, Weissleder R (2008). Chip-NMR biosensor for detection and molecular analysis of cells. Nat Med 14:869–874.

Leid JG, Ditto AJ, Knapp A, Shah PN, Wright BD,Blust R et al (2012). In vitro antimicrobial studies of silver carbene complexes: activity of free and nanoparticle carbene formulations against clinical isolates of pathogenic bacteria. J Antimicrb. Chemother 67:138–148.

Leimane V, Riekstina V, Holtz TH, Zarovska E, Skripconoka V, Thorpe LE, et al (2005). Clinical outcome of individualised treatment of multidrugresistant tuberculosis in Latvia: a retrospective cohort study. Lancet 365:318–326.

Longmire M, Choyke PL, Kobayashi H (2008). Clearance properties of nano-sized particles and molecules as imaging agents: Considerations and caveats. Nanomedicine 3:703–717.

Mamo T, Moseman EA, Kolishetti N, Morales CS, Shi J,Kuritzkes DR (2010). Emerging nanotechnology approaches for HIV/AIDS treatment and prevention. Nanomedicine 5:269–285.

Mannoor MS, Tao H, Clayton JD, Sengupta A, Kaplan DL, Naik RR et al (2012). Graphene-based wireless bacteria detection on tooth enamel. Nat Commun 3;763. doi: 10.1038/ncomms1767

Mansoori MA, Agrawal S, Jawade S, Khan MI (2012). A review on liposome. Int J Adv Res Pharm Bio Sci 1:453–464.

Matsumura Y, Yoshikata K, Kunisaki S, Tsuchido T (2003). Mode of bacterial action of silver zeolite and its comparison with that of silver nitrate. Appl Environ Microbiol 69: 4278–4281.

McCarthy JR, Kelly KA, Sun EY, Weissleder R (2007). Targeted delivery of multifunctional magnetic nanoparticles. Nanomedicine(Lond) 2:153–167.

McCarthy JR, Weissleder R (2008). Multifunctional magnetic nanoparticles for targeted imaging and therapy. Adv Drug Deliv Rev 60:1241–1251.

McNeil SE (2005), Nanotechnology for the biologist. J Leukoc Biol 78:585–594.

Medarova Z, Pham W, Farrar C, Petkova V, Moore A (2007). In vivo imaging of siRNA delivery and silencing in tumors. *Nat Med* 13:372–377.

Menon U, Jacobs IJ (2000). *Recent developments in ovarian cancer screening. Curr Opin Obstet Gynecol* 12:39–42.

Michalet X, Pinaud FF, Bentolila LA, Tsay JM, Doose S, Li JJ, et al (2005). *Quantum dots for live cells, in vivo imaging, and diagnostics. Science* 307:538–544.

Moyano DF, Rotello VM (2011). *Nano meets biology: Structure and function at the nanoparticle interface. Langmuir* 27:10376–10385.

Nagasaki Y, Ishii T, Sunaga Y, Watanabe Y, Otsuka H, Kataoka K (2004). *Novel molecular recognition via fluorescent resonance energy transfer using a biotin-PEG/polyamine stabilized CdS quantum dot. Langmuir* 20:6396–6400.

Nagy JO, Zhang Y, Yi W, Liu X, Motari E, Song JC, et al (2008). *Glycopolydiacetylene nanoparticles as a chromatic biosensor to detect Shiga-like toxin producing Escherichia coli O157:H7. Bioorg Med Chem Lett* 18:700–703.

Nam JM, Jang KJ, Groves JT (2007). *Detection of proteins using a colorimetric bio-barcode assay. Nat Protoc* 2:1438–1444.

Nath S, Kaittanis C, Ramachandran V, Dalal NS, Perez JM (2009). *Synthesis, Magnetic Characterization, and Sensing Applications of Novel Dextran-Coated Iron Oxide Nanorods. Chem. of Mater* 21:1761–1767.

NCI (2004) *Cancer Nanotechnology: Going Small for Big Advances – Using Nanotechnology toAdvance Cancer Diagnosis,Prevention and Treatment.* Washington, DC: U.S. Department Of Healthand Human Services, National Institutes of Health, National Cancer Institute.

Nederberg F, Zhang Y, Tan JPK, Xu KJ, Wang HY, Yang C et al (2011). *Biodegradable nanostructures with selective lysis of microbial membranes. Nat Chem* 2011;3:409–414.

Nguyen YH, Ma X, Qin L (2012). *Rapid identification and drug susceptibility screening of ESAT-6 secreting Mycobacteria by a NanoELIwell assay. Scientific Reports,* 2;635. doi: 10.1038/srep00635.

Nie S, Xing Y, Kim GJ, Simons JW (2007). *Nanotechnology applications in cancer. Annu Rev Biomed Eng* 9:257–288.

NNI (2005) *National Science and Technology Council Committee on Technology, The National NanotechnologyInitiative: Research and Development Leading to a Revolution in Technology and Industry, Office of Sciences and Technology Policy,* Washington, DC,USA.

NNI-FAQ (2013) *National Nanotechnology Initiative. Frequently asked questions.* Available at http://www.nano.gov/nanotech-101/nanotechnology-facts

O'Loughlin JO, Millwood IY, McDonald HM, Price CF, Kaldor JM, Paull JRA (2010). *Safety, tolerability, and pharmacokinetics of SPL7013 gel (VivaGel): a dose ranging, phase I study. Sex Transm Dis* 37: 100–104.

Pandey R, Ahmad Z (2011). *Nanomedicine and experimental tuberculosis: facts, flaws, and future. Nanomedicine.* 7:259–272.

Pandey R, Zahoor A, Sharma S, Khuller GK (2003). *Nanoparticle encapsulated antitubercular drugs as a potential oral drug delivery system against murine tuberculosis. Tuberculosis* 83:373–378.

Parboosing R, Maguire GEM, Govender P, Kruger HG (2012). *Nanotechnology and the treatment of HIV infection. Viruses* 4:448–520.

Park J, Fong PM, Lu J, Russell KS, Booth CJ, Saltzmam WM, et al (2009). *PEGylated PLGA nanoparticles for the improved delivery of doxorubicin. Nanomedicine 5:410–418.*

Peng CW, Li Y (2010). *Application of quantum dots-based biotechnology in cancer diagnosis: current status and future perspectives. J Nanomater2010:11. Available from: http://www.hindawi.com/journals/jnm/2010/676839/. Last accessed 29 November 2013.*

Perez JM, Josephson L, O'Loughlin T, Hogemann D, Weissleder R (2002). *Magnetic relaxation switches capable of sensing molecular interactions. Nat Biotechnol 20:816–820.*

Perez JM, Simeone FJ, Saeki Y, Josephson L, Weissleder R (2003). *Viral-induced self-assembly of magnetic nanoparticles allows the detection of viral particles in biological media. J Am Chem Soc 125:10192–10193.*

Qiao XF, Zhou JC, Xiao JW, Wang YF, Sun LD, Yan CH (2012). *Triple-functional core-shell structured upconversion luminescent nanoparticles covalently grafted with photosensitizer for luminescent, magnetic resonance imaging and photodynamic therapy in vitro. Nanoscale 4:4611–4623.*

Qin D, He X, Wang K, Tan W (2008). *Using fluorescent nanoparticles and SYBR Green I based two-color flow cytometry to determine Mycobacterium tuberculosis avoiding false positives. Biosens Bioelectron 24:626–631.*

Rathbun RC, Lockhart SM, Stephens JR (2006). *Current HIV treatment guidelines –an overview. Curr Pharm Des 12: 1045–1063.*

Ray S, Koshy NR, Reddy PJ, Srivastava S (2012). *Virtual Labs in proteomics: New E-learning tools. J Proteomics 75:2515–2525.*

Rhyner MN, Smith AM, Gao X, Mao H, Yang L, Nie S (2006). *Quantum dots and multifunctional nanoparticles: New contrast agents for tumor imaging. Nanomedicine (Lond)1:209–217.*

Richman DD, Margolis DM, Delaney M, Greene WC, Hazuda D, Pomerantz RJ (2009). *The challenge of finding a cure for HIV infection. Science 323:1304–1307.*

Rosengart AJ, Kaminksi MD, Chen H, Caviness PL, Ebner AD, Ritter JA (2005). *Magnetizable implants and functionalized magnetic carriers: A novel approach for non-invasive yet targeted drug delivery. J Magn Magn Mater293:633–638.*

Rosi NL, Mirkin CA (2005). *Nanostructures in biodiagnostics. Chem Rev 105:1547–1562.*

Rossi JJ, June CH, Kohn DB (2007). *Genetic therapies against HIV. Nat Biotechnol 25:1444–1454.*

Sakthivel T, Florence AT (2003). *Dendrimers and dendrons: Facets of pharmaceutical nanotechnology. Drug Deliv Technol 3:50–60.*

Santos-Magalhães NS and Mosqueira VC (2010). *Nanotechnology applied to the treatment of malaria. Adv Drug Deliv Rev 62,560–575.*

Sanvicens N, Marco MP (2008). *Multifunctional nanoparticles— properties and prospects for their use in human medicine. Trends Biotechnol 26:425–433.*

Sax PE, Cohen CJ, Kuritzkes DR (2007). *HIV Essentials. Physicians' Press; Royal Oak, MI, USA.*

Shim WB, Yang ZY, Kim JS, Kim JY, Kang SJ, Woo GJ, et al (2007). *Development of immuno-chromatography strip-test using nanocolloidal gold-antibody probe for the rapid detection of aflatoxin B1 in grain and feed samples. J Microbiol Biotechnol 17:1629–1637.*

Shin SH, Ye MK, Kim HS, Kang HS (2007). *The effects of nano-silver on the proliferation and cytokine expression by peripheral blood mononuclear cells. Int Immunopharmacol 7: 1813–1818.*

Shrivastava S, Dash D (2009). *Applying Nanotechnology to Human Health: Revolution in Biomedical*

Sciences. J Nanotechnol I D 184702 p14.

Singhal S, Nie S, Wang MD (2010). Nanotechnology applications in surgical oncology. Annul Rev Med 61:359–373.

Smith AM, Duan H, Mohs AM, Nie S (2008). Bioconjugated quantum dots for in vivo molecular and cellular imaging. Adv Drug Deliv Rev 60:1226–1240.

Soga O, van Nostrum CF, Fens M, Rijcken CJ, Schiffelers RM, Storm G, et al (2005). Thermosensitive and biodegradable polymeric micelles for paclitaxel delivery. J Control Release 103:341–353.

Sondi I, Salopek-Sondi B (2004). Silver nanoparticles as antimicrobial agent: a case study on E. coli as a model for Gram-negative bacteria. J Colloid Interface Sci 275: 177–182.

Storhoff JJ, Lucas AD, Garimella V, Bao YP, Muller UR (2004). Homogeneous detection of unamplified genomic DNA sequences based on colorimetric scatter of gold nanoparticle probes. Nat Biotechnol 22:883–887.

Strassert CA, Otter M, Albuquerque RQ, Hone A, Vida Y, Maier B et al (2009). Photoactive Hybrid Nanomaterial for Targeting, Labeling, and Killing Antibiotic-Resistant Bacteria Angew Chem Int Ed 48:7928–7931.

Tang S, Zhao J, Storhoff JJ, Norris PJ, Little RF, Yarchoan R, et al (2007). Nanoparticle-Based biobarcode amplification assay (BCA) for sensitive and early detection of human immunodeficiency type 1 capsid (p24) antigen. J Acquir Immune Defic Syndr 46:231–237.

Tian J, Wong KK, Ho CM, Lok CN, Yu WY, Che CM, et al (2007). Tropical delivery of silver nanoparticles promotes wound healing. Chem Med Chem 2: 129–136.

Tin S, Sakharkar KR, Lim CS, Sakharkar MK (2009). Activity of Chitosans in combination with antibiotics in Pseudomonas aeruginosa. Int J Bio Sci 5:153–160.

Torchilin VP, Lukyanov AN, Gao Z, Papahadjopoulos-Sternberg B (2003). Immunomicelles: Targeted pharmaceutical carriers for poorly soluble drugs. Proc Natl Acad Sci U S A100:6039–6044.

Uehara N (2010). Polymer-functionalized gold nanoparticles as versatile sensing materials. Anal Sci 26:1219–1228.

Valanne A, Huopalahti S, Soukka T, Vainionpaa R, Lovgren T, Harma H (2005). A sensitive adenovirus immunoassay as a model for using nanoparticle label technology in virus diagnostics. J Clin Virol 33:217–223.

Vatta LL, Sanderson RD, Koch KR (2006). Magnetic nanoparticles: Properties and potential applications. Pure Appl Chem 78:1793–1801.

Wang X, Li J, Wang Y, Koenig L, Gjyrezi A, Giannakakou P, et al (2011). A folate receptor-targeting nanoparticle minimizes drug resistance in a human cancer model. ACS Nano 5:6184–6194.

Wang X, Yang L, Chen ZG, Shin DM (2008). Application of nanotechnology in cancer therapy and imaging. CA Cancer J Clin 58:97–110.

Wu G, Datar RH, Hansen KM, Thundat T, Cote RJ, Majumdar A (2001). Bioassay of prostate-specific antigen (PSA) using microcantilevers. Nat Biotechnol19:856–860.

Yang F, Jin C, Subedi S, Lee CL, Wang Q, Jiang Y, et al (2012). Emerging inorganic nanomaterials forpancreatic cancer diagnosis and treatment. Cancer Treat Rev 38:566–579.

Yang J, Lee CH, Ko HJ, Suh JS, Yoon HG, Lee K, et al (2007). Multifunctional magneto-polymeric nanohybrids for targeted detection and synergistic therapeutic effects on breast cancer. Angew Chem Int Ed Engl 46:8836–8839.

Yellen BB, Forbes ZG, Halverson DS, Fridman G, Barbee KA, Chorny M, etal (2005). Targeted drug delivery to magnetic implants for therapeutic applications. J Magn Magn Mater 2005;293:647–654.

Zhang L, Gu FX, Chan JM, Wang AZ, Langer RS, Farokhzad (2008). Nanoparticles in medicine: Therapeutic applications and developments. Clin Pharmacol Ther 83:761–769.

Zhang S (2002). Emerging biological materials through molecular self assembly. Biotechnol Adv 20:321–339.

Zhao X, Hilliard LR, Mechery SJ, Wang Y, Bagwe RP, Jin S, et al(2004). A rapid bioassay for single bacterial cell quantitation using bioconjugated nanoparticles. Proc Natl Acad Sci U S A. 101:15027–15032.

Chapter 9

Infection with West Nile Virus: Opsoclonus-myoclonus Syndrome

Victoria Birlutiu[1], Rares-Mircea Birlutiu[1], Cristina Rezi[2]

1 Introduction

West Nile Virus (WNV) is transmitted mainly to humans by mosquitoes (especially Culex species), which get the virus by feeding on infected birds. WNV induces asymptomatic or symptomatic infections, with symptoms ranging from febrile syndrome (fever, muscle pain, headaches and exanthema) to neurological disease, the latter affecting only about 1% of the cases.

2 Epidemiology

WNV is a zoonotic arbovirus, belonging to the genus *Flavivirus* in the *Flaviviridae* family. It was first identified in Uganda, in 1937, in the blood culture of a woman with a febrile episode. It drew the attention of experts again in the 90s, when a high number of cases were identified throughout the whole world. In Southeastern Europe (Campbell GL, 2001), a large outbreak of meningoencephalitis took place in Romania (in Bucharest), in 1996 — almost 400 cases were confirmed — and in Russia, in 1999, with approximately 200 cases (in Volgograd).

In 1999 sporadic outbreaks of neuroinvasive infections occurred in New York City, followed by other cases in other regions of the United States, Central America, the Caribbean, Canada (Dauphin G, 2004).

Isolated cases are reported annually in Russia, the Czech Republic, France during

[1] Faculty of Medicine, "Lucian Blaga" University of Sibiu, Romania
[2] Polisano Medical Clinic, Sibiu, Romania

2000–2004 (Zeller H, 2004), Italy, and in the Mediterranean region — Algeria, Morocco (Schuffenecker I, 2005).

WNV has at least five different lineages (Mann BR, 2013). Lineage 1, spread worldwide, is subdivided into clades, 1a and 1b. Clade 1a was isolated in America, Africa, Asia, Europe and the Middle East, and was later divided into A and B sub-clades (Zehender G, 2011). Clade 1b, or the Kunjin virus (KUNV), is known to be endemic in Australia and only occasionally affects humans. Lineage 2 can be found in Sub-Saharan Africa, Madagascar, South Africa and in some countries in Europe such as (Sambri V, 2013) Russia, Hungary (Bakonyi T, 2006), Greece (Papa A, 2011), Italy (Bagnarelli P, 2011) (Magurano F, 2012). WNV lineage 2 from Europe has its origins in Africa and has become endemic in the last two decades (Ciccozzi M, 2013). Lineage 3 or Rabensburg virus, was isolated from *Culex pipiens* in the Czech Republic and South Moravia (Bakonyi T H. Z., 2005). Lineage 4 was isolated in the Caucasus region (Russia), from a Dermacentor tick and then from mosquitoes. WNV lineage 5 is considered to be clade 1c of lineage 1 and it was isolated initially in humans and mosquitoes in India. Some have discussed the existence of lineage 6 (Vazquez A, 2010), isolated from *Culex pipiens* in Spain, and also that of lineage 7, isolated from the Koutango virus in Senegal (King AMQ, 2011).

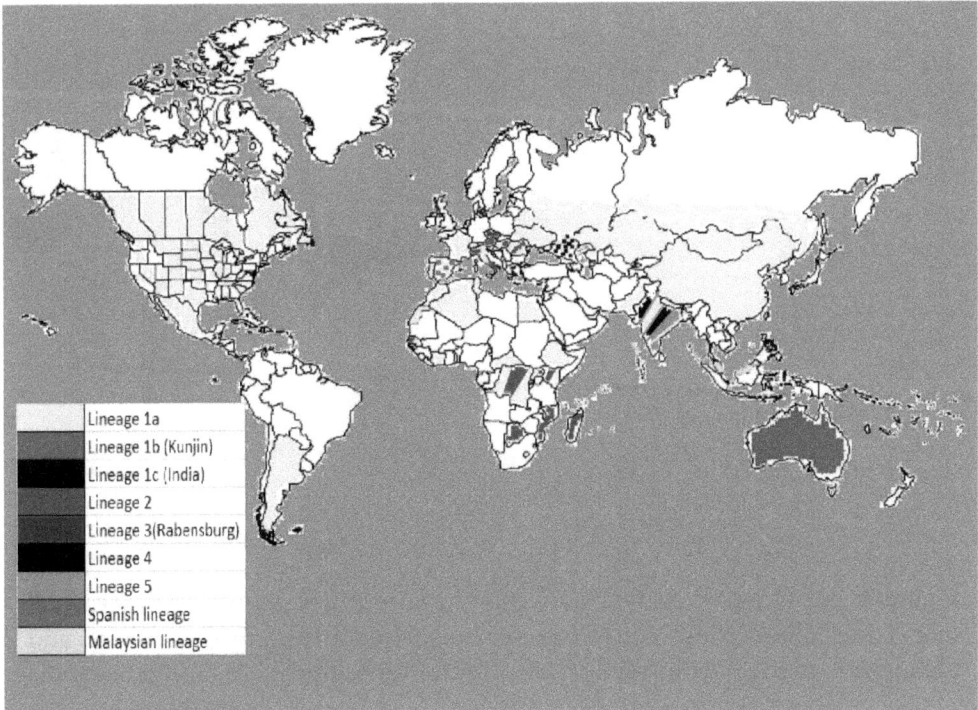

Figure 1: Worldwide distribution of WNV by lineage (after Ciota AT (2013)).

During 1999–2013, the Centers for Disease Control and Prevention (CDC) confirmed a number of 39 557 infections with WNV, 17 463 of which of the neuroinvasive kind (meningitis, encephalitis, acute flaccid paralysis), concluding that, in 2013, the WNV represented the most important cause of neuroinvasive infections produced by arboviruses. Recent studies suggest that WNV is currently the most important cause of viral encephalitis worldwide. (Chancey C, 2015)

In 2014, CDC reported a WNV incidence rate of over 1.00 to 100 000, i.e. 1 820 cases, 1070 of which were neuro-infections (59% of the confirmed cases) (Centers for Disease Control and Prevention National Center for Emerging and Zoonotic Infectious Diseases, 2014). According to the European Centre for Disease Prevention and Control (ECDC), up to 20/11/2014, there were only 74 cases in Europe and 136 in the Mediterranean region (ECDC, 2014) (Figure 2).

The most frequent way of transmission of WNV is from birds, especially *passerines* (though over 300 species of birds have been identified as being at risk of WNV infection), via *Aedes* and *Culex* genus mosquitoes, to humans or to other 30 species of vertebrates: horses, cats, dogs, skunks, rabbits, squirrels or reptiles — alligators, crocodiles, amphibians.

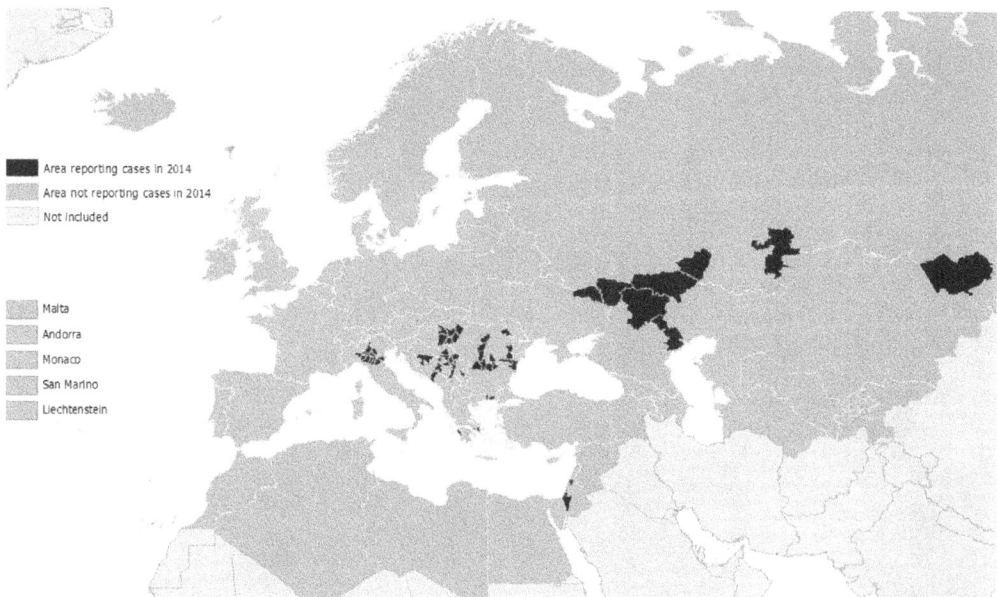

Figure 2: ECDC report on WNV infection in Europe and the Mediterranean region. Distributin of West Nile fever cases by affected areas, European region and Mediterranean basin. Transmission season 2014; latest update 20 November 2014.

The most frequent way of transmission of WNV is from birds, especially *passerines* (though over 300 species of birds have been identified as being at risk of WNV infection), via *Aedes* and *Culex* genus mosquitoes, to humans or to other 30 species of vertebrates: horses, cats, dogs, skunks, rabbits, squirrels or reptiles — alligators, crocodiles, amphibians.

Cases of vertical WNV transmission from mother to child during childbirth or breastfeeding have also been documented (Hayes EB, 2004). Transmission through blood transfusions was first confirmed in 2002 (Hayes EB, 2004) and in 2003 over 1000 collected samples which tested positive for WNV screening were eliminated from blood donation in North America . During the same period, 7 cases of blood transfusions with otherwise undetectable viral load were confirmed (Prevention, 2004).

Transmission is also possible from handling dead birds or infected vertebrates (Centers for Disease Control and Prevention National Center for Emerging and Zoonotic Infectious Diseases, 2014), by skin contamination or through aerosols in laboratories.

3 Etiology

WNV belongs to the genus *Flavivirus*, in the *Flaviviridae* family, together with Japanese encephalitis virus (JEV), yellow fever virus, dengue virus, and tick-borne encephalitis virus which produce a unique subgenomic flavivirus RNA (sfRNA) derived from the 3' untranslated region (UTR) (Roby JA, 2014), the product of incomplete degradation of the genomic RNA. The WNV virion has a diameter of 45–50 mm, with icosahedral symmetry and a structure similar to the one of Dengue fever virus. It has a lipid envelope with spike glycoprotein of surface M (membrane) and E (envelope), single-stranded genome, linear positive-sense RNA, containing between 11 000 and 12 000 nucleotides which encode seven nonstructural proteins (NS1, NS2A, NS2B, NS3, NS4A, NS4B, NS5) and three structural proteins: capsid protein C binds the viral RNA; pre-membrane protein (prM) blocks the viral fusion; and E protein. The viral genome is relieved by the noncoding variable regions – 3' and 5'. The nucleocapsid is formed from 12 kDa block proteins, while the capsid derives from the cellular membrane of the host, altered under the action of viral glycoproteins. The E protein is involved in the viral attachment to the host cell receptor and it facilitates the fusion at the cellular membrane; it is the site of hemagglutination and viral neutralization. Protein E consists of three domains: domain III is involved in the interaction with the host cell; domain II consists of a conservative region with 13 hydrophobic amino-acids involved in fusion by forming a fusion loop and domain I binds the other two domains (Nybakken GE, 2006). The nonstructural proteins are inolved in the process of transcription, translation, replication (NS1 and NS4a) and assembling of WNV (NS2a). sfRNA inhibits the INF α/β activity, has a role in the viral infection pathogenicity and possibly many other functions which are not yet elucidated; the defficiency in sfRNA is correlated itself with the reduction of the cytopathogenic effect in mice. Protein E is a major antigenic protein. Other structures, such as prM, NS1, NS3 and NS5, also have antigenic properties. At the same time, NS2A, NS2B, NS4A, and NS4B proteins act as co-factors for viral replication complex assembly and localization (Youn S, 2013).

Once the mosquito bite is produced, the saliva may produce vasoconstriction, coagulation, platelet aggregation, the altering of the immune response of the host, favoring a high viral load of the WNV and a severe form of the disease (Zeidner NS, 1999) (Schneider BS, 2007).

4 Pathogenesis

The virus is multiplying in the tegument, at the Langerhans cells level, in lymph nodes, the short time viral load being present before the central nervous system invasion. The asymptomatic infections are 300 times more frequent, compared with the symptomatic ones, due to the peripheral clearance of the virus, without neural invasion.

In the neural invasion, there are involved the Toll-like receptors 3, the CCR5 receptor and its ligand, CCL5, pushed by the WNV, with the local migration of the T CD4, CD8, NK1.1 lymphocytes and of the macrophages. The central nervous system invasion is produced from one cell to another, with the appearance of local inflammation, brain edema and encephalitis, especially by affecting the hippocampus, thalamus and temporal region, black substance and cerebellum. It is generally accepted that CNS invasion is the consequence of an inefficient systemic immune response, which allows a major viral replication whereby CNS is affected proportionally to the level and duration of the viremia (Stephanie ML, 2011). Several mechanisms of WNV entry into the CNS have been proposed, for which there is experimental evidence on mice: passive transport through the choroid plexus epithelial cells (Kramer-Hämmerle S, 2005), through the olfactory neurons or through the infected immune cells (Garcia-Tapia D, 2006). The CNS infection occurs most often in the cortex, cerebellum, basal ganglia and the brain stem, and rarely in the hippocampus or the olfactory bulb. WNV acts primarily at the neuronal level: at the level of microglia, astrocytes, endothelial cells, oligodendrocytes, and neuroblastoma cells but also at a spinal cord level, with the anterior gray column being affected most often.

The emergence of severe cases in immunocompromised persons and in the elderly seems to be explained by the decrease of the immune response to new antigens, which follows as a result of fewer T cells being produced by the thymus and the ineffective response of neutralizing IgM antibodies. LyCD4+ support a viral clearance response of LyCD8+ in the CNS, the latter being responsible for controlling the infection and preventing viral persistence in the tissue. IgM and IgG antibodies are responsible for controlling the viremia (Diamond MS, 2003) and for preventing a fatal outcome. The role of the microglia, astrocytes and oligodendrocytes (involved in the production of myelin) in the WNV infection has also been studied. Present in a ratio to neurons of 1.4 (Hilgetag CC, 2009), astrocytes represent the neuronal metabolic support and are essential to brain homeostasis. They play a limited part in the synthesis of acute phase proteins and proinflammatory cytokines but a crucial one in controlling leukocyte influx in the CNS, maintaining the integrity of the Blood-Brain-Barrier (BBB) through the glia limitans network. Microglia represent the CNS macrophages and are activated during inflammatory diseases or neuronal injuries. Their plasticity allows them to modify their cellularity numerically, morphologically and as an expression of surface receptors, as well as to synthesize proinflammatory cytokines and growth factors. After the viremia peaks, WNV enters into the CNS, where leukocyte recruitment takes place through the transmigration of peripheral leukocytes at the level of the BBB and at the vascular endothelium level. The leukocytes are then retained in the perivascular space. Leukocyte migration is influenced by not fully known mechanisms at the moment. The ability of TNF-α to increase vascular permeability is easy to see, as is the expression of the C-X-C motif chemokine 12 (CXCL12) (McCandless EE, 2006), and the effect of matrix metalloproteinases (MMP) produced by the astrocytes, which facilitate the leukocyte migration into the perivascular space and at the level of the glial limitans (Savarin C, 2010). The leukocyte migration in the brain parenchyma is the outcome of injuries that occurr at the level of glia limitans components such as collagen degradation under the action of cysteine protease cathepsins K, S, and L, the conversion of plasminogen into plasmin and the fibronectin and laminin degradation (Reijerkerk A, 2008). During the CNS invasion of WNV, there is an increase in the expression of two CXC chemokines-type, CXCL1 and CXCL2 that contribute to the neutrophil recruitment in the brain. Neutrophils are the most important immune cells involved in the early local defense (Bai F, 2010). WNV induces neuronal apoptosis through the caspase-3 (Samuel MA, 2007) and caspase-9 pathways, activated by the presence of capsidic WNV proteins in the CNS, but also by the activation of calphain and cathepsin (Hail N Jr, 2006) (Kroemer G, 2005). High levels of WNV structural proteins (NS2A, 2B, 4A, 4B) and E glycoprotein may induce apoptosis via endoplasmic reticulum (ER) stress (Yu CY, 2006). Research in the pathogenesis of WNV neuroinvazive infection highlights the hightened viral action that follows the release by neurons of proinflammatory cytokines such as IL-1β, -6, -8 and TNF-α (Kumar M, 2010) (Swarup V, 2007). Differences in virulence among strains of WNV is explained by the ability of virulent strains – for e.g. WNV-NY99 1999 New York, to act as a potent antagonist of alpha/beta interferon (IFN-α / β), mediated by Janus kinase — signal transducer and activator of transcription (JAK-STAT) (Laurent-Rolle M, 2010) by inhibiting JAK phosphorylation, by the intervention of nonstructural proteins NS2A, NS2B, NS3, NS4A, and NS4B.

In contrast to NY99, Kunjin virus subtype (KUN) currently endemic in Australia, occasionally produces illness in humans, the nonstructural protein NS5 not acting as an interferon antagonist (Liu WJ, 2005). It has also been hypothesised that the insufficiency of down-regulated TLR3 macrophages, present in the elderly, is responsible for the presence of high levels of proinflammatory cytokines with vasculogenic propertie (Kong KF, 2008). Among the WNV nonstructural proteins, NS1 plays an antagonist role in antiviral defense by inhibiting complement activation (Avirutnan P, 2010), TLR3 signal transduction (Wilson JR, 208)and by activating STAT1/STAT2 (Peña J, 2014).

5   Clinical Aspects

80% of the cases of WNV infection are asymptomatic. In the forms of the disease with-out neurological disease, or West Nile fever (WNF), the onset can be sudden, after a variable incubation period of about 2–15 days, with influenza-like syndrome — high fever,

headache, muscle pain, joint pain, lymph nodes enlargements and digestive manifestations like nausea, vomiting, loss of appetite, profuse transpiration.

Approximately one third to one half of the cases present skin rash (see Figure 3
and Figure 4 from patients we have treated). The skin eruption is described as punctate
exanthema , macula or papules, affecting mainly the extremities (Anderson RC, 2004), is
of a transitory nature — the rash disappears in 24 hours — and is more frequently associated with WNV encephalitis or meningitis (Ferguson DD, 2005), probably in direct
relation with the pro-inflammatory answer of the host. WNF appears mainly in younger
people (Pipperal C, 2003). Due to the digestive manifestations and fever there can appear different degrees of dehydration.

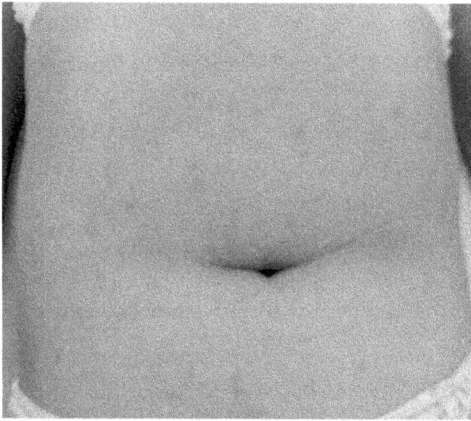

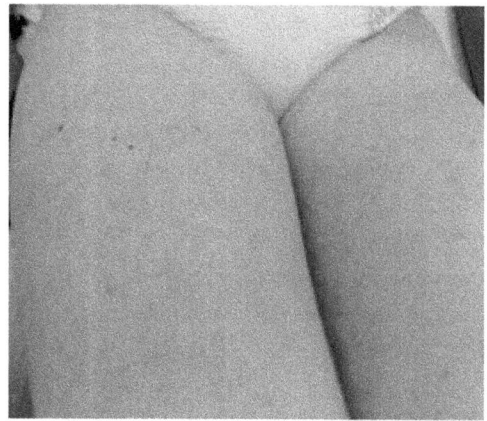

Figure 3: Exanthema on the abdomen   **Figure 4:** Exanthema on the hips

Other manifestations described in WNV infection include: hepatomegaly, sple-
nomegaly (Goldblum N, 1954), occasionally myocarditis and pancreatitis.

The central nervous system involvement appears in less than 1% of the cases,
mainly in men above 50, in patients infected with HIV, or patients immune-depressed
by co-morbidities (diabetes mellitus, arterial hypertension) or by recent immune-
suppressed therapy, as is the case, for example, in patients with organ transplants, for
whom the incidence of neurological disease can be 40 times higher compared to the
general population (Kumar D, 2004).

The CCR5 gene polymorphism, with defective alleles of the receptor for chemokine CCR5 (CCR5 Δ 52) is associated with a severe evolution of the WNV infection
(Glass WG, 2006).

The neurological involvement is preceded by a febrile episode, lasting 1–7 days,
sometimes the evolution being biphasic, associated with rash, eye pain, rarely lymph
node enlargement.

The central nervous system involvement consists of encephalitis, meningitis,
Guillain-Barre syndrome, optic neuritis, poliomyelitis-like paralysis. The mortality rate
is estimated at 10–30% of the cases, being influenced by age (over 50), the presence of

co-morbidities or of immune-deficiency (Burton JM, 2004), or by the presence of a motor deficit. The neurological recovery is slow, about 6 months to one year, sometimes incomplete, with the persistence of fatigability, asthenia, headache, muscle pain (Sejvar JJ, 2003).

Encephalitis is the most frequent neurological manifestation of the WNV infection, with lesions which can be found in different cerebral areas: basal ganglions, thalamus, cerebellum, cerebral trunk. It involves fever, headache and consciousness disturbances. In 30–50% of the cases, there can appear muscular weakness, peripheral motor neuron syndrome, flaccid paralysis, hypo-reflexes (Carson PJ, 2006) (Flores Anticona EM, 2012).

In a study performed by Hart et al, from a number of 55 confirmed cases with encephalitis with WNV, 93% presented neurological deficit, 70% presented cognitive disturbances/the alteration of the consciousness status, 49% presented muscle weakness, 35% tremor, 25% coma, 16% the crania nerves involvement (Hart J Jr, 2014). Other manifestations which were present in WNV encephalitis were: myoclonus with the upper limbs and facial involvement, parkinsonism, hypo-mimia, postural instability, abnormal movements with changes in the consciousness status, by affecting medulla, substantia nigra, cerebellum, thalamus. The central nervous system lesions consist in chronic inflammatory per vascular process, neuronal loss, necrosis or neuro-phagy, microglia nodules (KA, 2009).

The evolution of the cases with central nervous system involvement is slow, with the persistence of functional deficit in half of the cases upon discharge, only a third of whom will recover in one-year's time (Weiss D, 2001).

From our experience, the cases of WNV encephalitis in adults, presented fever or influenza-like syndrome, digestive manifestations in half of the cases, skin rash, localized especially in the lumbar or sacrum region in one third of the cases. The neurological manifestations were present in about half of the cases, and were dominated by dysmetria, tremor, nystagmus, problems with gait and balance. Other manifestations which were met were: motor deficit/hemiplegia, tonic-clonic seizures.

The laboratory exams revealed the presence in over 50% of the cases of neutrophilic leukocytosis, which appears also elsewhere in the literature (Nash D, 2001); high levels of C reactive protein and fibrinogen were also observed. The cerebrospinal fluid examination attests to the presence of low or moderate pleocytosis in about 50% of the cases, with the predominance of neutrophils (with a maximum of 56% from the cellularity), moderate protein levels in the cerebrospinal fluid, high levels of glucose in the cerebrospinal fluid in patients with normal glycemic levels (Birlutiu V, 2014) or normal values of glucose in the cerebrospinal fluid.

Until now there have been described five cases of WNV encephalitis, manifested as Opsoclonus Myoclonus Syndrome (OMS) (Khsola JS, 2005) (Shellenback L, 2012) (Aasim A, 2014) (Birlutiu V, 2014) (Cooper CJ, 2014), subject which will be discussed separately.

The WNV meningitis can be associated with encephalitis; symptoms include fever, headache, signs of meningeal irritation, photophobia, phonophobia. It cannot be clinically distinguished from other types of viral meningitis. The cerebrospinal fluid alterations are: pleocytosis with less than 500 elements/mm³, usually dominated by lymphocytes, but with the possible predominance of polinuclears, like in WNV encephalitis.

The poliomyelitis-like syndrome is caused by lesions of the anterior horn of spinal cord and it involves muscular weakness or asymmetric flaccid paralysis, monoparesis or quadriplegia, without sensorial or sensitivity alterations; the paralysis can appear in the absence of fever, sometimes affecting respiratory muscles and leading to acute respiratory insufficiency.

The Guillain-Barre syndrome presents with symmetric progressive ascending paralysis, with the involvement of the proximal and distal muscularity, paresthesia, loss of sensibility; the cerebrospinal fluid examination shows no pleocytosis, but an increased level of proteins, i.e. albuminocytological dissociation.

The evolution of the neurological manifestations does not correlate with the initial clinical appearance; cases with motor deficit, or coma may have a complete resolution in time, while cases with ataxia may present persistent abnormal movements, headache and tiredness. From the experience of the WNV breakout in New York, 37% of the patients with WNV encephalitis were considered cured in about one year after the acute episode (Klee AL, 2004).

The ocular manifestations, like chorioretinitis or vitritis can be associated both with WNF and with neurological manifestations, in the latter case with lesions of the optical nerve. On rare occasions there can occur hemorrhages in the retina or progressive eyesight loss (Adelman NA, 2003) (Bakeri SJ, 2004). Manifestations like myositis due to WNV, with rhabdomyolysis were observed in the absence of the WNV isolation from the muscle (Jeha LE, 2003).

In children, one can encounter neural infections with WNV such as meningitis, rarely encephalitis, rhombencephalitis, poliomyelitis-like paralysis, hepatitis; the prognosis is influenced by the immune-compromised status of the children.

6   Diagnosis

The laboratory diagnosis of WNV infection is performed routinely by serologic testing, using the ELISA method. The presence of specific IgM antibodies in serum and cerebrospinal fluid, respectively, in the cases with neurological involvement, confirm the diagnosis. Neurological impairment in WNV infection can be confirmed by a four-fold increase in the IgG titer in samples collected between the acute and convalescent period or by detecting the viral genome using reverse transcription-polymerase chain reaction with a sensitivity in the range of 10–40 genome copies/mL. The cerebrospinal fluid changes include lymphocytic pleocytosis, or characteristically neutrophilia (Tyler KL, 2006), increase in proteins and a normal level of glycorrhachia.

Some laboratories use indirect immunofluorescence technique in order to detect the specific antibodies, with a sensitivity of 95%. It should be noted that IgM can persist in the serum for up to 16 months in some cases (Rochrig JT, 2003), which brings about some problems of acuity of the etiological diagnosis.

Other tests, not routinely performed are hemagglutination-inhibition, the dosing of neutralized antibodies. Real time PCR is used in WVN screening in order to exclude positive samples from donation. One can identify WNV in cell cultures in case of a fatal outcome using sampled tissues, but this method is confined to reference laboratories. In the same situation, one can perform histopathology examination with immunohisto-chemistry and nucleic acid amplification. Through a multiplex enzyme-linked immuno-sorbent assay-based protein array (ELISA-array), an indirect ELISA, one can identify specific antibodies against WNV, Japanese B, tick-borne encephalitis, dengue and yellow fever viruses (Wang D, 2015).

7   Treatment. Prophylaxis.

The cases of WNV without neurological involvement need support with iv fluids and electrolites, fever and headache control. In the cases with neural infections, in the absence of a specific antiviral treatment, the patient is hospitalized and should avoid physical efforts, which may exacerbate the motor deficit. The cases with acute respiratory insufficiency benefit from mechanical ventilation.

In the WNV neural infection the administration of immunoglobulin seems to be beneficial (Shimoni Z, 2011), as well as the administration of monoclonal antibodies targeting WNV envelope protein (Oliphant T, 2005) (Morrey, Day, Julander, Blatt, Smee, & Sidwell, 2004); the administration of interferon alpha did not show any efficiency (Morrey JD, 2007). The antiviral therapy that uses inhibitors of NS3 proteases of the WNV flaviviruses is far from being usable now (Poulsen A, 2014) but remains a therapeutic possibility for the future.

There is no human vaccine on the market for now. In the US, horses are vaccinated with a formalin-inactivated vaccine or canarypox-vectored WNV vaccines. Some live attenuated vaccines (Hall RA, 2007) and combinations with Dengue virus vaccines are currently under evaluation for their degree of protection (Pletnev AG, 2004).

The general prophylaxis refers to the routine control of birds and the use of pesticides for maintaining the mosquito population at a low level in risk-prone areas. Veterinaries and public health authorities need to be informed regarding the appearance of deaths or diseases in birds or horses, the control of chemical products or the biological control of the transmission and need to drain pools of standing water. Personal protection measures against WNV include using insect repellent containing DEET, picaridin, oil of lemon eucalyptus, and IR3535 and wearing protective clothing to prevent mosquito bites, application of permethrin on clothes or avoiding direct contact with sick animals. In high-risk areas for WNV, the prevention of transmission through blood donation or organ transplants should be performed by real time PCR laboratory method.

8   Opsoclonus Myoclonus Syndrome

Opsoclonus myoclonus syndrome (OMS) also named Opsoclonus- Myoclonus Ataxia,

Dancing Eyes — Dancing Feet Syndrome, Dancing Eyes Syndrome, Kinsbourne syndrome, Myoclonic Encephalopathy of Infants, was described in the literature as a multi-etiological neurological disorder, responsible for approximate 60 diseases per year, worldwide.

In children, OMS is frequently a paraneoplastic syndrome, immune mediated, associated with neuroblastoma, with thoracic, abdominal, pelvic or cervical localizations, in over 50% of the cases, or with ganglioneuroblastoma, the manifestations starting early, between 1.5 and 2 years. There were extremely rare cases described which appeared before the age of 6 months; the gender repartition was equal. There has been a description of an exceptional association with a retroperitoneal tumor, prenatally diagnosed (Jamroz E, 2011).The evolution can be monophasic or chronic, with relapses, followed by motor, behavioural or cognitive disorders.

In adults, OMS appears as a paraneoplastic manifestation associated with breast, pulmonary, renal and pancreatic or gallbladder cancer. There are cases described in association with autoimmune diseases, in the presence of mainly type 2 antineural nuclear antibodies: Hashimoto disease, post streptococcal infections and the celiac disorder. Other cases of OMS have been reported during hydro-electrolytic imbalance, cerebral anoxia and cerebral hemorrhages.

More and more information appear related to the involvement of the viral infections in OMS unset: viral infections with Coxsackie virus (B2, B3), Epstein-Barr, herpes simplex virus (Klaas, et al., 2012) Saint Luis viral encephalitis, C virus hepatitis, rubella, mumps virus, cytomegalovirus, human immunodeficiency virus (HIV).

OMS was also described in infections with Mycoplasma pneumoniae, Rickettsia or Borrelia burgdoferi. There are also cases of OMS in which there wasn't any etiology identified.

8.1   Clinical Aspect

OMS in manifested by opsoclonus - rapid, multivectorial, conjugated movements of the eyes, which persist during sleep, without involving the alteration of the visual field, and by myoclonus — short involuntary movements of the body, limbs, and sometimes, but not mandatory associated with ataxia or other cerebellums signs, sleep disorders or dysphasia, strabismus, vomiting. In children, there can be irritability, excitability or lethargy. The signs and symptoms of OMS are extremely varied as frequency, the concomitant presence of all manifestations not being absolutely necessary: opsoclonus-myoclonus-ataxia.

8.2   OMS Physiopathology

Even though the etiology of OMS is not completely elucidated, the answer to the immune-suppressor treatment and the presence of auto-antibodies, both in children, and in adults, suggest an autoimmune mechanism, by the presence of anti-neural, Purkinje cerebellar antibodies, the intense activity of the B cells at the cerebrospinal fluid, suggesting a cross-over reaction between the antigens which are present in the tumor lesion (neuroblastoma) and the central nervous system. The immune answer explains the persistence of the lesions for a long time and implicitely of the neurological sequels.

The histological exam of the neuroblastoma, excised from the patients with OMS, reveals the presence of an interstitial and perivascular inflammatory infiltrate, which is rich in B and T lymphocytes. The B lymphocytes activation is secondary to the T lymphocytes answer to the presence of tumor antigen, with the antibodies production. Although the tumor is located remotely, the central nervous system involvement is due to the cerebellum lesions, sometimes cerebellum atrophy, demyelination or loss of Purkinje cells.

The OMS diagnosis cannot be sustained by the presence of a certain biomarker (Gorman, 2010); it is admitted that the appearance of the syndrome is due to an auto-immune mechanism, through the action of the T lymphocytes and of the auto-antibodies which are synthesized by the B lymphocytes on the cerebral structures, similar as characteristics to the tumor cells, more frequently at the level of the cerebral trunk, cerebellum and limbic system.

It was suggested, that the relative B cell expansion in CSF should be the marker of the OMS.; in these patients, the presence of an important percentage of CD19+ B cells can be observed in the cerebrospinal fluid, not in the serum, in comparison with the healthy population (Pranzatelli MR T. A., 2004).Compared to the patients with non-inflammatory neurological diseases, in the patients with OMS, previously to the immune-modulator treatment, high values of B-cell activation factor (BAFF) can be observed, which decrease dramatically in the serum after the treatment initiation (Pranzatelli MR T. E., 2008).

In OMS, we most frequently identify antineuronal nuclear antibody type 2, anti-Hu antibodies, anti-Ri antibodies (gynecologic cancers) or more rarely, anti-Yo, and anti-Ma-2 antibodies, IgG and IgM antibodies to neurofilament and peripheral nerve, anti-N-methyl-D-aspartate receptor encephalitis (Kurian M, 2010) with elevated IgG index, and positive oligoclonal banding.

The diagnosis is completed with the neurological evaluation of the case, by using cerebral MRI, EEG and the cerebrospinal fluid exam, by lumbar puncture in order to identify the white abnormal cells using the immunophenotyping technique. The B and T cells recruitment in the cerebrospinal fluid is associated with neurological manifestations and with relapses and the progression of the disease (Pranzatelli MR T. A., 2004).

The tumor identification needs both blood tests (the B cells population is most of the times over the normal ranges), urine tests, and imagistic exams, like body CT, PET and nuclear MIBG scans.

We illustrated a case from our casuistic from a patient with West Nile infection, in which the magnetic resonance scan of the brain showed: demyelination lesions and lacuna images in the left cerebellum, para-median in the right punt, and in the white substance per and supra ventricular bilateral. There were also described two lacuna zones per and supra-ventricular in the right, with the diameter of 4–5mm, with peripheral gliosis and restriction of peripheral diffusion (Figures 5, 6, 7 and 8).

In the cases associated with bacterial or viral infections, the confirmation is based on detecting the presence of specific antibodies type IgM in serum and concomitantly in

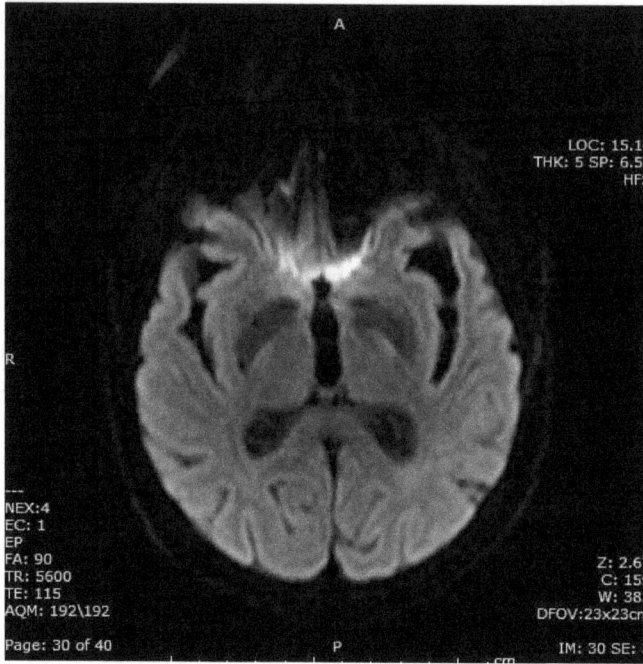

Figure 5: Magnetic resonance of the brain, T1-weighted image.

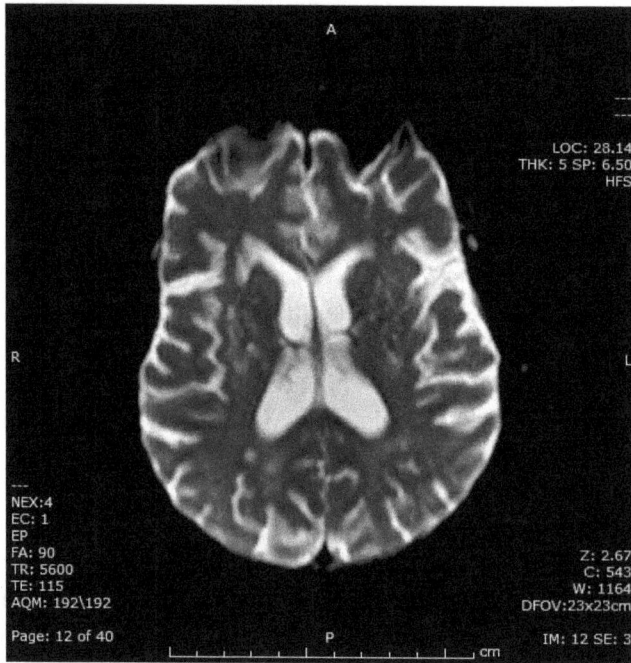

Figure 6: Magnetic resonance of the brain, T2-weighted image.

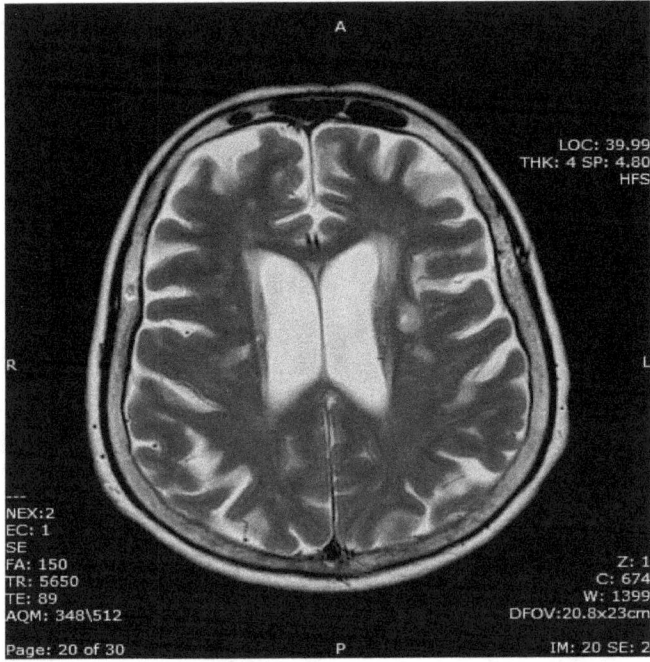

Figure 7: Magnetic resonance of the brain, T2-weighted image.

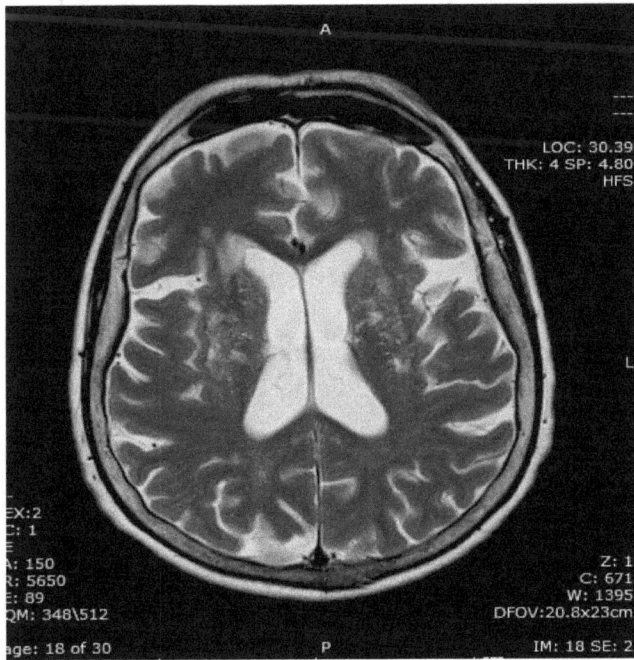

Figure 8: Magnetic resonance of the brain, T2-weighted image.

the LRC or detecting the infectious agent through RT PCR. In practice, we use the OMS scale as to evaluate the severity of the disease and the therapeutic response.

The confirmation in the cases which are associated with viral or bacterial infections, is based on the detection of specific IgM antibodies in the serum, and concomitant in the cerebrospinal fluid or on the detection of the infectious agent by using RT PCR.

In the clinical practice, there is used the OMS scale, for evaluating the disease's severity and also the therapeutic answer:

Scale Items	Normal	Mild	Moderate	Severe
Walking, side-to-side imbalance	0	1	2	3
Walking, front-to-back imbalance	0	1	2	3
Walking, wide base	0	1	2	3
Instability while standing (feet apart)	0	1	2	3
Difficulty achieving standing position	0	1	2	3
Truncal instability while sitting	0	1	2	3
Targeting difficulty	0	1	2	3
Difficulty grasping with one hand	0	1	2	3
Difficulty with pincer grasp	0	1	2	3
Abnormal eye movements while tracking (fixation)	0	1	2	3
Abnormal eye movements while resting	0	1	2	3
Speech abnormality (dysarthria)	0	1	2	3

Table 1: OMS scale.

The higher severity score of the neurological involvement in OMS is 36 points, the severe forms of disease being frequently correlated with intrathecal increasing of neopterine, as a marker of cellular immunity activation, especially by activating the T cells in this disease; there are also cases with important neurological manifestations which do not involve an increased level of the neopterine, possibly due to the immunomodulator therapy initiated before the dosing of this marker (Pranzatelli MR H. K., 2004).

8.3   Treatment

The conventional treatment is ACTH (adrenocorticotropic hormone), which is considered the gold standard, administrated intramuscularly, on a 20 week period. The side effects of the therapy should be monitored properly: the Cushing syndrome, the cardiovascular effects, the risk for diabetes mellitus, gastric ulcer, osteoporosis, psychical effects, medullar suppression, reversible at the therapy disruption, skin atrophy. The answer at the ACTH treatment is favorable in 80–90% of the cases, the treatment disruption being associated with the risk of relapse.

The glucocorticoids: prednisone, prednisolone, betamethasone, dexamethasone, hydrocortisone may be used in the OMS treatment instead of ACTH, with similar potential side effects. Prednisone or methylprednisolone is administrated in high doses — 500mg-2g/day, on a 3–5 days period, as an alternative of treatment in OMS.

The intravenous human immune-globulins (IVIG) are administrated in doses of 1–2g/kg/day 3–5 days/week, on a 6 week period. They associate a favorable answer in 40–60% from the cases, with less secondary effects in comparison with corticotherapy or ACTH, in 1–15% of the cases there can be fever, headache and flu-like symptoms. It is recommended to administer IVIG in children in whom neurological deterioration occur in the OMS evolution.

The patients who do not respond to the treatment, are candidates for the treatment with cyclophosphamide with dexamethasone, azathioprine or cyclosporine.

Azathioprine (Imuran®) is the most easily administered immune-suppressor in slowly progressive doses, with a prompt supervision of the leucocytes and platelets number, and of the liver tests. The therapeutic effects become evident at 6–12 months from the beginning of the treatment with azathioprine, the maximum benefits being observed in 2 years. The side effects presented in all cases are related to the medullar suppression; 10% of the cases present flu-like symptoms, being known the risk of malignity in time.

Chemotherapy, by administrating cyclophosphamide (Cytoxan®), methotrexate, cyclosporin or cellecept (therapy which is limited as general experience) in children with neuroblastoma, does not influence the neurological manifestations already appeared, but it is beneficial by its anti-tumor effect.

In the moderate or severe forms of idiopathic or paraneoplastic OMS, two or three etiological are recommended with different actions on the immune system: ACTH, IVIG and azathioprine or the association of cyclophosphamide (3–6 cycles), steroids and IVIG. The studies demonstrate the efficiency of associations based on ACTH, in comparison with those based on steroids (Tate ED, 2012). In viral encephalitis or in meningitis, the use of corticotherapy is rational.

The therapy with Rituximab monoclonal antibody against B cells (anti-CD20) 375–750 mg/m^2, is beneficial in the cases of OMS appeared as paraneoplastic manifestations, nonresponsive to the conventional therapy, as monotherapy, or in association with steroids and IVIG (Gorman, 2010) (Pranzatelli MR T. E., 2005) (Pranzatelli M.R, 2006) (Pranzatelli M.R T. E., 2010) (Battaglia T., 2012)(Battaglia T, 2012).

Other immune-modulating therapies in the OMS treatment are being evaluated for example Ofatumumab, a fully humanized anti-CD20 antibody, Alemtuzumab (with action on the T CD 52 cells), Daclizumab (inhibits the activation or proloferation of the T CD25 cells) and the inhibitor of mTOR Sirolimus, with promising results.

The treatment of the cases of OMS as manifestations of autoimmune N-methyl-D-aspartate receptor encephalitis by plasmapheresis, seems to be the best option (Smith JH, 2011), (Nunez-Enamorado N, 2012).

In the cases in which OMS in the consequence of the anti-epileptic medication, the change of this medication is imperative. The symptomatic treatment with Trazodone is efficient in the amelioration of irritability, sleep disorders, or with Clonazepam, which has the ability to link to the cerebral benzodiazepine receptors that facilitate inhibitory GABAergic transmission, valproic acid and 5-hydroxytryptophan.

According to the etiology, the OMS **prognosis** is variable, but it is admitted that the long term evolution is associated with neurological sequels in 80% of the cases — frequently manifested through speech disorders, learning problems, behavior problems, which can be controlled by a immune-modulating therapy (Brunklaus A, 2011).

8.4   Therapeutic Apheresis

Apheresis is a method used in different severe diseases, with an autoimmune mechanism, in which the patient's stabilization is needed; one can perform plasmapheresis, leukocytapheresis or lymphocytapheresis, in a limited number of 5–6 episodes, with a clinical improvement which is evident in the next 2 months. The disadvantages are related to the risk of hypotension and the impossibility of using it in small children. Immunoadsorption, a type of apheresis, uses an immunoabsorbant column for antibodies, using for example, as antigen, the staphylococcal A protein; this method is also limited, as clinical experience, in children.

8.5   Prognosis

The OMS prognosis depends on the clinical severity at the moment of therapeutic initialization, on the period from the diagnosis to the therapeutic answer, and also on the presence of relapses.

The easy forms of diseases remit completely. In the mild or severe forms of the disease, although the myoclonus has the tendency of diminish in time, the incongruity persists. The surgical ablation of the tumor in children (of the neuroblastoma, most frequently), is not associated with the remission of the neurological manifestations. The problems related to the behavior and learning disorders, the attention deficit and even the obsessive-compulsive disorders need specific medication in association with the immunomodulatory one.

A favorable evolution is associated with the viral infections, in the meningoencephalitis produced by the enteroviruses or EBV or in the idiopathic forms of OMS. In the severe forms of OMS, with the persistence of neurological manifestations and of the diminished intellect, the dependence of these children on adults is definitive.

8.6   Relapses

The reappearance or augmentation of the symptoms is known as being associated with some special affective situations, with febrile episodes, during surgical interventions, after anesthesia, immune-prophylactic therapy, or with the attempt of immune therapy suppression. The cases which present a relapse will repeat these episodes several times, at short intervals, exceptionally after long periods of slack time (several years). The relapses therapy is similar to the first episode, with one or more therapeutic agents.

8.7   Treatment of Failures

The lack of therapeutic answer to immune-therapy in children, requires completing the investigations in order to identify the tumor or viral cause; a combined therapy with two or more therapeutic agents, plasmapheresis, etc. is also necessary.

8.8   Treatment of Complications

The complications are most of the time associated with immune-suppression, produced by chemotherapy or immune-therapy. It is necessary to carefully monitor the medullar suppression and the risk of severe infections which can appear in the immune-suppressed patient.

References

Aasim A, S. A. (2014). *Opsoclonus Myoclonus syndrome: an unusual presentation for West Nile.* Proc (Bayl Univ Med Cent), 27(2), 108–110.

Adelman RA, M. J. (2003). *West Nile virus chorioretinitis.* Retina, 23, 100–101.

Anderson RC, H. K. (2004). *Punctate exanthem of West Nile Virus infection: report of 3 cases.* J Am Acad Dermatol, 5(51), 820–3.

Avirutnan P, F. A. (2010). *Antagonism of the complement component C4 by flavivirus nonstructural protein NS1.* J Exp Med(207), 793–806.

Bagnarelli P, M. K. (2011). *Human case of indigenous West Nile virus lineage 2 infection in Italy.* Euro Surveill(16).

Bai F, K. K. (2010). *A paradoxical role for neutrophils in the pathogenesis of West Nile virus.* J Infect Dis(202), 1804–12.

Bakonyi T, H. Z. (2005). *Novel flavivirus or new lineage of West Nile virus, central Europe.* Emerg Infect Dis(11), 225–31.

Bakonyi T, I. E. (2006). *Lineage 1 and 2 strains of encephalitic West Nile virus, central Europe.* Emerg Infect Dis, 12, 618–23.

Bakri SJ, K. P. (2004). *Ocular manifestation of West Nile virus.* Curr OPin Ophtalmol, 15, 537–540.

Battaglia T, d. G.-B. (2012). *Response to rituximab in 3 children with opsoclonus-myoclonus syndrome resistant to conventional treatments.* European Journal of Paediatric Neurology, 16(2), 192–195.

Birlutiu V, B. R. (2014). *Neurological manifestations of the West Nile virus infection in some cases found in the clinic of infectious diseases in Sibiu, Romania.* BMC Inf Dis, 14(Supl 7), P47.

Birlutiu V, B. R. (2014). *Opsoclonus-myoclonus syndrome attributable to West Nile encephalitis:a case report.* Journal of Medical Case Report, 8(232).

Brunklaus A, P. K. (2011). *Outcome and prognosis features in opsoclonus-myoclonus syndrome from infancy to adult life.* Pediatrics, 128(2), 388–94.

Burton JM, K. R. (2004, May). *Neurological manifestations of West Nile virus infection.* Can J Neurol Sci, 31(2), 189–93.

Campbell GL, C. C. (2001). *Epidemic West Nile encephalitis in Romania: witing for history to repeat itself.* Ann N Y Acad Sci, 951, 94–101.

Carson PJ, K. P. (2006). *Long-term clinical and neuropsychological outcomes of West Nile virsu infection.* Clin Infect Dis, 723–30.

Centers for Disease Control and Prevention National Center form Emerging and Zoonotic Infectious Diseases. (2014). *West Nile virus.* Atlanta: Home page CDC.

Chancey C, G. A. (2015). *The Global Ecology and Epidemiology of West Nile Virus.* Biomed Res Int, 20. doi:10.1155/2015/376230

Ciota AT, K.L. (2013). *Vector-Virus Interactions and Transmission Dynamics of West Nile Virus.* Viruses, 5(12), 3021–3047.

Ciccozzi M, P. S. (2013). *Epidemiological history and phylogeography of West Nile virus lineage 2.* Infect Genet Evol(17), 46–50.

Cooper CJ, S. S. (2014). *West Nile virus encephalitis induced opsoclonus-myoclonus syndrome.* Neurol Int, 6(2), 5359.

Dauphin G, Z. S. (2004). *West Nile: worldwide current situation in animals and humans.* Comp Immunol Microbiol Infect Dis, 27, 343–55.

Dauphin G, Z. S. (2004). *West Nile: worldwide current situation in animals and humans.* Comp Immunol Microbiol Infect Dis, 27, 343–55.

Diamond MS, S. E. (2003). *A critical role for inducing IgM in the protection against West Nile virus infection.* J Exp Med(198), 1853–62.

ECDC. (2014, 11 20). *West Nile fever maps.* Retrieved 12 1, 2014, from European Centre for Disease Prevention and Control: http://www.ecdc.europa.eu/en/healthtopics/west_nile_fever/West-Nile-fever-maps/pages/index.aspx

Ferguson DD, G. K. (2005). *Characteristics of the rash associated with West Nile virus fever.* Clin Infect Dis, 41, 1204–07.

Flores Anticona EM, Z. H. (2012). *Two case reports of neuroinvasive West Nile virus in the critical care unit.* Case Rep Infect Dis, 839458.

Garcia-Tapia D, L. C. (2006). *Replication of West Nile virus in equine peripheral blood mononuclear cells.* Veterinary Immunology and Immunopathology, 110(3–4), 229–244.

Glass WG, M. D. (2006). *CCR5 deficiency increases risk of symptomatic West Nile virus infection.* Journal of Experimental Medicine, 1(203), 35–40.

Goldblum N, S. V. (1954). *West Nile fever: The clinical features of the disease and the isolation of West Nile virus from the blood of nine human cases.* Am J Hyg(59), 89–103.

Gorman. (2010). *Update on diagnosis, treatment, and prognosis in opsoclonus-myoclonus-ataxia syndrome.* Curr Opin Pediatr, 22(6), 745–50.

Hail N Jr, C. B. (2006). *Apoptosis effector mechanisms: a requiem performed in different keys.* Apoptosis(11), 889–904.

Hall RA, K. A. (2007). *ChimeriVax-West Nile vaccine.* Curr Opin Mol Ther, 9, 498–504.

Hart J Jr, T. G. (2014). *West Nile neuroinvasive disease:neurological manifestations and prospective longitudinal outcomes.* BMC Inf Diseases, 14(248), 1–10.

Hayes EB, O. D. (2004). *West Nile virus infection: a pediatric perspective.* Pediatrics(113), 1375–81.

Hilgetag CC, B. H. (2009). Are there ten times more glia than neurons in the brain? Brain Struct Func(213), 356–6.

Jamroz E, G. E. (2011, Apr-Jun). Opsoclonus-myoclonus syndrome in a 2 year old boy with prenatally diagnosed retroperitoneal tumor. Med Wieku Rozwoj, 15(2), 151–6.

Jeha LE, S. C. (2003). West NIle virus infection: A new acute paralytic ilnness. Neurology, 41.

Jeha LE, S. C. (2003). West Nile virus infection:A new acute paralytic ilness. Neurology, 61, 55–59.

KA, G. (2009, oct). West Nile virus infections. J Neuropathol Exp Neurol, 68(10), 1053–60.

Khsola JS, E. M. (2005, Mar 22). West Nile virsu presenting as opsoclonus-myoclonus cerebellar ataxia. Neurology, 64(6), 1095.

King AMQ, A. M. (2011). Virus Taxonomy: Ninth Report of the International Committee on Taxonomy of Viruses. (1st ed.). San Diego, CA, USA: Elsevier.

Klass JP, A. J. (2012). Adult Onset Opsoclonus Myoclonus Syndrome. Arch Neurol, 12(69), 1598–1607.

Klee AL, M. B. (2004). Long-term prognostic for clinical West Nile virus infection. Emerg Infect Dis, 10, 1405–11.

Kong KF, D. K. (2008). Dysregulation of TLR3 impairs the innate immune response to the West Nile virus in the elderly. j vIROL(82), 7613–23.

Kramer-Hämmerle S, R. I.-W. (2005). Cells of the central nervous system as targets and reservoirs of the human immunodeficiency virus. Virus REs(111), 194–213.

Kroemer G, M. S. (2005). Caspase-independent cell death. Nat Med(11), 725–30.

Kulstad EB, W. M. (2003). West Nile encephalitis presenting as a stroke. Ann Emerg Med, 41.

Kumar D, P. G. (2004). Community-acquired West Nile virus infection in solid-organ transplant recipients. Transplantation(77), 399–402.

Kumar M, V. S. (2010). Pro-inflammatory cytokines derived from the West Nile virus (WNV)-infected SK-N-SH cells mediate neuroinflammatory markers and neuronal death. J Neuroinflammation(31), 73.

Kurian M, L. P. (2010). Opsoclonus-myoclonus syndrome in anti-N-methyl-D-aspartate receptor encephalitis. Arch Neurol, 67(1), 118–21.

Laurent-Rolle M, B. E.-S. (2010). The NS5 Protein of the Virulent West Nile Virus NY99 Strain Is a Potent Antagonist of Type I Interferon-Mediated JAK-STAT Signaling. J Virol(84), 3503–15.

Liu WJ, W. X. (2005). Inhibition of Interferon Signaling by the New York 99 Strain and Kunjin Subtype of the West Nile Virus Involves Blockage of STAT1 and STAT2 Activation by Nonstructural Proteins. J Virol(79), 1934–42.

Magurano F, R. M. (2012). Circulation of West Nile virus lineage 1 and 2 during an outbreak in Italy. Clin Microbiol Infect(18), E545–47.

Mann BR, M. A. (2013). Molecular Epidemiologi and evolution of West NIle virus in North America. Int. J. Environ. Res. Public Health(10), 5111–29. doi:10.3390/ijerph10105111

McCandless EE, W. Q. (2006). CXCL12 limits inflammation by localizing mono-nuclear infiltrates to the perivascular space during experimental autoimmune encephalomyelitis. J Immunol(177), 8053–64.

Morrey JD, D. C. (2004). Effect of interferon-alpha and interferon-inducers on West Nile virus in mouse and hamster animal models. Antivir Chem Chemother, 15, 101–109.

Morrey JD, S. V. (2007). Defining limits of humanized neutralizing monoclonal antibody treatment for

West Nile virus neurological infection in a hamster model. Antimicrob Agents Chemoter, 51, 2396–2402.

MP, G. (2010). Update on diagnosis, treatment, and prognosis in opsoclonus-myoclonus-ataxia syndrome. Curr Opin Pediatr, 22(6), 745–50.

MP, G. (2010). Update on diagnostic, treatment, and prgnosis in opsoclonus-myoclonus-ataxia syndrome. Curr Opin Pediatr, 22(6), 745–50.

Nash D, M. F. (2001). The outbreak of West Nile virus infection in the New York area in 1999. N Engl J Med, 344, 1807–14.

Nunez-Enamorado N, C.-S. A.-H.-C.-D.-D.-S.-M. (2012, Apr). Fast and spectacular clinical response to plasmapheresis in a paediatric case of anti-NMDA encephalitis. Rev Neurol, 54(7), 420–4.

Nybakken GE, N. C. (2006). Crystal structure of the West Nile virus envelope glycoprotein. J Virol(80), 11467–74.

Oliphant T, E. M. (2005). Development of humanized monoclonal antibody with therapeutic potential against West Nile virus. Nat Med, 11, 522–30.

Papa A, X. K. (2011). Detection of West Nile virus lineage 2 in mosquitoes during a human outbreak in Greece. Clin Microbiol Infect(17), 1176–80.

Peña J, P. J.-A. (2014). Multiplexed digital mRNA profiling of the inflammatory response in the West Nile Swiss Webster mouse model. PLoS Negl Trop Dis(8), e3216.

Pike. (2013). Opsoclonus-myoclonus syndrome. Handb Clin Neurol, 112, 1209–11.

Pipperal C, R. N. (2003). West Nile virus infection in 2002: Morbidity and mortality among patients admitted to hospital in southcentral Ontario. Can Med Assoc J, 168, 1399–1405.

Pletnev AG, P. R. (2002). West Nile virus/dengue type 4 virus chimeras that are reduced in nerovirulence and peripheral virulence without loss of immunogenicity or protective efficacity. Proc Natl Acad Sci USA, 99, 3036–3041.

Poulsen A, K. C. (2014). Drug design for flavivirus proteases: what are we missing? Curr Oharm Des(20), 3422–7.

Pranzatelli MR, H. K. (2004). Evidence of cellular immune activation in children with opsoclonus-myoclonus:cerebrospinal fluid neopterin. Journal of Child Neurology, 19(12), 919–24.

Pranzatelli MR, T. A. (2004, May 11). B-and T-cell markers in opsoclnus-myoclonus syndrome. Immunophenotyping of CSF lymphocytes. Neurology, 62(9), 1526–1532.

Pranzatelli MR, T. A. (2004). CSF B-cell expansion in opsoclonus-myoclonus syndrome: a biomarker of disease activity. Movement Disorders, 19(7), 770–777.

Pranzatelli MR, T. E. (2005). Immunologic and clinical responses to rituximab in a child with opsoclonus-myoclonus syndrome. Pediatrics, 115(1), e115–119.

Pranzatelli MR, T. E. (2006). Rituximab (anti-CD20) adjunctive therapy for opsoclonus-myoclonus syndrome. Journal of Pediatrics Hematology/Oncology, 28(9), 585–93.

Pranzatelli MR, T. E. (2008). Therapeutic down-regulation of central and peripheral B-cell-activating factor (BAFF) production in pediatric opsoclonus-myoclonus syndrome. Cytokine, 44(1), 26–32.

Pranzatelli MR, T. E. (2010). Long-term cerebrospinal fluid and blood lympohocyte dynamics after rituximab for pediatric opsoclonus-myoclonus. Journal of Clinical Immunology, 30(1), 106–113.

Prevention, C. f. (2003). Possible dialysis-related West Nile virus transmision. MMWR Morb Mortal Wkly

Rep , Georgia.

Prevention, C. f. (2004). Transfusion-associated transmission of West Nile virus. MMWR Morb Mortal Wkly Rep, Arizona.

Reijerkerk A, K. G. (2008). Tissue-type plasminogen activator is a regulator of monocyte diapedesis through the brain endothelial barrier. J Immunol(181), 3567–74.

Roby JA, P. G. (2014, Jan 27). Noncoding subgenomic flavivirus RNA:multiple functions in West Nile virus pathogenesis and modulation of host responses. Viruses, 6(2), 404–27.

Rochrig JT, N. D. (2003). Persistence of virus-reactive serum immunoglobulin M antibody in confirmed WEst NIle encephalitis cases. Emerg Infect Dis, 3, 185–93.

Sambri V, C. M. (2013). West Nile virus in Europe: emergence, epidemiology, diagnosis, treatment, and prevention. Clin Microbiol Infect.(19), 699–704.

Samuel MA, M. J. (2007). Caspase 3-dependent cell death of neurons contributes to the pathogenesis of the West Nile virus encephalitis. J Virol(81), 2614–23.

Savarin C, S. S. (2010). Monocytes regulate T cell migration through the glia limitans during acute viral encephalitis. J Virol(84), 4878–88.

Schneider BS, M. C. (2007). Prior exposure to un infected mosquitoes enhances mortality in naturally-transmitted West Nile virus infection. PLoS ONE 2, 2(11), e1171.

Schneider BS, M. C. (2007). Prior exposure to uninfected mosquitoes enhances mortality in naturraly-transmitted West Nile virus infection. e1171.

Schneider BS, S. L. (2006). Potentiation of West Nile encephalitis by mosquito feeding. Viral Immunol, 1(19), 74–82.

Schuffenecker I, P. C. (2005). West Nile virus in Morocco. Emerg Inf Dis, 11, 306–9.

Sejvar JJ, H. M. (2003). Neurologic manifestations and outcome of West NIle virus infection. JAMA, 290(4), 511–515.

Shellenback L, P. J. (2012). 1240: West Nile encephalitis presenting as opsoclonus-myoclonus and alteration of consiousness in apost-liver transplant patient receiving immunosupression. Critical Care Medicine, 40(12), 1–328.

Shimoni Z, N. M. (2001). Treatment of West NIle encephalitis with intravenous immunoglobulin. Emerg Infect Dis, 7, 759.

Smith JH, D. R. (2011, Aug). N-methyl-D-aspartate receptor autoimmune encephalitis presenting with opsoclonus-myoclonus: treatment response to plasmapheresis. Arch Neurol, 68(8), 1069–72.

Stephanie ML, P. K. (2011). West Nile Virus: Immunity and Pathogenesis. Viruses(3), 811–28.

Styer LM, B. K. (2006). Enhanced early West Nile virus infection in young chickens infected by mosquito bite: effect of viral dose. Am. J. Trop. Med. Hyg, 2(75), 337–45.

Swarup V, D. S. (2007). Tumor necrosis factor receptor-1-induced neuronal death by TRADD contributes to the pathogenesis of Japanese encephalitis. J Neurochem(103), 771–83.

Tate ED, P. M. (2012). Active comparator-controlled, rater-blinded study of corticotropin-based immunotherapies for opsoclonus-myoclonus syndrome. J Child Neurol, 27(7), 875–884.

Tyler KL, P. J.-D. (2006). CSF findings in 250 patients with serologically confirmed the West Nile virus meningitis and encephalitis. Neurology(66), 361–5.

Vazquez A, S.-S. M. (2010). Putative new lineage of west nile virus, Spain. Emerg Infect Dis.(16), 549–52.

doi:10.3201/eid1603.091033

Wang D, Z. Y. (2015). A multiplex ELISA-based protein array for screening diagnostic antigens and diagnosis of Flaviviridae infection. Eur J Clin Microbiol Infect Dis(34), 1327–36.

Weiss D, C. D. (2001). Clinical finding of West Nile virus infection in hospitalized patients, New York and New Jersey,2000. Emerg Infect Dis, 7, 654–658.

Wilson JR, d. S. (208). West Nile virus nonstructural protein 1 inhibits TLR3 signal transduction. J Virol(82), 8262–71.

Youn S, A. R. (2013). Non-structural protein-1 is required for West Nile virus replication complex formation and viral RNA synthesis. Virol J(10), 339. doi:10.1186/1743-422X-10-339

Yu CY, H. Y. (2006). Flavivirus infection activates the XBP1 pathway of the unfolded protein response to cope with endoplasmic reticulum stress. J Virol(80), 11868–80.

Zehender G, E. E. (2011). Phylogeography and epidemiological history of West Nile virus genotype 1a in Europe and the Mediterranean basin. Infect Genet Evol(11(3)), 646–53. doi:10.1016/j.meegid.2011.02.003

Zeidner NS, H. S. (1999). Mosquito feeding modulates Th1 and Th2 cytokines in flavivirus susceptibile mice: an effect mimicked by injection of sialokinins, but not demonstrated in flavivirus resistant mice. Parasite Immunol., 1(21), 35–44.

Zeller H, Z. S. (2004, Oct 7). West Nile outbreak in horses in southern France. p. 8.

Zeller HG, S. I. (2004). West Nile: an overview of its spread in Europe and the Mediterranean basin in contrast to its spread in the Americas. Eur J Clin Microbiol Inf Dis, 23, 147–56.

Chapter 10

Histological Image Mosaicing: Application to Microbiology

Wei-Yen Hsu[1]

1 Introduction

In medical and biological research, the microscope is an indispensable tool that is used widely in various investigations and evaluations (Feddema *et al.*, 1998; Hsu, 2011 & 2012). However, in providing high magnification for the observation of specimens, most microscopes suffer from a limited field of view. Therefore, microbiology research requiring information from large tissue areas has a need to overcome this limitation. A common solution is to move the sample platform around, and then cut and paste the images together to create a panoramic image of a unified view of the specimen. However, this method, known as image mosaicking, is tedious and time-consuming. An automatic image-mosaicking system is thus an essential requirement for effectively and efficiently handling these types of microscopic images.

Three main methods are available for the traditional mosaicking technique, as follows: the interactive method, the "brute force" parallel method, and the Fourier method. The interactive method (Williams *et al.*, 1993; Hu & Brown, 2002) provides a short-term solution by using a software package for manual patching and verification. In this approach, individual images are aligned interactively by the user. Additional capabilities include the ability to zoom in for detailed observation and zoom out to view the entire sample. This method is user-friendly but tedious. The second approach is the "brute force" parallel method (Inampudi, 1998), which calculates the sum of the squared difference errors for all possible overlapping zones between two adjacent images, and then chooses the minimum as the desired solution. However, this procedure

---

[1] Department of Information Management & Advanced Institute of Manufacturing with High-tech Innovations, National Chung Cheng University, Taiwan

is also time-consuming, and all data are mostly batch-processed. This mosaicking process, while considered parallel, is still very slow. The last method is the Fourier autocorrelation method (Hibbard *et al.*, 1986 & 1992). This technique replaces convolution-based template matching by applying the Fourier transform to the source and template images, multiplying one by the complex conjugate of the other, and then calculating the inverse Fourier transform to produce the resultant image. The result should, ideally, provide a single peak at the point of correlation. Here, in order to mosaic two images together, one image is considered the basis image and the corresponding image is considered the reference. If the adopted area in the reference image is much larger than the real matching region, the precise determination of correlation will be greatly confused and result in erroneous matching. Hence, the reference must be a small region, and thus this application of the spectrum-based method is severely restricted. Investigations of this technique show its difficulty in identifying suitable peaks of correlation (Hibbard *et al.*, 1986 & 1992). This is why Fourier autocorrelation methods were inappropriate for these applications. In all three of the methods described above, the parameters of translation are adjusted only to align the field of microscopic images. If the XY table is interfered with, such that misalignment consists of translation, rotation, and scaling factors, these methods are no longer effective, and the results of matching become imperfect.

In this study, we have developed an automatic system to manage all the problems noted above. In the acquisition step, this system sequentially captures high-resolution (HR) images from the microscope. Each HR image is arranged to overlap with the adjacent images at the boundary areas where the two images are to be mosaicked together. These images are acquired horizontally or vertically, sequentially capturing the whole specimen. The mosaicking step is then used to match these partially overlapped image pairs into a complete image that includes all the areas in the input images. Cut-lines between each pair of adjacent images are precisely aligned after the images are registered by the proposed method. Due to the congenital sampling characteristic and the optical effects of microscopy, the registered images have a visible seam line on the side of the overlapping zone, which will be made invisible by the image-blending technique. In addition to the registration and blending problems, inconsistent CCD characteristics and/or non-homogeneous illumination conditions during microscopic imaging may also result in color differences between adjacent images and/or color degradation in each acquired image frame. Although these are commonly encountered in microscopic images, they can hardly be resolved by manual adjustment or by motor-driven optics and electronics, and they are seldom addressed by image-processing software, since the latter are designed for general rather than microscopic images. Hence, the "lattice" phenomenon on the mosaicked images may remain and cause the result to look unnatural. The proposed system takes into consideration both color differences and color degradation to achieve more "natural-looking" mosaicked images using simple, effective steps. Image blending is the final but important step to make the seam lines invisible. Traditionally, this was handled by applying a weighting average with a sigmoid function within the transition zone. However, the seam lines were rarely invisible after using this method. The multi-resolution concept with spline technique was reported to achieve more successful image blending (Burt & Adelson,

1983); it is more flexible for handling images with transition zones of various widths. Human visual sensitivity responds to different transition zones with different resolutions that are proportional to the size of smoothing filters. Due to a better analogy to a multiscale visual system and more-efficient computation, Daubechies discrete wavelet transform (DWT) is adopted in this approach for image blending and achieves good results in the experiments with different types of images. After all, the design concept of these mosaicking steps is to retain as many of the global characteristics of all input images with as little misalignment and distortion as possible.

The remainder of this paper is organized as follows: in Section 2, the image-mosaicking technique is described in detail; the experimental studies conducted with different medical specimens are described in Section 3, and discussions on different results are included; conclusions are addressed in Section 4.

2 Method

In this section, we will illustrate the system designed for automatically mosaicking microscopic images. It consists of several important steps including feature extraction, image matching, matching refinement, and image blending. Each of these steps will be described in detail in the following subsections.

2.1 Feature Extraction

Feature extraction involves the extraction of sharp or key content information from the original image data. It is usually crucial for feature-based image matching, especially for accuracy in matching results. The most important aspect of feature extraction is how to simultaneously extract representative features, which exist at the overlapping zone in both the basis and reference images, in order to effectively provide the geometrical and photometric information for the image matching.

Multi-resolution image decomposition is a useful approach for analyzing the information within an image. Hence, we have developed a method based on wavelet-based edge correlation to obtain the feature points that have strong and consistent responses for different scales within a local area (Mallat & Zhong, 1992; Xu *et al.*, 1994; Hsieh *et al.*, 1997; Hsu, 2013). Based on this property, feature points usually have larger values on the product of gradient moduli in multiscales, while the noise points will not last for different scales.

It is possible to express 2D wavelet transform in each level as the tensor product of two 1D wavelet transforms, i.e., $\varphi(x,y) = \varphi(y)\varphi(y)$, that are orthogonal to each other due to their separable characteristics, with the formulae:

$$\varphi^H(x,y) = \frac{\partial S(x,y)}{\partial x} \text{ and } \varphi^V(x,y) = \frac{\partial S(x,y)}{\partial y},$$

where $S(x,y)$ is a 2D smoothing function representing two 1D wavelet functions in x and

y directions, respectively. We denote:

$$\xi_j(x,y) = \frac{1}{2^{2j}}\xi(\frac{x}{2^j},\frac{y}{2^j}),$$

which is the dilation by a scaling factor j of any 2D function $\xi(x,y)$. Then, we can have:

$$\varphi_j^H(x,y) = \left(\frac{1}{2^{2j}}\right)\varphi^H\left(\frac{x}{2^j},\frac{y}{2^j}\right),$$

$$\varphi_j^V(x,y) = \left(\frac{1}{2^{2j}}\right)\varphi^V\left(\frac{x}{2^j},\frac{y}{2^j}\right),$$

$$S_j(x,y) = \left(\frac{1}{2^{2j}}\right)S\left(\frac{x}{2^j},\frac{y}{2^j}\right),$$

which are the dilated versions of $\varphi^H(x,y)$, $\varphi^V(x,y)$ and $S(x,y)$, respectively. The related mathematical expressions for 2D wavelet transform of an image $f(x,y)$ are described as follows:

$$W_j^H f(x,y) = f * \varphi_j^H(x,y) = f*(2^j \cdot \frac{\partial S_j}{\partial x})(x,y) = 2^j \cdot \frac{\partial}{\partial x}(f*S_j)(x,y),$$

and

$$W_j^V f(x,y) = f * \varphi_j^V(x,y) = f*(2^j \cdot \frac{\partial S_j}{\partial y})(x,y) = 2^j \cdot \frac{\partial}{\partial y}(f*S_j)(x,y), \tag{1}$$

where $W_j^H f(x,y)$ and $W_j^V f(x,y)$ represent the gradient of image $f(x,y)$ in the x and y directions at level j respectively. Then, the modulus can be derived as:

$$M_j f(x,y) = \sqrt{\left| W_j^H f(x,y)\right|^2 + \left| W_j^V f(x,y)\right|^2} \tag{2}$$

All the edge points in image $f(x,y)$ at level j can be located after applying a predefined threshold to the detected local maxima of $M_j f(x,y)$. Generally speaking, noise is a major factor resulting in the false detection of edge points and can be easily filtered by a multiscale edge confirmation process. The criterion of edge correlation (Xu *et al.*, 1994) is used to detect feature points that are more reliable and suppress the influence of noise, as follows,

$$R_n(j,x,y) = \prod_{i=0}^{n-1} M_{j+i} f(x,y), \tag{3}$$

where n is the scale number in multiplication, and j is the initial level for the expression. By means of edge correlation, significant feature points can be obtained and distinguished from noise. The well-known concept noting that features can exist in multiscales, while noise cannot continue, is employed to detect feature points in this technique. The product of the gradient moduli in multiscales is used to determine the true feature points of the microscopic images. Usually, the number of levels for the multiplication is chosen as two or three; this is because the edge delocalization property of wavelet transform in multiscale becomes more noticeable and is a serious problem when it becomes too large. In the detection process, an additional constraint is used to filter out some noises and adjust the number of feature points; the point in its gradient modulus must be the local maximum within a window and must also be greater than a threshold. The window is uniformly sampled with a fixed size from the two given images, and the window size will greatly affect the number of feature points. When it is large, fewer feature points will be extracted in the image. Conversely, more feature points will be extracted when the window is smaller. The results of feature-point extraction are shown in Figure 1. A test image sequence with partial overlapping is shown in Figure 1(a). Figure 1(b) shows the results of feature-point extraction.

2.2   Image Matching

After feature points are extracted from the two images, we then search for all the possible matching pairs. The two images can usually be aligned well when there is a sufficient number of resulting matching pairs. However, when the total feature points or matching pairs are inadequate, an alternative method based on the correlation of projection profiles must be used to obtain the parameters for geometric transform. In most cases, sufficient matching pairs can be obtained from the two images. The following method can be used to obtain the transform for image alignment. There are four steps in the proposed method, as follows;

1. Selecting feature points: At this step, several key feature points must be selected from the basis image in advance. These feature points not only have higher edge magnitude but also are closer to the seamed boundary. In most cases, the overlapping is within a small region, about 20 to 30 percent of the image size. Feature selection helps to reduce erroneous matching caused by using the wrong features.

2. Finding all possible matching pairs: For each key feature point in the basis image, we search for all the possible matching points from the reference image, based on the normalized correlation coefficient. Of course, the measured coefficient between each pair of matched feature points should be larger than a predefined threshold in order to avoid incorrect matching. All possible matching feature pairs from both images are obtained in this step.

3. Extracting reliable matching pairs: Based on the assumption that only slight rotation and scaling may exist between adjacent images, each matching feature pair can define a simple geometric transform, i.e., translation, to align the two adjacent images. Then, a consistency test is devised to measure the similarity between each possible matching feature pair, and a count of matched feature.

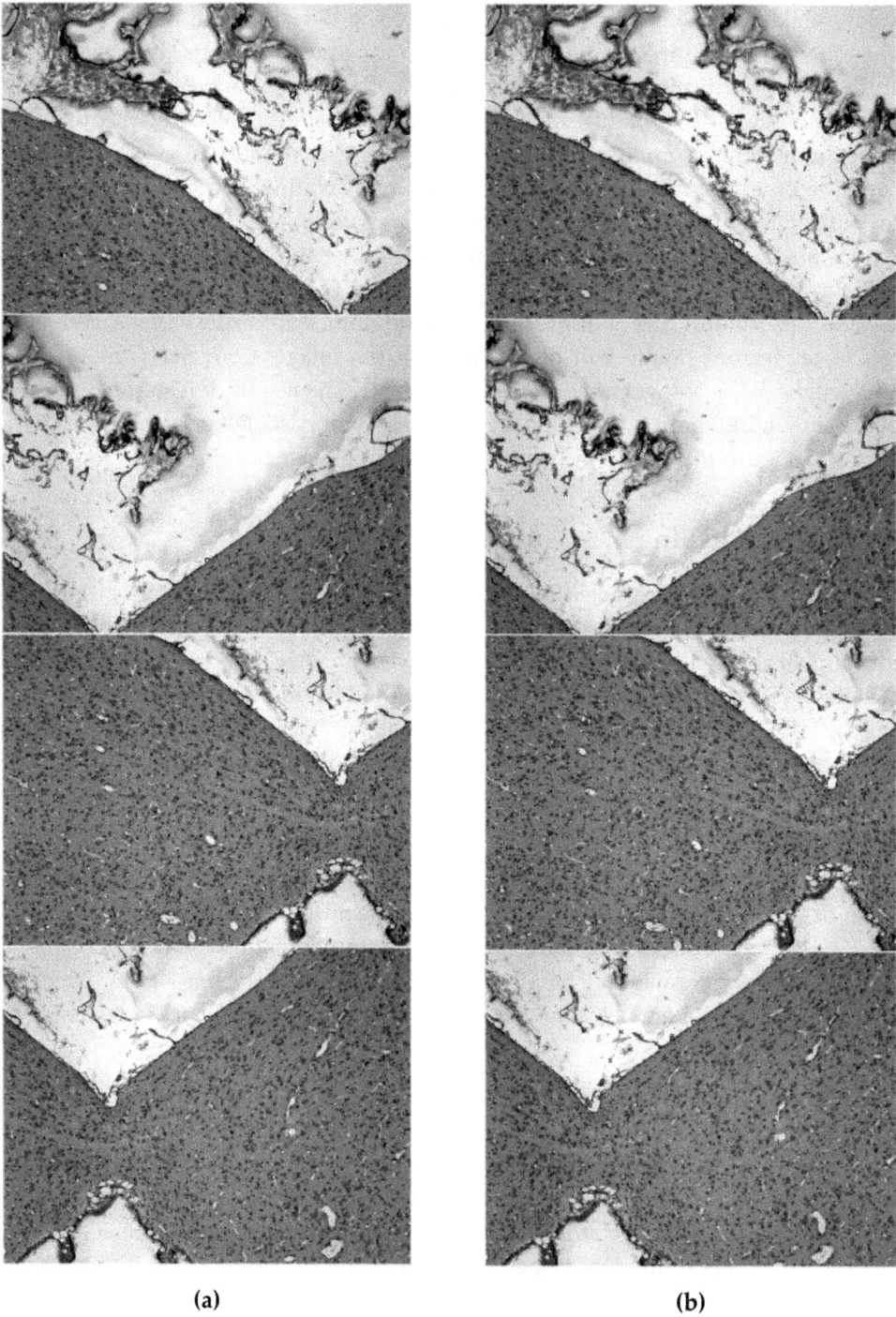

(a)   (b)

Figure 1. Feature point extraction, (a) a test image sequence with partially over-lapping, (b) extracted feature points.

pairs is computed for each of the possible feature pairs obtained in step 2 above. The feature pair with the largest matching count is chosen as the reliable matching pair. Here, we expect this count to be at least three. When the count is less than three, registration based on projection profiles will be adopted instead

4. Refined geometric transform: All the matching pairs associated with the reliable matching pair are then applied in order to estimate the parameters of the refined geometric transform by using the singular value decomposition (SVD) method (Arun *et al.*, 1987).

Because the refined geometric transform covers all the parameters for translation, rotation, and scaling, it usually achieves more-accurate image matching for each pair of adjacent images.

2.3   Matching Refinement

In order to make the matching result more reliable and accurate, a refining step for image matching is necessary. A feature-based modified Levenberg-Marquardt (MLM) method (Thevenaz *et al.*, 1998) is adopted to achieve this. Since the optimization problem is reformulated so that the Hessian matrix no longer needs to be recomputed at each iteration, the modified algorithm is much more efficient than the conventional one. In our case, the MLM method is slightly modified to fit the requirements for image mosaicking, where the rigid transformation is adopted instead of the original affine transformation. Because the acquired images have hardly any affine distortion, the simplification speeds the processing time and reduces the occurrence of unexpected geometric warping. In addition, by using feature points only instead of total pixels, this refining step is efficient and robust. Due to the nonlinear characteristic of the MLM method, it converges much faster than most other methods, as long as the initial estimation is close to the global optimal solution. The sums of the squared intensity errors for feature-point blocks are minimized to measure the similarity between adjacent and overlapping images. The ε^2, which is the sum of squared intensity error, is adopted as the optimization criterion and defined by:

$$\varepsilon^2 = \sum_{fp} \left(f(x) - C_p \left(g(x) \right) \right)^2 , \tag{4}$$

where C_p is the geometric transform between $f(x)$ and $g(x)$ for mosaicking. For the adaptive geometric transform $C_p(.)$, we consider the general transformation parameterized by the translation vector T_t, rotation angle R_ϑ, and scaling factor S_s. After decomposition, the respective operators are written as:

$$\left\{ \begin{array}{l} T_t \left(g(x) \right) = g(x+t) \\[2mm] R_\theta \left(g(x) \right) = g(\tilde{\theta}x) = g(\begin{bmatrix} \cos\theta & -\sin\theta \\ \sin\theta & \cos\theta \end{bmatrix} x) \\[2mm] S_s \left(g(x) \right) = g(sx) \end{array} \right. . \tag{5}$$

Using these operators, the geometric transform for mosaicking can be represented by:

$$C_p\big(g(x)\big) = C_{t,s,\theta}\big(g(x)\big) = T_t\Big(S_s\Big(R_\theta\big(g(x)\big)\Big)\Big) = g(s\tilde{\theta}x + t),\tag{6}$$

and using the MLM algorithm, we then obtain the following equations:

$$\varepsilon^2 = \frac{1}{s^2}\sum_{fp}\Big(T_{-t}\Big(S_{s^{-1}}\Big(R_{-\theta}\big(f(x)\big)\Big)\Big) - T_{\Delta t}\Big(S_{1+\Delta s}\Big(R_{\Delta\theta}\big(g(x)\big)\Big)\Big)\Big)^2,\tag{7}$$

where $C_{\Delta p} = (T_{\Delta t}, S_{\Delta s}, R_{\Delta\theta})$ is the update of transformation operators for the geometric transform. By minimizing equation (7) with respect to Δp, the parameter $\hat{p}$ is recursively updated with the estimated component Δp, as

$$\hat{p}^{(k+1)} = \hat{p}^{(k)} + \Delta p \ \text{ with } \ \Delta p = \big(\hat{A} + \lambda I\big)^{-1}\hat{b},\tag{8}$$

where λ is a positive parameter adjusted according to the variation of the sum of the squared error. When the error decreases, the parameter λ decreases, and the next estimated update Δp tends to the Newton method. Conversely, the parameter λ increases, and the next estimated update tends to the gradient descent approach while the error increases. The MLM method is updated iteratively until either the relative error

$$\frac{\big(\varepsilon^2\big)^{(t)} - \big(\varepsilon^2\big)^{(t-1)}}{\big(\varepsilon^2\big)^{(t-1)}}$$

is under a given threshold, or the number of iterations reaches a predefined value.

2.4   Image Blending

When two adjacent images are mosaicked together, the chromatic deviation around the seam area, even after color adjustment and degradation compensation, is still slightly visible or even obvious. Traditionally, within the transition zone, the intensity of each pixel is usually obtained as the weighting average of the corresponding pixels from the two overlapping images. In practice, weighted average is good for image blending when the differences between the corresponding features in the two images are small. However, the mosaicked zones usually become unnatural or blurred when the feature variations are large. Although the weighting function is carefully selected, the seam is not guaranteed to be invisible, since image variations are sometimes large. The multi-resolution spline technique was reported to achieve successful results for image blending (Burt & Adelson, 1983). In addition, the multiscale concept is more flexible for handling images with transition zones of various widths. In this method, human visual sensitivity responding to different widths of transition zone can be handled with different filters of spatial resolution. Due to a good analogy with the human visual system, it obtains natural-looking results with successful seam-line removal. We utilize the Daubechies discrete wavelet transform (DWT) to design the multiscale image blending, and it results in well-mosaicked images with a natural appearance and invisible seams.

Multiresolution characteristics of wavelet transform have proven useful in analyzing image content in many applications. One of the principal concepts in wavelet transform is to decompose the image into a multiscale structure. The component in each level can later be processed based on its distinct frequency property. Although many wavelet transforms have been developed, Daubechies wavelet (in 2nd family) is adopted in this paper because it obtains the most-reliable results in these experiments. The scaling and wavelet functions of Daubechies wavelet transform are represented as:

$$\varphi_{2^j}(x-2^{-j}k) = \sum_n \left\langle \sqrt{2^{-j-1}}\,\varphi_{2^{j+1}}(u-2^{-j-1}n), \varphi_{2^j}(u-2^{-j}k) \right\rangle \cdot \sqrt{2^{-j-1}}\,\varphi_{2^{j+1}}(x-2^{-j-1}n),$$
$$\psi_{2^j}(x-2^{-j}k) = \sum_n \left\langle \sqrt{2^{-j-1}}\,\psi_{2^{j+1}}(u-2^{-j-1}n), \psi_{2^j}(u-2^{-j}k) \right\rangle \cdot \sqrt{2^{-j-1}}\,\varphi_{2^{j+1}}(x-2^{-j-1}n),$$

$$(9)$$

where $\varphi_{2^j}(x-2^{-j}k)$ and $\psi_{2^j}(x-2^{-j}k)$ are the dilated and translated forms of the scaling function $\varphi(x)$ and the wavelet function $\psi(x)$, respectively. It could be rearranged to obtain

$$\varphi_{2^j}(x-2^{-j}k) = \sum_n \frac{1}{\sqrt{2}} h(n-2k)\varphi_{2^{j+1}}(x-2^{-j-1}n),$$
$$\psi_{2^j}(x-2^{-j}k) = \sum_n \frac{1}{\sqrt{2}} q(n-2k)\varphi_{2^{j+1}}(x-2^{-j-1}n),$$

$$(10)$$

where

$$h(n-2k) = \sqrt{2}\left\langle \varphi_{2^{-1}}(u), \varphi(u-(n-2k)) \right\rangle = h_{n-2k}$$
$$q(n-2k) = \sqrt{2}\left\langle \psi_{2^{-1}}(u), \varphi(u-(n-2k)) \right\rangle = (-1)^{n-2k} h_{(2N-1)-(n-2k)}$$

where $h(n-2k)$ and $q(n-2k)$ stand for the low-pass filter and high-pass filter of the wavelet, respectively. N represents the number of levels. Instead of the symbols used in (10), G represents signal function, and S and D are the approximation and detail spaces of G, respectively. The expression is the continuous version of Daubechies wavelet transform, and it can be further adjusted to the discrete form:

$$S_k = \sum_{m=0}^{2N-1} h_m \cdot G_{2k+m-1},$$
$$D_k = \sum_{m=0}^{2N-1} (-1)^m h_{(2N-1)-m} \cdot G_{2k+m-1}.$$

$$(11)$$

Daubechies wavelet transform can be directly applied to the images. Let $G_{M,N}$ be the original image with size M x N. After Daubechies DWT and rearrangement, the image $G_{M,N}$ is transformed to:

$$\begin{bmatrix} S_{\frac{M}{2}\times\frac{N}{2}} & D^{H}_{\frac{M}{2}\times\frac{N}{2}} \\ D^{V}_{\frac{M}{2}\times\frac{N}{2}} & D^{D}_{\frac{M}{2}\times\frac{N}{2}} \end{bmatrix},$$

where

$$S_{\frac{M}{2}\times\frac{N}{2}}, \ D^{H}_{\frac{M}{2}\times\frac{N}{2}}, \ D^{V}_{\frac{M}{2}\times\frac{N}{2}}, \ D^{D}_{\frac{M}{2}\times\frac{N}{2}}$$

represent the low-frequency part and high-frequency part in the horizontal direction, the high-frequency part in the vertical direction, and the high-frequency part in the diagonal direction, respectively.

In other words, 2D wavelet transform applied to images can be regarded as the tensor product of two orthogonal 1D wavelet transforms along the vertical and horizontal directions. A multiscale Daubechies DWT-based image-blending method consists of the following three steps:

a) Decomposing both the basis and reference images to the pyramids by means of Daubechies DWT. We sample the image data outside the current boundary by adopting samples from the other side of the image in the DWT implementation:

$$S_k = \sum_{m=0}^{2N-1} h_m \cdot G_{2k+m-1 \bmod M}$$

$$D_k = \sum_{m=0}^{2N-1} (-1)^m h_{(2N-1)-m} \cdot G_{2k+m-1 \bmod M}$$

(12)

b) Merging all the corresponding subimages at each resolution level; and

c) Reconstructing the resultant image according to inverse Daubechies DWT:

$$G_k = \sum_{m=0}^{N-1} \left(h_{(2N-2)-2m+(k-1 \bmod 2)} \cdot S_{\left(2N-3+\left\lfloor \frac{k-1}{2}\right\rfloor \bmod \frac{M}{2}\right)+1} \right.$$

$$\left. +(-1)^{k-1} h_{1+2m-(k-1 \bmod 2)} \cdot D_{\left(2N-3+\left\lfloor \frac{k-1}{2}\right\rfloor \bmod \frac{M}{2}\right)+1} \right)$$

(13)

With the test image sequence shown in Figure 1(a), the rough and refined image-matching results are shown in Figures 2(b) and 2(c), respectively. Figure 2(c) illustrates the excellent results of image blending using Daubechies DWT. By making use of the periodic image extension property, the boundary problems can be overcome.

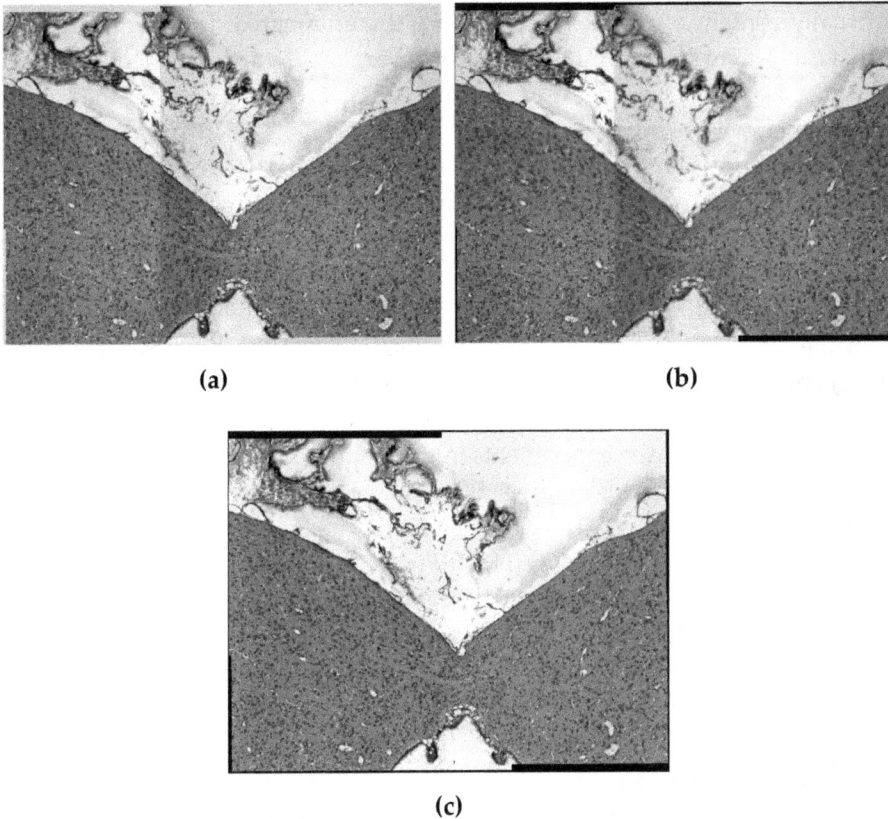

(a)   (b)

(c)

Figure 2. Procedure for image mosaicking, (a) rough image matching, (b) refined image matching, (c) image blending with multiscale wavelet.

3   Experimental Results and Discussion

In this research, we have developed a complete image mosaicking system that automatically mosaics all microscopic images acquired from the specimen. Its results on the mosaicked areas have as little distortion as possible with respect to the areas in the original. When microscopic images are acquired, the platform moves horizontally from the left-most to right-most for the first row, and then from the right-most to left-most for the second row. It then goes from left to right followed by right to left sequentially as it moves down row by row. The process of image mosaicking is repeated on each pair of neighboring images till the whole specimen is scanned thoroughly. In contrast to conventional methods, the proposed method is automatic, efficient, and insensitive to poor image quality.

A test image sequence with partial overlapping is shown in Figure 1(a). Figure 1(b) shows the result of feature point extraction. The edge points, which are usually in the borders of rat brain and blood vessels, are extracted as features. These edges are retained on the multiscale wavelet-based edge correlation, while the edges of neuron cells, which usually contain only a couple of pixels, are eliminated. In other words, feature points that can retain consistent responses for several scales are extracted and others are regarded as noise and discarded. A reliable feature detector is crucial for the subsequent image matching.

Figure 2 shows the procedure for image mosaicking. Figure 2(a) and 2(b) show image matching based on the detected feature points with rough and refined geometric transform respectively. Figure 2(c) shows the image blending with multiscale wavelet. Comparing resulting images in Figure 2(b) and 2(c), stitching lines are obviously visible along the edge of overlapping zones in the former image, while those lines become invisible in the latter. After blending with multiscale wavelet, the mosaicked results in Figure 2(c) appear natural and without all the defects appearing in Figure 2(b). The color difference adjustment and color degradation compensation techniques proved very simple and effective in all the experiments in this paper.

In the experiments, several differently stained image sequences are used to evaluate the proposed mosaicing method. They are illustrated in Figure 3. Among them, the rat brains are stained by Haematoxylin (H) in Figure 3. Figure 3(a) shows the image sequence captured by the microscopy with higher magnification. Figure 3(b) shows the results of rough alignment based on the detected feature points or the correlation of projection profiles. Figure 3(c) shows the resulting image after refined matching. Figure 3(d) shows the final results after image blending with multiscale wavelet. Figure 3(e) shows the low-magnified image corresponding to the mosaicked high-magnified image in Figure 3(d). The image shown in Figure 3(d) is in fact around one twentieth of the real size of mosaicked high-magnified image. Comparing the two images, the fine details of biomedical specimens are much better revealed and less blurred in the mosaicked image even after it has been shrunk to the same size as the low-magnified one. The detailed features throughout the specimen can be clearly depicted under the original high resolution when browsing the mosaicked images. Besides, the global appearance in Figure 3(d) is almost identical to that of Figure 3(e). It thus indicates that the proposed mosaicked method is precise and capable of compensating for the optical degradations in microscopic images.

4   Conclusion

Image mosaicking is one of the most critical functions required in microscopic image analysis. In this paper, an automatic and complete system is proposed for microscopic image mosaicking. Based on the discrete wavelet transform, this system consists of several processing steps including feature extraction, matching and blending. In addition, a modified Levenberg-Marquardt method is designed to achieve more superior accuracy in registration by efficient computation. They resolve the inherent problems in microscopic image acquisition, obtain more consistent image quality, and make the mosaicking results with more natural appearance. In the experimental studies, the proposed system achieves very good visual results as well as error measures in various types of image sequences. It affords a convenient and accurate tool for biologists and medical doctors in managing microscopic images for various studies and researches.

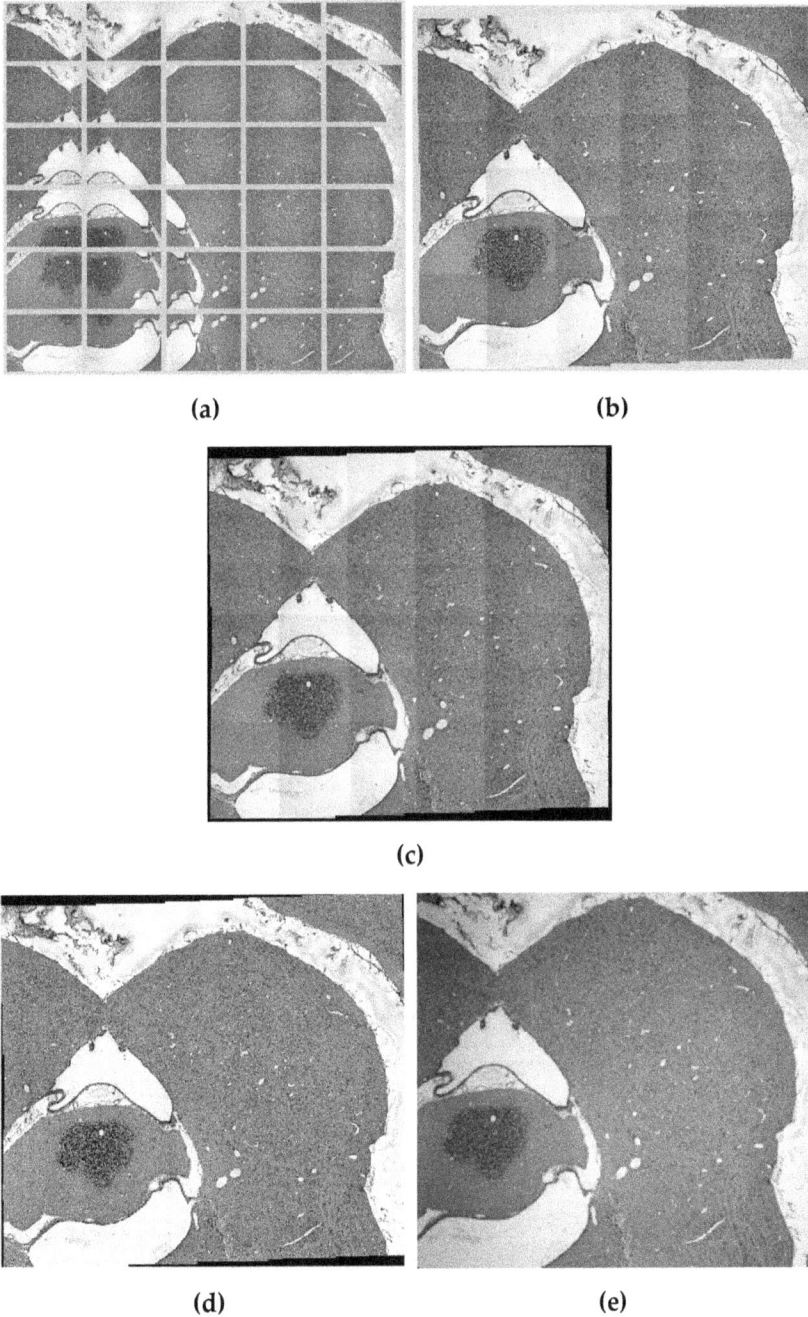

Figure 3. Image mosaicking example, (a) image sequence of rat brain stained by H, (b) result of rough geometric transform, (c) result after refined image matching, (d) final result after image blending with multiscale wavelet, and (e) low-magnified image corresponding to the mosaicked high-magnified one.

Acknowledgement

The author would like to express his sincere appreciation for grant partially from NSC102-2633-E-194-002, MOST103-2410-H-194-070-MY2, NSC103-2622-E- 194-003-CC2, MOST105-2410-H-194-059-MY3, Ministry of Science and Technology, Taiwan.

References

Arun, K. S., Huang, T. S., & Blostein, S. D. (1987). Least-square fitting of two 3-D points sets. IEEE Trans. Pattern Analysis and Machine Intelligence, PAMI-9, 698–700.

Burt, P. J., & Adelson, E. H. (1983). A Multiresolution spline with Application to Image Mosaics. ACM Trans. On Graphics, 2, 217–236.

Feddema, J. T., Keller, C. G., & Howe, R. T. (1998). Experiments in micromanipulation and CAD-driven microassembly. Proceedings of SPIE: Microroboticsand Microsystem Fabrication, 3202, 98–107.

Hibbard, L. S., Hartman, B. J. D., & Page, R. B. (1986). Three-dimensional reconstruction of median eminence microvascular modules. Computational Biology, 16, 411–421.

Hibbard, L S, et al. (1992). Computed alignment of dissimilar images for three-dimensional reconstructions. Journal of Neuroscience Methods, 41, 133–152.

Hsieh, J. W., Liao, H. Y. M., Fan, K. C., Ko, M. T., & Hung, Y. P. (1997). Image Registration Using a new Edge-Based Approach. Computer Vision and Image Understanding, 67, 112–130.

Hsu, W. Y. (2011). Analytic differential approach for robust registration of rat brain histological images. Microscopy Research and Technique, 74, 523–530.

Hsu, W. Y. (2012). Registration Accuracy and Quality of Real-Life Images. PLoS ONE, 7, e40558.

Hsu, W. Y. (2013). A practical approach based on analytic deformable algorithm for scenic image registration. PLoS ONE, 8, e66656.

Hu, B., & Brown, C. (2002). Interactive indoor scene reconstruction from image mosaics using cuboid structure. Workshop on Proceedings of Motion and Video Computing 2002 (pp. 208–213).

Inampudi, R. B. (1998). Image mosaicing. IEEE International on Geoscience and Remote Sensing Symposium Proceedings 1998, 5, 2363–2365.

Mallat, S., & Zhong, S. (1992). Characterization of Signals form Multiscale edges. IEEE Trans. Pattern Analysis and Machine Intelligence, 14, 710–732.

Thevenaz, P., Ruttimann, U. E., & Unser, M. (1998). A Pyramid Approach to Subpixel Registration Based on Intensity. IEEE Trans. On Image Processing, 7, 27–41.

Williams, J., Hills, D., & Okazaki, D. (1993). An interactive swath mosaic editor in a visual programming environment. OCEANS 93: Proceedings of Engineering in Harmony with Ocean (pp. III462–467).

Xu, Y., Weaver, J. B., Healy, D. M., & Lu, J. (1994). Wavelet Transform Domain Filters: A Spatially Selective Noise Filtration Technique. IEEE Trans. Image Processing, 3, 747–757.

Chapter 11

Parallel Phylogenetics in Personal Computers

Leandro Roberto Jones[1], Julieta M. Manrique[1]

1 Summary

Phylogenetic analysis provides a powerful tool for incorporating historical information into biological hypothesis testing. During the last decades, there was an exponential proliferation of phylogenetic studies due to the sustained development and improvement of molecular methods and the advance of computer algorithms and hardware. Parallel computing entered the scene several years ago but, until recently, parallel computers were unavailable for everyone. However, thanks to relatively recent advances in processor technologies, multicore processors are nowadays within easy reach. In this chapter, the problems related to phylogenetic tree searches, sequence alignment, and phylogenetic uncertainty estimation are briefly reviewed. In addition, parallel approaches to these issues are outlined, and examples are provided of their use with microbial datasets. The chapter thus covers basic aspects of phylogenetic analysis and provides a general introduction to parallel phylogenetics.

2 Why Phylogenetic Analysis is So Popular?

Phylogenetics is the study of evolutionary histories of living beings. The publication of revealing studies such as those on the natural history of the three domains of life (Cedergren et al., 1988; Woese, Kandler, and Wheelis, 1990) and the epidemiology of influenza viruses (Buonagurio et al., 1986; Fitch et al., 1991), triggered a spectacular domino effect that resulted in the more than 40,000 articles containing the words "virus"

---

[1] Laboratory of Virology and Molecular Genetics, Faculty of Natural Sciences, Trelew branch, National University of Patagonia "San Juan Bosco", Argentina

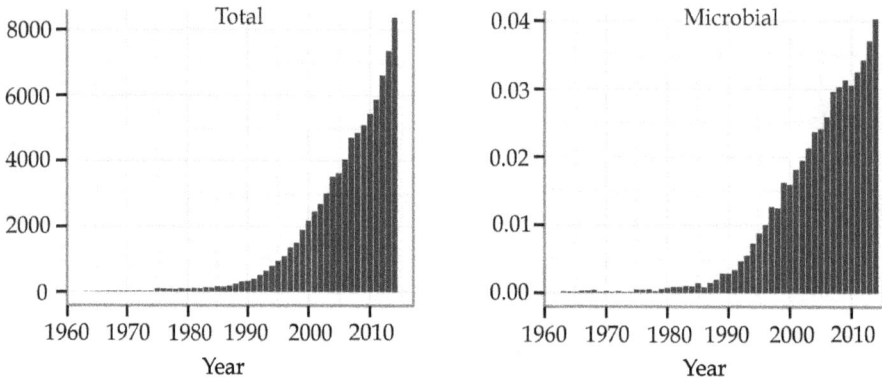

Figure 1: Number of publications indexed in PubMed that contain the world "phylogenetic" (total; n=81,636), and the proportion of the papers indexed in the database that contain the words "virus" or "bacteria" or "fungi" (n=2,375,701) and also contain the word "phylogenetic" (n=41,014) (microbial). The data include works published between the years 1963 and 2014.

or "bacteria" or "fungi", and "phylogenetic" that are indexed in Pubmed (Figure 1).

Phylogenetics is a field full of never ending debates and uncertainties, such as if probabilistic approaches are better than cladistic ones, or if data partitions should or should not be combined. Nevertheless, there is common agreement in that phylogenies are relevant for taxonomic classification (Menezes, Bonvicino, and Seuanez, 2010; Olvera *et al.*, 2010; Schleifer, 2009; Voigt and Kirk, 2011) and dealing with phylogenetic nonindependence in comparative data (Dilernia *et al.*, 2008; Felsenstein, 1985b; Freckleton, Cooper, and Jetz, 2011). Furthermore, phylogenetic analysis is of key importance for rapidly evolving microorganisms, such as viruses, for which the time scales of evolution and epidemiology are almost equivalent (Pybus and Rambaut, 2009; Rasmussen, Boni, and Koelle, 2013).

3   Complexity in Phylogenetic Analysis

Phylogeneticists usually face a spectrum of challenges including selecting the techniques that best fit their needs, choosing adequate phylogenetic markers, and designing sampling strategies that fit both their scientific goals and technical capabilities. But perhaps the most complicated aspect of phylogenetics is tree inference itself, which involves issues that, in computational complexity theory, are classified among the hardest-to-solve known problems (Bodlaender *et al.*, 1992). These issues are briefly reviewed below.

3.1   Tree Inference

Phylogenies are inferred by the use of optimality functions. These are functions of a dataset (generally a sequence alignment) and a tree. Every optimality function is linked to an optimality criterion, which corresponds to a series of theoretical considerations that allow to objectively assess the quality of alternative evolutionary trees. The most popular optimality criteria used in phylogenetics are Maximum Likelihood (ML; Cavalli-Sforza and Edwards, 1967; Huelsenbeck and Crandall, 1997), Parsimony (Camin and Sokal, 1965; Crisci, 1982; Farris, 1970) and Minimum Evolution or "Distance" (Edwards, 1996). There are many works, such as for example (Blair and Murphy, 2011; Felsenstein, 2004; Holder and Lewis, 2003; Olvera et al., 2010; Wheelan, 2008), in which these criteria, as well as the corresponding optimality functions, are described in detail. From a practical point of view, the inference of phylogenies consists of applying an optimality function to alternative trees, and selecting the tree for which this function reaches a maximum. This may seem trivial but, actually, exact solutions are not attainable in polynomial time due to the disproportionate amount of possible phylogenetic trees, which makes it impossible to find the best tree by means of exhaustive searches even for relatively small datasets (Figure 2) (Cavalli-Sforza and Edwards, 1967; Felsenstein, 1978; Swofford and Olsen, 1996; Wheelan, 2008; Chor and Tuller, 2005; Chor and Tuller, 2006; Edwards, 1996; Graham and Foulds, 1982).

Thus, several heuristic methods have been developed that allow exploring tree spaces with reasonable intensities and in affordable times (Goloboff, 1999; Goloboff and Farris, 2001; Guindon et al., 2010; Guindon and Gascuel, 2003; Moilanen, 1999; Nixon, 1999; Stamatakis, 2006; Stamatakis, Hoover, and Rougemont, 2008; Stamatakis, Ludwig, and Meier, 2005). In essence, these techniques progressively refine a candidate tree by iterative topological rearrangements (Felsenstein, 2004; Swofford and Olsen, 1996; Wheelan, 2008).

If optimality increases after a rearrangement, the old tree is discarded and the refined one is saved and submitted to further topological rearrangements. In this way, the optimality space is progressively "climbed", up to a point in which the tree can no longer be improved. Given that tree spaces can be very complex (Chor et al., 2000; Maddison, 1991; Steel, 1994), tree searches must proceed from many independent starting trees in order to avoid settling for a local optimum (Figure 3).

3.2   Statistical Support

Uncertainty is a commonplace issue in science. Phylogeneticists are interested in monophyletic groups and thus much effort has been put in developing statistical support measures for tree branches or nodes. The most popular approaches used to this end are resampling methods and Bayesian phylogenetics. Bootstrapping is a statistical procedure aimed at estimating the sampling distribution of a random variable of interest by resampling (Efron, 1979). Joseph Felsenstein has devised a bootstrap approach (here after phylogenetic bootstrap) for placing confidence values on phylogenies (Felsenstein, 1985a). In phylogenetic bootstrap, resampling is performed from a sequence alignment until the pseudoreplicates have the same number of alignment positions than the real alignment. Given that resampling is made with replacement, some alignment columns can be duplicated in each pseudoreplicate and some others can be missing. This procedure is repeated many times (e.g. 100–1000), and trees are inferred, independently, from

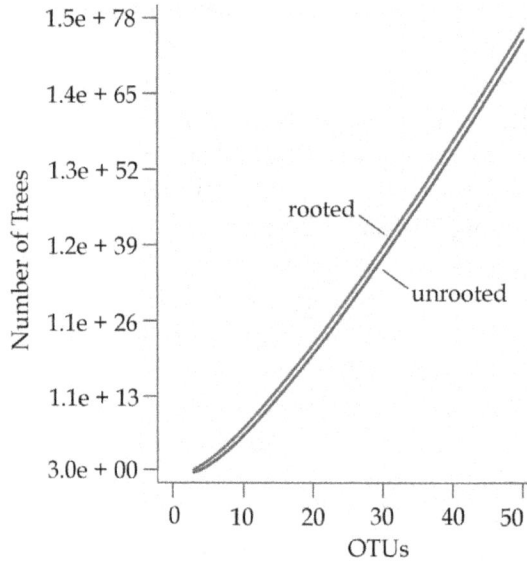

Figure 2: Number of rooted and unrooted phylogenetic trees, in function of the number of operational taxonomic units (OTUs) under study. The scale of the y axis is logarithmic.

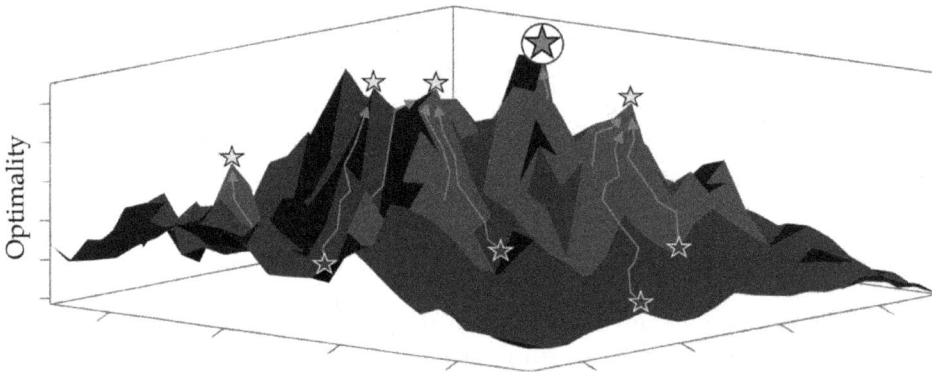

Figure 3: Graphical representation of a hypothetical search space and a heuristic search. Points in the x-y plane correspond to different topologies, and the z axis to the corresponding optimality values. The purple surface represents the search space. The blue stars represent initial trees. The red arrows describe the optimality paths followed by each individual rearrangements series. The encircled, red star represents the optimal topology. Local optima (aka islands), are indicated by green stars. The real analyses usually result in many optimal trees, and actual islands can have lots of topologies.

the obtained pseudoreplicates. The results are usually displayed by trees in which branches/splits are labeled by numbers indicating the frequencies at which that branches/splits appeared among the trees inferred from the resampled datasets. The complete procedure is outlined in Figure 4. The Bayesian approach is somewhat more sophisticated than the bootstrap (Huelsenbeck *et al.*, 2001). The approach is grounded on Bayes' theorem, which is focused in the posterior probability of a hypothesis, which in phylogenetic analysis is an evolutionary tree (Eddy, 2004; Huelsenbeck *et al.*, 2001; Ronquist, Huelsenbeck, and van der Mark, 2005). Under the probabilistic paradigm, phylogenetic trees are viewed as random variables. Thus, the majority of Bayesian phylogenetic studies are grounded on random walks through posterior tree distributions. Trees are sampled from this distribution, and branch posterior probabilities are obtained by computing the proportion of sampled trees that show the branch of interest. Posterior distributions are explored by a technique called Markov chain Monte Carlo (MCMC), for which a detailed explanation can be found in (Altekar *et al.*, 2004).

In phylogenetic bootstrap, complexity is given by the number of resampled datasets to be obtained; that is, the larger the number of pseudoreplicates, the higher the time needed to perform the analyses. Bayesian phylogenetics have extra complications. The posterior space of trees must be thoroughly explored, which means running many generations of the MCMC chains (in the order of the millions). As running an MCMC chain involves complex calculations, the procedure can spend much computing resources, specially with big datasets. Furthermore, MCMC chains could need to be run for a long time in order to achieve stationarity, depending on the size and intrinsic characteristics of the dataset. In order to deal with these difficulties, Bayesian computer programs such as MrBayes (Ronquist and Huelsenbeck, 2003) and BEAST (Drummond and Rambaut, 2007) use a variant of the MCMC algorithm called Metropolis-coupled Marcov chain Monte Carlo (MCMCMC), which consists of running *n* MCMC chains, *n-1* of which are *heated*. In heated chains, the possibilities of exploring the tree space by traversing valleys of low optimality is exacerbated, in comparison to the cold one, by a factor directly proportional to *n* (Huelsenbeck and Ronquist, 2001). Swaps between the cold and heated chains are attempted every certain number of generations of the MCMC chains. This greatly enhances the capability of exploring the posterior distribution. However, it carries a computational cost, since an extra set of complex calculations must be performed for every additional MCMC chain.

3.3   Sequence Alignment

Sequence alignment, despite being NP-hard (Just, 2001), has received little attention in comparison to tree searching and branch support. When sequences are similar to each other, their alignment is generally a straightforward process. However, as the divergence between the sequences increases, so does alignment uncertainty. Sequence alignments are the basis upon which phylogenetic trees are inferred. Therefore, poor quality alignments result in phylogenies with a series of problems, which can range from lack of support to topological errors (Feng and Doolittle, 1987; Loytynoja and Goldman, 2008; Phillips, Janies, and Wheeler, 2000; Wong, Suchard, and Huelsenbeck, 2008).

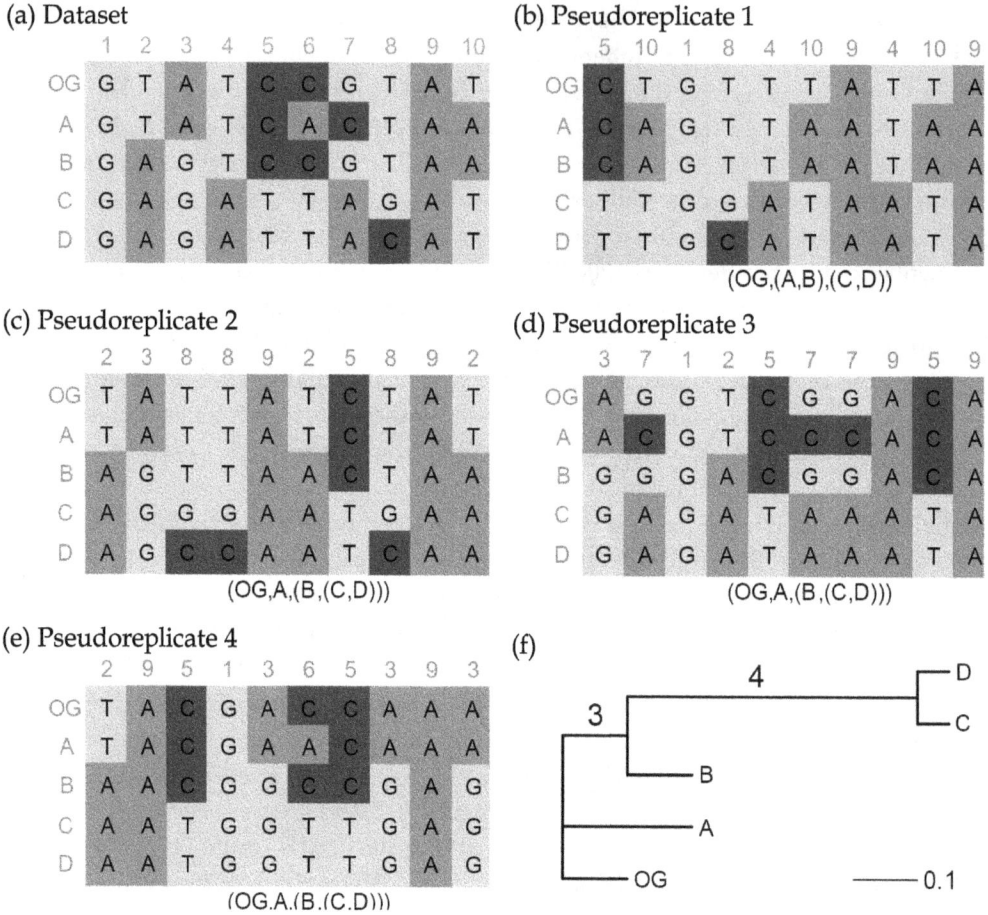

Figure 4: Toy phylogenetic bootstrap analysis (n = 4). An imaginary dataset is shown (a), together with 4 resampled datasets or pseudoreplicates (b–e). The numbers above the pseudoreplicates' positions indicate which alignment positions they correspond to [as indicated in (a)]. Phylogenetic trees, in parenthetic format, are drawn under each pseudoreplicate. These are Minimum Evolution trees obtained with Desper & Gascuel's algorithm (Desper and Gascuel, 2002), as implemented in the Ape package (Paradis, Claude, and Strimmer, 2004). Panel (f) displays the Minimum Evolution tree corresponding to the real dataset. Numbers on branches correspond to the toy bootstrap supports.

The progressive alignment method has been the most used algorithm so far. This heuristic technique consists of the three following steps: (i) Obtaining pairwise distances for every pair of sequences; (ii) Making a guide tree based on the obtained distances; and (iii) Aligning the sequences following the relationships suggested by the guide tree. The greedy nature of progressive alignment implies that when a suboptimal alignment is made in a given step of the alignment process, this error cannot be corrected in posterior steps (Feng and Doolittle, 1987; Pirovano and Heringa, 2008; Wong, Suchard, and

Huelsenbeck, 2008). To overcome this problem, new techniques have been developed that can go back in the alignment timeline and introduce modifications for improving the alignment optimality. The optimality functions used for evaluating the alignment are based on the quality and consistency of the alignments. Consistency is evaluated with respect to a set of paired alignments that are obtained before the multiple alignment process itself, which, ideally, must match with the final multiple alignment (Notredame, 2007).

Both progressive and consistency guided alignment have a low complexity in comparison to tree inference. Nevertheless, with very large datasets, complexity in time and memory can be significant or even limiting.

4   Parallel Phylogenetic Analysis

To be suitable for parallelization, a given problem must be divisible into independent subproblems. The resolution of any of these subproblems should not depend on the earlier resolution of any of the others so that, instead of solving one subproblem after another, they can be solved simultaneously, in separate processors. This entails a cost economy that is proportional to the number of subproblems that can be simultaneously solved. However, a second factor that must be considered is overhead, which consists of bookkeeping to manage message passing and interprocessor communication time. In this context, it is obvious that writing parallel programs is a challenging task for most programmer. Likewise, there are many kinds of parallel hardware architectures available, such as graphic processing units and cloud computer services, that can be used in phylogenetic studies. The details of parallel programming and hardware are beyond the scope of the present chapter. The readers interested in these matters can find solid introductory material in the classical book by Sterling et al. (Sterling et al., 1999) or Blaise Barneys et al.'s "Introduction to Parallel Computing".

Parallelization has been used in biology for several years now (Trelles, 2001). However, traditional parallel computing architectures, such as computer clusters, were not within the reach of everybody for three main reasons: First, its use required specific technical skills; second, they required a quite large space and third, they were quite expensive. However, recent advances in processor technologies made multicore CPUs available for the wide audience (Chaichoompu, Kittitornkun, and Tongsima, 2007). A multicore CPU combines two or more independent processors into a single unit, allowing a single computing device (for example a notebook computer) to perform parallel calculations.

An example of a parallelized bootstrap analysis is shown in Figure 5. In this example, the four pseudoreplicates displayed in Figure 4 were generated and analyzed simultaneously in four separate processors. Afterwards, the obtained bootstrap trees were passed back to a master processor that was in charge of creating a tree from the actual dataset, counting the number of times this tree clades were represented among the bootstrap trees, and annotate the optimal tree branches with these data. The black lines in the figure represent interprocessor communication, which is very slow relative

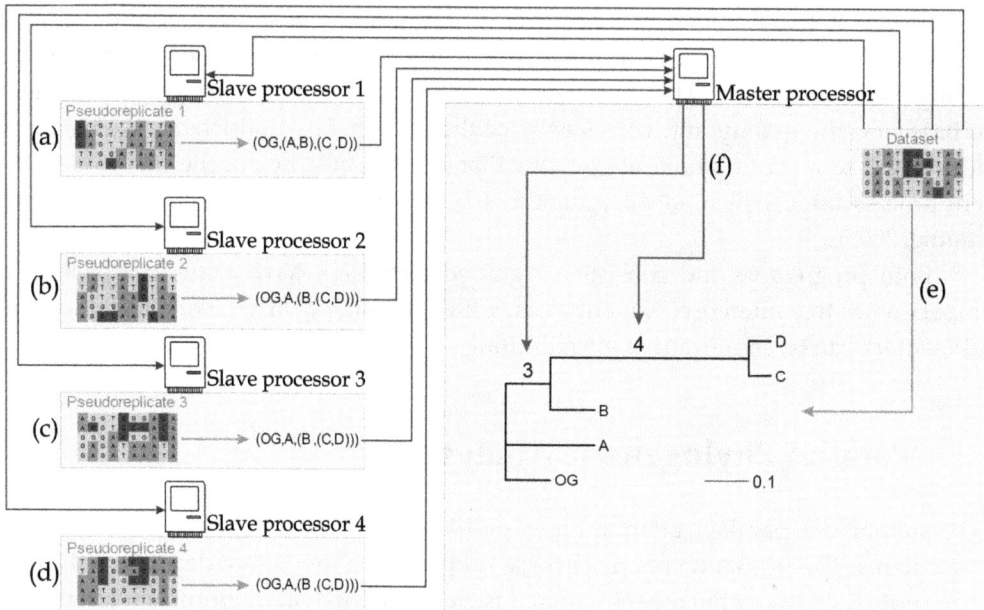

Figure 5: Toy parallel bootstrap. The imaginary analysis depicted in Figure 4 was divided into six subproblems: resampling and phylogenetic analysis of the obtained pseudoreplicates (*a–d*), phylogenetic analysis of the actual dataset (*e*) and calculation of bootstrap support (*f*). Phylogenetic analysis from the actual dataset was performed by the master processor and phylogenetic analyses of the resampled datasets were performed by slaves processors 1 to 4 concurrently. The black lines depict inter-processor exchange of information; *i.e.* the master processor sent the actual dataset to each of the four slave processor, which after resampling and phylogenetic analysis sent the bootstrap trees back to the master processor.

to CPUs' processing rates, and thus significantly contribute to the overall process overhead. There are several problems in phylogenetic analysis that can be parallelized. These are explained in the following subsections.

4.1   Parallel Tree Search

Tree search costs can be reduced by building and refining the starting trees (Figure 3) in separate processors. Furthermore, it is also possible to use medium- and fine-grained parallelization for each individual starting tree, and to combine all of these strategies (Olsen *et al.*, 1994; Stamatakis, 2006). Two examples illustrating the improvements that can be achieved by parallelizing Maximum Likelihood analyses are shown in Figure 6.

In the first example, a dataset of 120 Pestivirus sequences (Jones *et al.*, 2004) was analyzed with RAxML (Stamatakis, 2006) using different numbers of processor cores. The corresponding sequential analysis required an over-night run, whereas an equivalent analysis made using six cores could be done in less than 3 hours (Figure 6). The se-

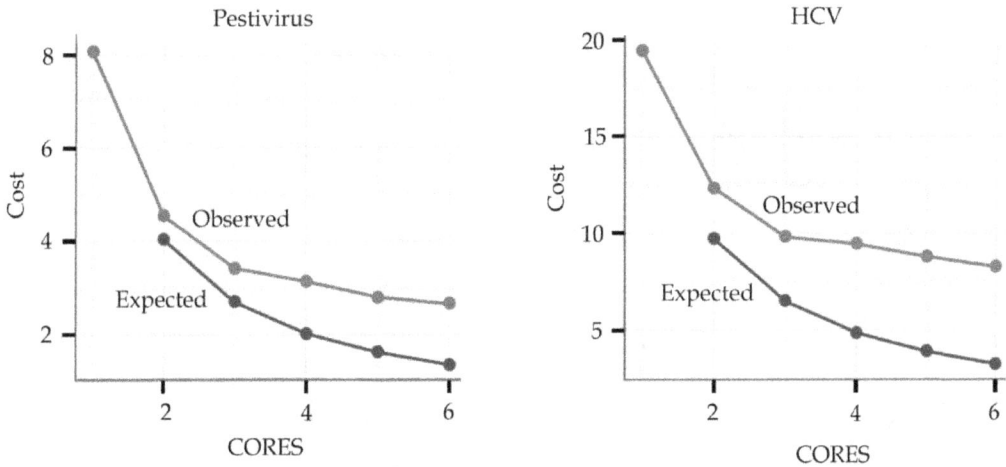

Figure 6: Costs (in hours) of Maximum Likelihood analyses performed using different numbers of cores. The left panel corresponds to an analyses of 120 *Pestivirus* sequences for which ML searches based on one thousand starting trees were performed with the program RAxML. The right panel shows an equivalent analyses of 322 HCV sequences. Observed and expected costs are shown. The analyses were performed on a 3.3 GHz six core processor, running Ubuntu server 10.04.

cond example corresponds to Maximum Likelihood analyses of 322 Hepatitis C Virus (HCV) sequences (Golemba *et al.*, 2010) made with 1 to 6 processor cores. The linear analysis taken almost 20 hours to complete, whereas it ran to completion in approximately 8 hours when the calculations were distributed among six processor cores (Figure 6). The parallelization of the Pestivirus analysis scaled better than the HCV ones, which can be explained by the fact that larger trees requires exchanging larger amounts of data, which results in greater overheads.

Figure 7 depicts a parallel Parsimony analysis of 1358 subtype B HIV-1 sequences compiled from (Jones *et al.*, 2012) and (Dilernia *et al.*, 2007) performed with TNT (Goloboff, 2008). The tree searches consisted of cyclic iterations of Tree Fusing, Ratchet, Tree Drift and Sectorial Search (Goloboff, 1999) that were run for 5 hours. The search engine (left panel of Figure 7) was implemented with either 1 or 6 cores, with the consequent six times increment of the search intensity. Every iteration, the trees found by the search engine were fused to each other and to previously found trees, which were saved in a tree pool (Figure 7, left panel). Parallel searches resulted in shorter trees and greater climbing efficiencies (Figure 7, right panel).

4.2 Parallel Analysis of Phylogenetic Uncertainty

In the bootstrap, the pseudoreplicate analyses can be distributed among different processors or processor cores, as implemented in the program PhyML (Guindon *et al.*, 2010)

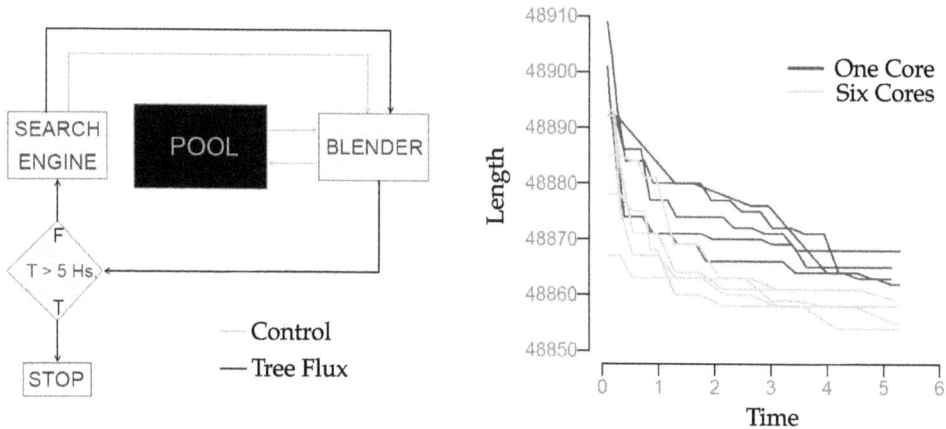

Figure 7: Parsimony analysis of 1358 subtype B HIV-1 sequences using sequential and parallel tree searches. The left panel describe the search strategy. In each iteration, trees obtained by a combination of Ratchet, Tree Drift and Sectorial Search (Search Engine) were fused to each other and to the trees found in previous iterations (Blender), which were saved in a tree pool. The algorithm was ran for 5 hours. Ten independent searches were performed using either one or six cores. The right panel shows the tree lengths found along these searches.

and depicted in Figure 5. Besides, it is also possible to distribute independent task within each pseudoreplicate analysis, and to combine both strategies, as implemented in RAxML. In the MCMCMC processes of Bayesian analyses, the cold and heated chains can be run in separate processors, though the use of finer-grain approaches is difficult because of the high communication costs carried by exchanging tree data structures and the associated conditional likelihoods among processors or processor cores (Altekar *et al.*, 2004).

Figure 8 depicts the effect of parallelizing a bootstrap analysis of 1358 subtype B HIV-1 sequences compiled from references (Dilernia *et al.*, 2007) and (Jones *et al.*, 2012), and a Bayesian analysis of 58 *Paracoccidioides brasiliensis* strains (Salgado-Salazar *et al.*, 2010). The bootstrap analysis took around 38 hours when a single processor core was used, whereas it ran in approximately 8.5 hours when six cores were used. The Bayesian analysis took 41 hours to complete with a single core, whereas it only took 10 hours to complete when 6 cores where used.

Table 1 shows how the MCMCMC chains were distributed among processor cores relative to the number of cores used. As mentioned above, state information can be very large (several megabytes) for Bayesian analyses. Thus, exchanging tree data structures and the associated, conditional likelihoods among processors carries significant costs that can counteract the benefits of parallelization. The program MrBayes avoids this problem by exchanging heats rather than states (Altekar *et al.*, 2004). This carries the impossibility of redistributing MCMCMC chains from overloaded cores to idle ones. That is why the computational costs were almost equivalent for 4 and 5 processor cores (Figure 8, Table 1).

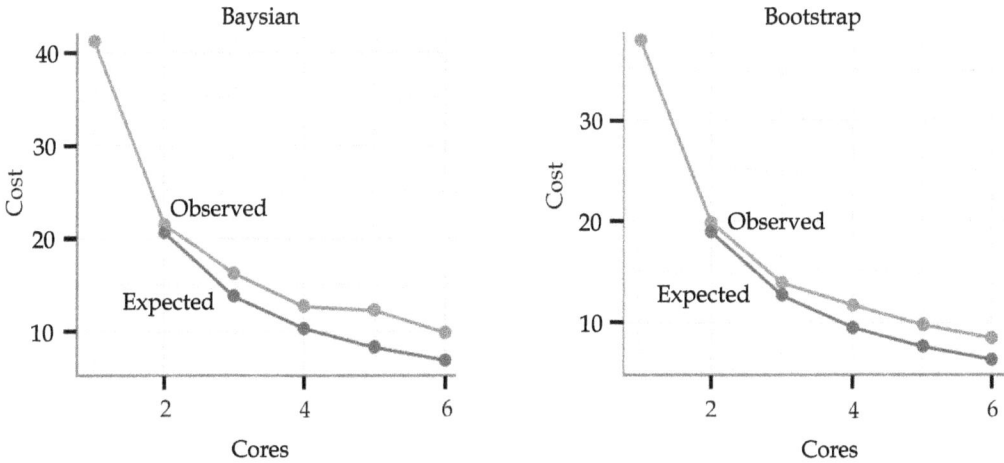

Figure 8: Costs (in hours) of Bayesian and bootstrap analyses made using diffe-rent numbers of processor cores. In the Bayesian analyses, a dataset of 58 *Paracoc-cidioides brasiliensis* strains was examined using 16 MCMCMC chains (*i.e.*, nchains=8; nruns=2) that were run for 10E7 generations. The bootstrap analyses (n = 100) were performed with a dataset of 1358 subtype B HIV-1 sequences using the rapid bootstrap algorithm implemented in RAxML. Observed and expected costs are shown. The analyses were performed on a 3.3 GHz six core processor, running Ubuntu server 10.04.

		Core					
		1	2	3	4	5	6
Number of cores	1	16	0	0	0	0	0
	2	8	8	0	0	0	0
	3	6	5	5	0	0	0
	4	4	4	4	4	0	0
	5	5	3	3	3	3	0
	6	3	3	3	3	2	2

Table 1: Processor loads (number of MCMCMC chains per core) corresponding to the Bayesian analyses depicted in Figure 8.

The times spent for aligning 167 ribosomal gene sequences (Manrique *et al.*, 2012) with ClustalW-MPI and the parallel version of MAFFT using different numbers of pro-cessor cores are shown in Figure 9. With a single core, ClustalW-MPI finished the job in 10.2 minutes, whereas with six cores it finished in just 2.3 minutes. It took 8.1 minutes to align the sequences with MAFFT using a single core, and just 1.6 minutes with six cores. ClustalW-MPI uses a master/slave design such that when it is run with a single proces-

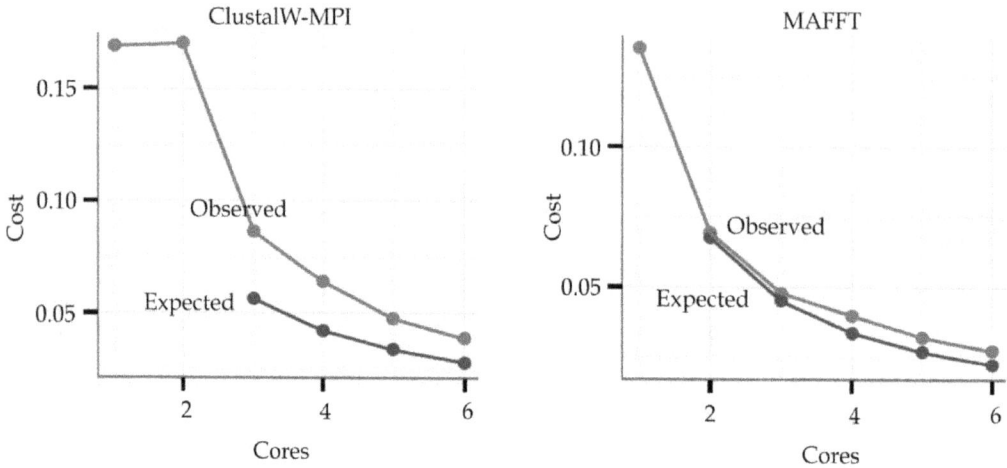

Figure 9: Costs (in minutes) required to align 167 *16S* gene sequences with ClustalW-MPI and the parallel version of MAFFT using different numbers of CPU cores. The sequences were obtained as described elsewhere (Manrique *et al.*, 2012). The purple lines corresponds to expected costs and the red ones to the observed costs. The analyses were performed on a 3.3 GHz six core processor, running Ubuntu server 10.04.

sor, the MPI master and slave are invoked on the same physical CPU core. When two processors are used, the master MPI process is invoked on the first CPU core, while the slave one performs the main alignment computation. That is why there was no improvement when the program was provided with a second processor core (Figure 9). The small time increment observed for the analysis performed with two cores with respect to the analysis done with a single core, is due to communication overhead.

5 Final remarks

The availability of affordable parallel computers has brought phylogenetics practitioners important technical improvements. Although the usefulness of parallelization is indisputable, the greatest advancements so far are due to the development of highly efficient algorithms (Goloboff, 1999; Goloboff and Farris, 2001; Guindon *et al.*, 2010; Guindon and Gascuel, 2003; Moilanen, 1999; Nixon, 1999; Stamatakis, 2006; Stamatakis, Hoover, and Rougemont, 2008; Stamatakis, Ludwig, and Meier, 2005). Notwithstanding this, it is very likely that many future developments in phylogenetics involve the implementation of new parallel algorithms. Since multicore processors are common in modern PCs (Chaichoompu, Kittitornkun, and Tongsima, 2007), the dissemination of parallel programs is guaranteed.

Acknowledgement

The authors are members of the Scientific Career of the National Council of Scientific and Technical Research (CONICET, Argentina). This work was partially supported by grants PIP 11220130100255CO (CONICET) and PICT PRH-2008-120 (National Agency for the Promotion of Science and Technology, ANPCyT, Argentina).

References

Altekar, G., Dwarkadas, S., Huelsenbeck, J. P., and Ronquist, F. (2004). Parallel Metropolis coupled Markov chain Monte Carlo for Bayesian phylogenetic inference. Bioinformatics 20(3), 407–15.

Blair, C., and Murphy, R. W. (2011). Recent trends in molecular phylogenetic analysis: where to next? J Hered 102(1), 130–8.

Bodlaender, H., Fellows, M., and Warnow, T. 1992. Two strikes against perfect phylogeny. Lecture Notes in Computer Science 623, 273–283.

Buonagurio, D. A., Nakada, S., Parvin, J. D., Krystal, M., Palese, P., and Fitch, W. M. (1986). Evolution of human influenza A viruses over 50 years: rapid, uniform rate of change in NS gene. Science 232(4753), 980–2.

Camin, J., and Sokal, R. (1965). A method for deducing branching sequences in phylogeny. Evolution 19, 311–326.

Cavalli-Sforza, L. L., and Edwards, A. W. (1967). Phylogenetic analysis. Models and estimation procedures. Am J Hum Genet 19(3 Pt 1), 233–57.

Chaichoompu, K., Kittitornkun, S., and Tongsima, S. (2007). Speedup bioinformatics applications on multicore-based processor using vectorizing and multithreading strategies. Bioinformation 2(5), 182–4.

Chor, B., Hendy, M. D., Holland, B. R., and Penny, D. (2000). Multiple maxima of likelihood in phylogenetic trees: an analytic approach. Mol Biol Evol 17(10), 1529–41.

Chor, B., and Tuller, T. (2005). Maximum likelihood of evolutionary trees: hardness and approximation. Bioinformatics 21 Suppl 1, i97–106.

Chor, B., and Tuller, T. (2006). Finding a maximum likelihood tree is hard. Journal of the ACM 53, 722–744.

Crisci, J. (1982). Parsimony in evolutionary theory: law or methodologycal prescription? Journal of Theoretical Biology 97, 35–41.

Desper, R., and Gascuel, O. (2002). Fast and accurate phylogeny reconstruction algorithms based on the minimum-evolution principle. J Comput Biol 9(5), 687–705.

Dilernia, D. A., Jones, L., Rodriguez, S., Turk, G., Rubio, A. E., Pampuro, S., Gomez-Carrillo, M., Bautista, C. T., Deluchi, G., Benetucci, J., Lasala, M. B., Lourtau, L., Losso, M. H., Perez, H., Cahn, P., and Salomon, H. (2008). HLA-driven convergence of HIV-1 viral subtypes B and F toward the adaptation to immune responses in human populations. PLoS One 3(10), e3429.

Dilernia, D. A., Lourtau, L., Gomez, A. M., Ebenrstejin, J., Toibaro, J. J., Bautista, C. T., Marone, R., Carobene, M., Pampuro, S., Gomez-Carrillo, M., Losso, M. H., and Salomon, H. (2007). Drug-resistance surveillance among newly HIV-1 diagnosed individuals in Buenos Aires, Argentina. Aids 21(10), 1355–60.

Drummond, A. J., and Rambaut, A. (2007). BEAST: Bayesian evolutionary analysis by sampling trees. BMC Evol Biol 7, 214.

Eddy, S. R. (2004). What is Bayesian statistics? Nat Biotechnol 22(9), 1177–8.

Edwards, A. W. F. (1996). The origin and early development of the method of minimum evolution for the reconstruction of phylogenetic trees. Systematic Biology 45, 79–91.

Efron, B. (1979). Bootstrap methods: another look at the jackknife. The Annals of Statistics 7, 1–26.

Farris, J. (1970). Methods for computing wagner trees. Systematic Zoology 19, 83–92.

Felsenstein, J. (1978). The number of evolutionary trees. Systematic Zoology 27, 27–33.

Felsenstein, J. (1985a). Confidence limits on phylogenies: an approach using the bootstrap. Evolution 39.

Felsenstein, J. (1985b). Phylogenies and the comparative method. The American Naturalist 125, 1–15.

Felsenstein, J. (2004). "Inferring Phylogenies." Sinauer Associates, Inc., Sunderlands, Massachusetts.

Feng, D. F., and Doolittle, R. F. (1987). Progressive sequence alignment as a prerequisite to correct phylogenetic trees. J Mol Evol 25(4), 351–60.

Fitch, W. M., Leiter, J. M., Li, X. Q., and Palese, P. (1991). Positive Darwinian evolution in human influenza A viruses. Proc Natl Acad Sci U S A 88(10), 4270–4.

Foulds, L., and Graham, R. (1982). The Steiner problem in phylogeny is np-complete. Advances in Applied Mathematics 3, 43–49.

Freckleton, R. P., Cooper, N., and Jetz, W. (2011). Comparative methods as a statistical fix: the dangers of ignoring an evolutionary model. Am Nat 178(1), E10–7.

Golemba, M. D., Di Lello, F. A., Bessone, F., Fay, F., Benetti, S., Jones, L. R., and Campos, R. H. (2010). High prevalence of hepatitis C virus genotype 1b infection in a small town of Argentina. Phylogenetic and Bayesian coalescent analysis. PLoS One 5(1), e8751.

Goloboff, P. (1999). Analizing large data sets in reasonable times: Solutions for composite optima. Cladistics 15, 415–428.

Goloboff, P., and Farris, J. (2001). Methods for quick consensus estimation. Cladistics 17, S26–S34.

Goloboff, P. A., Farris, J. S. and Nixon, K. C. (2008). TNT, a free program for phylogenetic analysis. Cladistics 24, 774–786.

Graham, R., and Foulds, L. (1982). Unlikelihood that minimal phylogenies for a realistic biological study can be constructed in reasonable computational time. Mathematical Biosciences 60, 133–142.

Guindon, S., Dufayard, J. F., Lefort, V., Anisimova, M., Hordijk, W., and Gascuel, O. (2010). New algorithms and methods to estimate maximum-likelihood phylogenies: assessing the performance of PhyML 3.0. Syst Biol 59(3), 307–21.

Guindon, S., and Gascuel, O. (2003). A simple, fast, and accurate algorithm to estimate large phylogenies by maximum likelihood. Syst Biol 52(5), 696–704.

Holder, M., and Lewis, P. (2003). Phylogenetic estimation: traditional and bayesian approaches. Nature Reviews 4, 275–284.

Huelsenbeck, J., Ronquist, F., Nielsen, R., and Bollback, J. (2001). Bayesian inference of phylogeny and its impact on evolutionary biology. Science 294, 2310–2314.

Huelsenbeck, J. P., and Crandall, K. A. (1997). Phylogeny estimation and hypothesis testing using maximum likelihood. Annual Review of Ecology and Systematics 28, 437–466.

Huelsenbeck, J. P., and Ronquist, F. (2001). MRBAYES: Bayesian inference of phylogenetic trees. *Bioinformatics* 17(8), 754–5.

Jones, L. R., Cigliano, M. M., Zandomeni, R. O., and Weber, E. L. (2004). Phylogenetic analysis of bovine pestiviruses: testing the evolution of clinical symptoms. *Cladistics* 40, 443–453.

Jones, L. R., Moretti, F., Calvo, A. Y., Dilernia, D. A., Manrique, J. M., Gomez-Carrillo, M., and Salomon, H. (2012). Drug resistance mutations in HIV pol sequences from Argentinean patients under antiretroviral treatment: subtype, gender and age issues. *AIDS Res Hum Retroviruses* 28, 949–955.

Just, W. (2001). Computational complexity of multiple sequence alignment with SP-score. *J Comput Biol* 8(6), 615–23.

Katoh, K., Asimenos, G., and Toh, H. (2009). Multiple alignment of DNA sequences with MAFFT. *Methods Mol Biol* 537, 39–64.

Katoh, K., and Toh, H. (2008). Recent developments in the MAFFT multiple sequence alignment program. *Brief Bioinform* 9(4), 286–98.

Katoh, K., and Toh, H. (2010). Parallelization of the MAFFT multiple sequence alignment program. *Bioinformatics* 26(15), 1899–900.

Li, K. B. (2003). ClustalW-MPI: ClustalW analysis using distributed and parallel computing. *Bioinformatics* 19(12), 1585–6.

Loytynoja, A., and Goldman, N. (2008). Phylogeny-aware gap placement prevents errors in sequence alignment and evolutionary analysis. *Science* 320(5883), 1632–5.

Maddison, D. (1991). The discovery and importance of multiple islands of most-parsimonious trees. *Systematic Zoology* 40, 315–328.

Manrique, J. M., Calvo, A. Y., Halac, S. R., Villafane, V. E., Jones, L. R., and Walter Helbling, E. (2012). Effects of UV radiation on the taxonomic composition of natural bacterioplankton communities from Bahia Engano (Patagonia, Argentina). *J Photochem Photobiol B* 117, 171–8.

Menezes, A. N., Bonvicino, C. R., and Seuanez, H. N. (2010). Identification, classification and evolution of owl monkeys (Aotus, Illiger 1811). *BMC Evol Biol* 10, 248.

Moilanen, A. (1999). Searching for Most Parsimonious Trees with Simulated Evolutionary Optimization. *Cladistics* 15, 39–50.

Nixon, K. (1999). The parsimony ratchet, a new method for rapid parsimony analysis. *Cladistics* 15, 407–414.

Notredame, C. (2007). Recent evolutions of multiple sequence alignment algorithms. *PLoS Comput Biol* 3(8), e123.

Olsen, G. J., Matsuda, H., Hagstrom, R., and Overbeek, R. (1994). fastDNAmL: a tool for construction of phylogenetic trees of DNA sequences using maximum likelihood. *Comput Appl Biosci* 10(1), 41–8.

Olvera, A., Busquets, N., Cortey, M., de Deus, N., Ganges, L., Núñez, J., Peralta, B., Toskano, J., and Dolz, R. (2010). Applying phylogenetic analysis to viral livestock diseases: Moving beyond molecular typing. *The Veterinary Journal* 184, 130–137.

Paradis, E., Claude, J., and Strimmer, K. (2004). APE: Analyses of Phylogenetics and Evolution in R language. *Bioinformatics* 20(2), 289–90.

Phillips, A., Janies, D., and Wheeler, W. (2000). Multiple sequence alignment in phylogenetic analysis. *Mol Phylogenet Evol* 16(3), 317–30.

Pirovano, W., and Heringa, J. (2008). Multiple sequence alignment. In "Bioinformatics, Volume I: Data, Sequence Analysis, and Evolution" (J. Keith, Ed.). Humana Press.

Pybus, O., and Rambaut, A. (2009). Evolutionary analysis of the dynamics of viral infectious disease. Nature Reviews 10, 540–550.

Rasmussen, D. A., Boni, M. F., and Koelle, K. (2013). Reconciling phylodynamics with epidemiology: The case of dengue virus in southern Vietnam. Mol Biol Evol.

MrBayes 3.1 Manual

Ronquist, F., and Huelsenbeck, J. P. (2003). MrBayes 3: Bayesian phylogenetic inference under mixed models. Bioinformatics 19(12), 1572–4.

Salgado-Salazar, C., Jones, L. R., Restrepo, A., and McEwen, J. G. (2010). The human fungal pathogen Paracoccidioides brasiliensis (Onygenales: Ajellomycetaceae) is a complex of two species: phylogenetic evidence from five mitochondrial markers. Cladistics 26, 613–624.

Schleifer, K. H. (2009). Classification of Bacteria and Archaea: past, present and future. Syst Appl Microbiol 32(8), 533–42.

Stamatakis, A. (2006). RAxML-VI-HPC: maximum likelihood-based phylogenetic analyses with thousands of taxa and mixed models. Bioinformatics 22(21), 2688–90.

Stamatakis, A., Hoover, P., and Rougemont, J. (2008). A rapid bootstrap algorithm for the RAxML Web servers. Syst Biol 57(5), 758–71.

Stamatakis, A., Ludwig, T., and Meier, H. (2005). RAxML-III: a fast program for maximum likelihood-based inference of large phylogenetic trees. Bioinformatics 21(4), 456–63.

Sterling, T. L., Salomon, J. , Becker, D. J., and Savarese, D. F. (1999). How to build a Beowulf. The MIT Press. Cambridge, Massachusetts; London, England.

Steel, M. (1994). The maximum likelihood point for a phylogenetic tree is not unique. Systematic Biology 43, 560–564.

Swofford, D., and Olsen, G. L. (1996). Phylogenetic reconstructions. In "Molecular Systematics" (D. Hillis, and C. Moritz, Eds.). University of Illinois Press.

Trelles, O. (2001). On the parallelisation of bioinformatics applications. Briefings in Bioinformatics 2, 181–194.

Voigt, K., and Kirk, P. M. (2011). Recent developments in the taxonomic affiliation and phylogenetic positioning of fungi: impact in applied microbiology and environmental biotechnology. Appl Microbiol Biotechnol 90(1), 41–57.

Wheelan, S. (2008). Inferring trees. In "Bioinformatics, Volume I: Data, Sequence Analysis, and Evolution" (J. Keith, Ed.), pp. 287–309. Humana Press.

Woese, C. R., Kandler, O., and Wheelis, M. L. (1990). Towards a natural system of organisms: proposal for the domains Archaea, Bacteria, and Eucarya. Proc Natl Acad Sci U S A 87(12), 4576–9.

Wong, K. M., Suchard, M. A., and Huelsenbeck, J. P. (2008). Alignment uncertainty and genomic analysis. Science 319(5862), 473–6.

www.ingramcontent.com/pod-product-compliance
Lightning Source LLC
Chambersburg PA
CBHW081101220326
41598CB00038B/7177